AF702084

AMBIVALENT PLEASURES

AMBIVALENT PLEASURES

SOFT DRUGS AND EMBODIED ANXIETY IN EARLY MODERN EUROPE

SCOTT K. TAYLOR

CORNELL UNIVERSITY PRESS
Ithaca and London

Copyright © 2024 Cornell University Press

All rights reserved. Except for brief quotations in a review, this book, or parts thereof, must not be reproduced in any form without permission in writing from the publisher. For information, address Cornell University Press, Sage House, 512 East State Street, Ithaca, New York 14850. Visit our website at cornellpress.cornell.edu.

First published 2024 by Cornell University Press

Library of Congress Cataloging-in-Publication Data

Names: Taylor, Scott K., 1969- author.
Title: Ambivalent pleasures : soft drugs and embodied anxiety in early modern Europe / Scott K. Taylor.
Description: Ithaca : Cornell University Press, 2024. | Includes bibliographical references and index.
Identifiers: LCCN 2023058422 (print) | LCCN 2023058423 (ebook) | ISBN 9781501775468 (hardcover) | ISBN 9781501775475 (pdf) | ISBN 9781501775482 (epub)
Subjects: LCSH: Substance abuse—Social aspects—Europe—History. | Substance abuse—Europe—History—17th century. | Substance abuse—Europe—History—18th century. | Psychotropic drugs—Social aspects—Europe—History. | Psychotropic drugs—Europe—History—17th century. | Psychotropic drugs—Europe—History—18th century.
Classification: LCC HV5000.E85 T395 2024 (print) | LCC HV5000.E85 (ebook) | DDC 362.29094/09032—dc23/eng/20240131
LC record available at https://lccn.loc.gov/2023058422
LC ebook record available at https://lccn.loc.gov/2023058423

For my parents

Contents

Acknowledgments

This book has been long in the making, and it would have taken me longer still had I not had the help of many.

Early on in the project the American Council of Learned Societies awarded me a fellowship that helped me begin the research, and the National Endowment for the Humanities awarded me a summer stipend that I stretched into two summers' worth of visits to European libraries.

When I began this book, there were many fewer early modern printed books available online than there are now, so I am grateful for the patient support of the staff of several research libraries in Europe, including: the Biblioteca Apostolica Vaticana; Biblioteca Marciana; Biblioteca Nacional de España (especially in the Sala de Cervantes); Biblioteca Nazionale Braidense; Biblioteca Nazionale Centrale di Firenze; Biblioteca Nazionale Centrale di Roma; Biblioteque National de France; Biblioteca Provinciale Giulio e Scipione Capone; British Library; Koninklijk Biblioteek; Onderzoekzaal of the Allard Pierson; Universiteit van Amsterdam; Wellcome Library; and, here in the United States, the National Library of Medicine. The staff at the libraries at the University of Kentucky have been crucial, especially in the interlibrary loan office.

I conceived of this book while teaching at Siena College. I am grateful for the people there who made it a place where I believed I could pursue such an ambitious research agenda while teaching at a liberal arts college, especially Ralph Blasting, Jim Harrison, and Karen Mahar. The Schaffer Library at nearby Union College allowed me to visit and access Early English Books Online and Eighteenth Century Collections Online. When I arrived at the University of Kentucky I found more allies, including Mark Kornbluh and Karen Petrone, who were then the dean of the College of Arts and Sciences and the chair of the history department. They and others in the dean's office supported my research with time off from teaching and more funding for travel, both to European libraries and to conferences where I could try out my initial thoughts.

Anastasia Curwood, the current department chair, helped me get to the end. Everything was made easier by the indispensable Tina Hagee, the department manager for the Department of History.

Also at the University of Kentucky, I am grateful to David Olster for advice, as well as students in various graduate courses that helped me think through ideas. Many colleagues, especially Jeremy Popkin, gave me helpful commentary on papers I presented that drew from this project, and Jonathan Glixon helped me with Italian sources. Gretchen Starr-LeBeau allowed me to workshop material in her graduate course and introduced me to the Premodern Spanish History Association of the Midwest. Claire Clark welcomed me into the community of historians of drugs and alcohol, especially through her NEH Summer Institute. Coteaching a course with her on dependency behavior helped me think through the meaning of addiction; thanks also to the students in that course.

Outside of the university, I wish to thank Tom Cohen, Carlos Eire, Robert Ingram, Julie Landweber, Erik Midelfort, Steve Norris, and Duane Osheim for advice and encouragement. I am grateful to Phil Withington for allowing me to join his series of panels at the Renaissance Society of America conference in Boston in 2016. Christine Jones, Julie Landweber and Julia Sarreal asked me to join their panel at the Alcohol and Drugs History Society in Mexico City in 2022, helping to integrate me into that scholarly community. At ADHS meetings and elsewhere David Courtwright has always been eager to talk with me about drug and alcohol history—he and Claire Clark have made me feel welcome in this field of history that was brand new to me. Thanks also to An Castangia, who helped me learn early modern Dutch.

Thanks to Joel Harrington, Marcy Norton, and the members of the Premodern History Association of the Midwest for commenting on various papers spun off from this book. A very special thanks to Jim Amelang, David Clemis, Elizabeth S. Cohen, Joe Clark, Mark Hailwood, Emily Michelson, Mary Noll Venables, and Steven Shapin for reading and commenting on parts of the manuscript.

At Cornell University Press, thanks to Emily Andrew for bringing me in, and to Mahinder Kingra for keeping me, and for providing editorial guidance. Thanks also to the two anonymous readers who, along with Mahinder, made insightful interventions into the direction and shape of this project. All errors and omissions in this book are, of course, entirely my own.

Thanks to Ashgate Publishing and *Eighteenth-Century Studies* for permitting me to reuse already published material.

Thanks to my children, Katie and Alex, for their patience with me when I could not be with them, especially on those trips to Europe when they were very young.

I feel special gratitude to Amy Murrell Taylor for setting her own career aside at times to help me. She made summer travel to Europe possible during the first years of this project by taking care of the girls, the house, and the dog by herself for weeks on end. During the past several years she took on more than her share of stewarding our household through the teenage years and through at-home schooling during the coronavirus pandemic, all to allow me to focus on writing. As a scholar, she has also been a source of inspiration for me and a model, as well as a reader who commented on several sections of this book. She gives me hope and a reason to keep going, every day.

Amy's parents, Joyce and Darwin Murrell, who always wanted to talk about my research, have been inspiring to me as well. They helped materially, too, by donating air miles for one of my trips abroad. I regret deeply that Joyce is no longer with us to celebrate the completion of this project; as a book lover, she would have been delighted to see and hold it in its physical form.

My own parents and stepmother, Susan Taylor, Gary Taylor, and Beverly Monnens, have also been a source of guidance and enthusiasm. Their faith in me set me on the path to a career in history, and in the beginning they made everything possible. Their love for me and my family have added great joy to my life. It is to them that I dedicate this book.

Note on Transcription and Translation

Spelling and syntax have been left in the original, except for a few changes of orthography for clarity's sake—for example, a *j* at the end of a word changed to *i*.

All translations by the author unless otherwise noted.

AMBIVALENT PLEASURES

Introduction

A Unified Drug Culture

In the seventeenth and eighteenth centuries, the psychotropic drugs tobacco, chocolate, tea, coffee, distilled spirits (like gin), sugar, and opium all either became available to western Europeans for the first time or were newly available in mass quantities. As novelties, these soft drugs forced Europeans to come to terms with their effects on both individual consumers and on society and to pin them down into categories, such as gender, class, religion, race, medicine, governmental regulation, market value, and moral worth. Not least of all, they had to confront the new sensory experiences, bodily changes, and mood shifts accessed through these drugs. As use of these substances became integrated into everyday life in European cities, Europeans found that their use sometimes became compulsive, a surprising and strange discovery in an era that was increasingly emphasizing self-discipline, initiating an embryonic understanding of addiction. While ingesting psychotropic drugs, early modern Europeans consumed tangible symbols of the intangible forces that were changing their societies such as urbanization, global trade, and capitalism. Starting with the beginnings of significant importation into Spain of tobacco and chocolate around 1600 and ending with Thomas De Quincey's publication of *Confessions of an English opium-eater* in 1821, the early modern period established the broad cultural patterns for fitting modern drugs and alcohol into modern life.

One critic of the new soft drugs and their effects on consumers was the British naval physician Thomas Trotter, an advocate of the view, newly prominent in his day among western European physicians, that nerves and their disorders were the key to understanding both physical and mental health.[1] In 1807 Trotter published *A view of the nervous temperament*, which connected the alarming rise in nervous disorders to wider changes in England: he believed that nervous disorders afflicted only societies in an advanced state of civilization, like his own Georgian England, where he estimated they made up two-thirds of all ailments.[2] Indeed it was the increasing wealth of English society, Trotter argued, and the ensuing luxury and excess that was fueling the increase in "the nervous temperament." In general his concerns reflected a general turn against overcivilization, in which nervous disorders embodied the anxiety felt about the decadence thought to be brought on by excessive wealth and the consumption of exotic novelties.[3] In particular, the use of tea, coffee, opium, and distilled spirits like gin appeared to be the chief causes of nervous diseases, and once someone made a habit of using of one or more of these drugs there was little hope for a cure. Elsewhere Trotter asserted that "the habit of drunkenness is a disease of the mind," an idea analogous to today's understanding of addiction that he applied not just to alcohol but to all the new exotic drugs.[4] Because it was so hard to stop consuming psychotropic drugs, Trotter emphasized prevention over treatment, and if it was too late to prevent the development of a nervous disposition, then "the only means of cure lie in a total abstinence from every species of spirit or fermented liquor; from every thing that bears any analogy to them, such as tea, coffee, opium, and all other narcotics."[5] Not only did these drugs cause nervous diseases, but they also fed on each other: "The use of tea often paves the way to habitual dram-drinking."[6] Some consumers were ingesting opium with the hope of curing the problems that other drugs had caused, leading to opium dependency: "The bodily complaints of the human race, when enervated by luxury and refinement," that is, drinking tea and gin, "seem to produce more acute pain. . . . The spirits are apt to flag, as if the mind had no resting place. Opium alone gives relief, though it must feed the disease. . . . When opium happens to be soothing to weak nerved people from their quick sensations it is apt to be the more craved for, and converted into habit. The languor and dejection which follow its operation pave the way for the repetition of the dose, till general debility succeeds."[7] Trotter was also sympathetic to the British antislavery movement, and he combined these two interests when reminding his readers that the rise of ancient Rome to a position of wealth and power led to luxury, decadence, and then ruin: "Let Great Britain look to this example. The East and West Indies . . . are a theatre of oppression and slavery, to gorge her with commercial wealth" while Africa "is made a field of blood" to provide enslaved labor on plantations "whose produce only tends to weaken [Britain's] manly character, and overwhelm her with nervous infirmities!"[8] Britain had built an empire of slavery to quench its thirst for luxury and refinement, which then led to effeminacy, feeble health, and anxiety at home.

Trotter's apprehension revealed many of the assumptions that undergirded Europeans' attitudes toward the new stimulants. Like other observers, he incorporated them all into a single threat, treating them not as separate issues but as different facets of the same problem. In Trotter's view, there was a unity to the early modern soft drugs, including alcohol. Further, he linked drugs to luxury; the nervous temperament was a result of the burgeoning consumer society that characterized newly wealthy England, which gave English consumers the ability to spend money not just on necessities like food and shelter but on unnecessary trifles from abroad. What is more, drugs brought the malign results of foreign luxury directly into the bodies of the consumer. Physical and mental health therefore suffered in new ways as a direct consequence of Europe's deepening ties to the rest of the world. Ingesting psychotropic drugs also brought social and moral consequences. Drinking tea and gin made men effeminate, and purchasing these exotic goods connected the consumer to the violence and oppression by which they were produced. Lastly, there was a strange circularity to the consumption of these drugs. Their use became a craving, and indulging in the desire for the drugs led only to a desire for even more, an observation that gestured toward the modern understanding of addiction. In short, Trotter's deep unease about the moral and physical consequences of consuming drugs for both individuals and society sums up the main theme of this book: that early modern drugs and alcohol catalyzed profound social and cultural changes, and that they also provided conspicuous symbols of those changes.

The enormous influx of drugs into Europe accelerated to new heights during the eighteenth century. Sugar, a rare luxury until the development of plantation slavery in the Americas, saw its consumption in Europe rise by 1800 to almost 245,000 tons per year.[9] Chocolate and tobacco were wholly unknown in Europe until 1492, but by 1800 15 million pounds of chocolate and well over 100 million pounds of tobacco

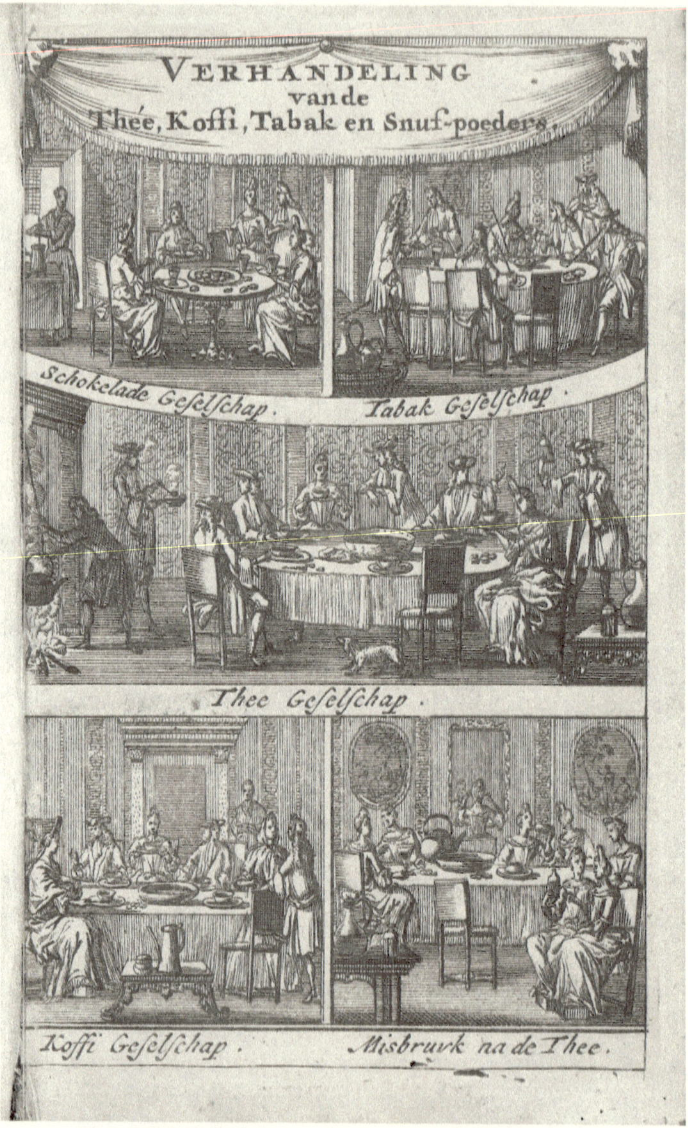

FIGURE I.1. R. V. N., *Natuur-kundige verhandeling van de thee, koffee, tabak, en snoef-poeders* (Amsterdam: J. ten Hoorn, 1701), frontispiece. The illustration demonstrates the use of the new exotic stimulants at home in an elite Netherlandish home, with different modes of socializing for each different drug, including the "Abuse of Tea" in the lower right-hand corner featuring a disordered gathering of women. Reproduced courtesy of Harvard Libraries.

per year were taxed as they entered Europe, with unknowable extra amounts smuggled in.[10] Coffee was first brewed into a drink in the area around the Red Sea around the same time that Columbus reached the Caribbean, although Europeans soon transplanted it to their colonies in the Americas and Asia. Just before the Haitian Revolution, the French colony Saint-Domingue had become the largest single producer of coffee in the world, exporting 89 million pounds in 1789. Meanwhile imports into Europe of tea, which continued to be grown only in East Asia during this period, rose from zero to perhaps 40 million pounds by the 1790s, although it is hard to know exactly how much, thanks to pervasive smuggling.[11] Europe produced its own distilled spirits, but hard liquor was merely an alchemist's plaything until the seventeenth century. By 1800 millions of gallons of gin, whiskey, brandy, fortified wine, and rum were produced in Europe and throughout the Atlantic World each year.[12] Opium had been a medicine in Europe since antiquity, but its availability grew as Europe's ties strengthened with the Middle East and India, which produced most of the world's opium. In sum, by the time the wars of the French Revolution and Napoleon disrupted global trade, the cities and towns of western Europe had become well acquainted with these previously unknown or rare commodities. Sugar, tobacco, tea, coffee, and spirits in particular were all becoming accessible as regular, even daily, items of consumption for all but the most poor in towns of any size, and they were beginning to make their way into rural areas as well.

The use of the term "drugs" requires some explanation. There is no good word to describe all the substances under consideration here in their early modern form. This book will use the terms "drugs," "drugs and alcohol," "psychotropic drugs," "soft drugs," "exotic drugs," and "stimulants" somewhat interchangeably. Chocolate and sugar are not always considered drugs today, but early modern Europeans certainly thought of them in the same terms as the rest, forming a bounded field whose constituents shared broad similarities. Gin, made in Europe, was not "exotic" but it was new. Yet this field excluded substances that were foreign and strange like sarsaparilla or quinine, medicants that were new to Europeans at the time and attracted attention, appearing in medical handbooks, but were rarely used in ways that would be called "recreational" today. Nor does the category include items like coca, hallucinogens like peyote and mushrooms, qat, and cannabis, which are certainly considered drugs today, because while some adventuresome Europeans ingested them in their native lands they did not adopt them at any scale back in Europe.[13] The term "soft drugs" will be used simply to distinguish them from the drugs considered "hard" today like morphine, heroin, fentanyl, cocaine, and amphetamines. This is not to downplay the dependence and the pain that tobacco, alcohol, and opium can cause and have caused, then and now. By today's definition, opium and alcohol are not thought of as "stimulants," but like the other terms it will be used here as a catch-all, for the sake of convenience, to describe the psychotropic nature of the drugs.

This book is concerned with trying to understand the cultural and social meaning of drugs in the past rather than adhering to today's ideas of how the drugs "really worked." Early modern consumers noticed the ability of coffee and tea to promote wakefulness, but they were also concerned with their power to cause sterility and infertility; the thoughts of early modern Europeans are more pertinent here than trying to trace the origins of scientific knowledge about these psychotropics. Surely they were not quite the same then as now. Gin was more akin to grain alcohol than the sophisticated, botanical-infused liquor of today, while chocolate was not served in solid form, and mixing it with milk was a novelty in the eighteenth century. Proportions are hard to discern, as well. Cornelis Bontekoe, the Dutch "tea doctor," sometimes drank up to two hundred cups of tea in a day; certainly the cups were smaller than those used today, but it is hard to know exactly how much tea that would have been.[14] The purpose of this book will instead to be explore the social and cultural construction of the meaning of these items in Europe.

Thus, this book addresses not so much how or how much Europeans consumed drugs but rather the discourse that arose to determine the meaning of that consumption. Drug consumption fostered sharp debates over its medical, social, moral, cultural, and political consequences, much of them finding their way into publication in an era when print culture was also rapidly increasing. Most of that commentary was critical of the use of the new drugs. This was obviously an unpopular view in light of the rapid expansion of their use in Europe, and there were plenty of defenders of the new drugs, too, especially for their curative powers as newly available medicines. There were also writers who remarked on the pleasures of psychotropic drug use, on their usefulness in regulating emotions, and the number of people who found that their impulsive sampling of the new exotic drugs became a compulsive habit. This commentary both reflected the experience of the users and helped shape the expectations, the "set and setting," of the new drugs.

Historians have studied each of these stimulants, but their work tends to treat them as commodities—that is to say, as subjects of economic history—and to treat each of them individually. This book will consider them all together, as Thomas Trotter did, and less for their economic importance and more for how they changed European society and culture. David Courtwright calls the impact of drugs and alcohol on early modern Europe "the psychoactive revolution," as Europeans discovered and developed a taste for some (but not all) of the stimulants they encountered during their travels through the rest of the world. They gained control of the transportation and, in the case of sugar, chocolate, tobacco, and coffee, the production of the new exotic stimulants, which, combined with home-grown distilled alcohol, fueled enormous profits, unprecedented government intervention into markets, and great changes in the daily habits of European consumers.[15] Daniel Lord Smail has called the long eighteenth century "the century of addiction," by which he means that drugs and alcohol began to replace religion and ritual as the main way that western Europeans regulated their emotional states.[16] Both Courtwright and Smail point to large changes taking place not just in the economic world of commodities but in the intimate lives of early Europeans. This book aims to expand on their ideas and examine what it meant for Europeans to consume large quantities of psychotropic drugs for the first time.

The first reason for studying the encounters with all these drugs together is that sugar, chocolate, tobacco, coffee, tea, gin, and opium compelled early modern Europeans to confront deep changes taking place in their society. The seventeenth and eighteenth centuries saw a rapid increase in the number and intensity of ties between Europe and the rest of the world. Europeans were gaining political control over much of the Americas and of slices of Asia and sending people on the move to and from all these different regions, all while buying and trading items from around the world, including new exotic drugs. What did it mean for Europeans to live in this new globalized world? How would the consumption of the products of exotic cultures affect Europe? Drugs like chocolate seemed to weaken consumers' control over their bodies, minds, and identities, threatening to affect them in racial, gendered, class, and religious ways. Perhaps most surprisingly to contemporaries, the new stimulants seemed to impair the ability of consumers to exercise free will; once they began using substances like tobacco they found themselves unable to stop. The new drugs made their most profound marks on urban life, at a time when the cities of western Europe were undergoing significant and unsettling changes and a few, like London and Paris, were growing to unprecedented size. Stimulants like coffee became a part of the new consumer culture, which included a niche for substances that provided users a new blend of luxury, comfort, and medicine—an early modern wellness industry. They also changed the way that city dwellers interacted with one another, creating new sites and rituals of sociability like the tea table. New forms of social interaction threatened institutions like the alehouse and disrupted old, familiar rituals of social life while reshaping social relations around use of the new drugs. In the backdrop of all these changes was the growing and changing economy, as Europeans wrestled with the consequences of early capitalism. New drugs like gin were enormously profitable, but at what cost, if they led to an increase in disorder? Could anyone ethically profit from drugs that hurt the broader community? All of these issues were compounded by the fact that, unlike other products of the consumer revolution, purchasers ate, drank, or breathed these substances into their bodies. Could the sweetness and pleasure of a substance like sugar be divorced from the physical suffering of the enslaved people who produced it?

The new soft drugs were catalysts for these changes. Their production, purchase, and transportation helped tie the early modern world together more tightly, and the profits they produced helped fuel the growth of capitalism. They changed the way people behaved in the new modern cities, and their dense presence in urban areas made cities even more attractive for country people on the move. They were also conspicuous symbols of those changes, especially since they were, unlike older, more commonplace stimulants like beer and wine, brand new, arriving in Europe with little context or familiarity. All of these new drugs caused controversy, with some observers celebrating them and the changes they brought, and many more condemning them. An argument about sugar might be an argument about which comestibles were pleasant and which were disgusting, and why. A debate over chocolate could also be a debate about race, gender, religion, and class. Thinking about tobacco meant thinking about volition and self-control. Criticizing coffee was a way to attack the growth of a consumer-oriented health-care market. Complaining about tea was a means of expressing misgivings over changing social relations. Attacking gin was a way to question capitalism, and so on. The novelty of these drugs, plus the fact that they were ingested into the body, made them perfect emblems for the social and cultural changes that accompanied the birth of global capitalism.

This book will feature the critics of the new drugs more than the apologists, in part because so much more of what was printed about them was critical. But all of these drugs were popular and saw their use explode in the seventeenth and eighteenth centuries. Despite the disapproval of many commentators, consumers were voting with their spending power, and with their mouths and noses. The criticism was not an accurate representation of how most western Europeans thought about the new stimulants but rather of the elite, especially from medicine and science, who expressed a mix of resistance and approval to their adoption. Even if unrepresentative of general opinion, their writings are still valuable as reminders of the powerful anxieties surrounding the new drugs, even while historians have downplayed contemporaries' fears in the face of the drugs' overwhelming success. Also, by discussing their encounters with the new soft drugs, writers gave testimony about their hopes and fears for consequences of globalization, urbanization, capitalism, and modernity. Long before modern legal and medical regimes codified society's unease about the balance of harms and benefits of drugs and alcohol by dividing them into legal medicines and illegal drugs, early modern Europeans felt and expressed a deep ambivalence about them.

Among historians studying early modern globalization and capitalism, the Atlantic World tends to draw the most attention. Of course, Europe's growing engagement with the world extended well beyond the Atlantic, into the Mediterranean region, the Indian Ocean, Southeast Asia, and East Asia as well, and there would be no coffee, tea, or opium without these ties. This history often gets pulled into the category of "imperial" history, but outside of a few ports and islands there was very little empire east of the Cape of Good Hope until the late eighteenth century. While sugar, tobacco, and rum were produced in the context of Caribbean and Chesapeake plantation slavery, the rest of the psychotropic drugs did not depend on coercion or political hegemony to find their way to Europe. Atlantic World history rests on the assumption that the concept "includes and connects the entire region," as Alison Games put it, but in truth most of the work—almost all of it—treats Europe as a mover and the rest of the world as moved by the actions and decisions of Europeans.[17] Work on global history east of the Cape of Good Hope follows the same pattern, at least through 1800. A second reason for studying drug use and what Europeans thought and felt about it is to place Europe itself under the scrutiny of Atlantic World and global history—to situate Europeans, not just Native Americans or Africans, as people affected by early modern global capitalism. The "encounters" featured in this book took place in Europe, not among explorers, sailors, creoles, or botanists roving through the Americas, Africa, and Asia.

The most profound ambivalence centered on the effects of drugs and alcohol on the will. A third reason for studying the encounters with drugs is the fact that early modern drugs and alcohol provided a radically destabilizing threat to self-mastery at precisely the same time that, if influential social theorists are to be believed, western European began to increasingly prize that virtue. Max Weber, Norbert Elias, Gerhard Oestreich, Jürgen Habermas, and Michel Foucault have all argued that the early modern period in Europe saw the origin of the modern ideal of self-discipline—indeed in one way or another they have all made this history central to their thought. For Weber, the rise of capitalism depended on religiously motivated self-denial and dedication to hard work, ideals that moved from the monastery into the outside world via Protestantism. Regulating one's consumption and one's time was crucial to the development of the modern economy and also for modern rationality.[18] For Elias, the civilizing process that enabled Europeans to shed their primitive emotional states and allow for state formation depended on a shift from external control to an ever-tightening self-discipline. Complexity and competition in the increasingly urban, commercial society led to self-restraint, including a sense of self-awareness of the body, and a distancing of the self from the body.[19] Oestreich argued that the revival of Stoicism by Justus Lipsius and others, who used Roman writers like Seneca and Tacitus to encourage men to inhibit their emotions and behavior, helped install discipline in the new militaries of the gunpowder age and then society as a whole. Neostoic social discipline first took the form of a variety of church and town ordinances governing everyday behavior, and then through education it took the form of self-discipline.[20] For Habermas, coffeehouses provided spaces for the rational discussion of public affairs, places where men were free to speak without oversight from the state or the church. Self-restraint was key to maintaining this new public sphere as a civil and productive space. Foucault detected an increasing control emanating on the one hand from institutions like the clinic or the prison and on the other, from physicians and other professionals who reshaped language into discourses that buttressed their own growing authority. Initially starting as constraint from without, discipline shifted from simply constraining behavior to teaching people eventually to constrict their own speech, thought, and behavior.[21] Taken together, the influence of these theorists is hard to overstate—they portray early modern

Europe as the crucible where the state, the church, and the elite professional classes tightened their grip on the everyday lives of their subjects through social discipline, which then generated the stifling confines of self-discipline.

None of these writers were historians, and their real concerns lay in trying to understand the experience of their own time and place, but they all looked to the early modern period to explain the problems of modernity. Indeed they helped invent the idea that the time span between the Protestant Reformation and the French Revolution constituted a discrete era, an "early modern" Europe in which the qualities that created modern Europe first appeared. Historians have largely disputed the details and even the broad claims of their conclusions, but the general sentiment that the early modern period was one of increasing self-discipline lingers in the historical imagination. That this same period saw a dramatic increase in the use of new drugs and types of alcohol, as well in waves of anxiety about how those drugs affected the control of users over their bodies, minds, and behavior, complicates this story. As Trotter's assessment demonstrates, Europeans felt a deeply rooted ambivalence about the tensions between the self-discipline they desired and the disorder—and freedom—fostered by the use of drugs and alcohol.

All of these stimulants have been studied individually, but usually singly and in a specific country. Other scholars have studied each of them as commodities (the rise of sugar and the plantation complex, for example) or as they changed the societies and cultures of individual countries (such as the coffeehouse in Restoration England, or the Gin Craze of eighteenth-century London).[22] This book will be the first to treat all of these drugs together, in all of Europe west of the Rhine, and not as economic commodities but in terms of their social and cultural impact. All of them created controversy, and the books and pamphlets published in response—over six hundred total in English, Dutch, French, Italian, and Spanish—form the evidentiary basis for this monograph. These five languages were chosen because they represent the regions where drugs were most prominent and the amount of printed material focusing on them was the greatest. Latin is left out to avoid featuring scholarly discussions that would exclude the reading public who read only their vernacular languages, a public that was growing throughout the period.[23] Half or more of the sources are in English, thanks in part to England playing perhaps the largest role in the accommodation of the new drugs into western Europe and in part to its thriving publishing business.[24] Nevertheless western Europe formed a unified drug culture, where scholars learned from and quoted one another while sharing the same kinds of drugs. Chocolate was more popular in the Mediterranean, and tea found more drinkers in Britain and the Netherlands, but all of these substances were noticeable, and commented on, throughout western Europe. The drugs were used together, too—coffeehouses served tea, chocolate, and liquor, and Europeans did not drink coffee, tea, and chocolate (the so-called "hot drinks") without sugar. Tobacco was used alone or with other drugs, finding a home in taverns, alehouses, and coffeehouses.

One last reason for studying multiple drugs across several countries is to demonstrate that early modern Europe set important patterns for how drugs and alcohol would fit into modern culture and society. Templates established in the seventeenth and eighteenth centuries repeat themselves in the twentieth and twenty-first, too. Some of these patterns are already well known, such as that drugs continue to get stronger and more fast-acting as time goes on—for example, from opium to morphine to heroin to fentanyl, or coca leaves to power cocaine to crack cocaine. Another is that recreational drugs all began as medicines.[25] Drugs today continue to inspire both pleasure and loathing, and observers continue to critique their use in racialized, gendered, and class-based terms. The contemporary understanding of addiction finds its origins in the early modern understanding of compulsive behavior, and the use of drugs today continue to shape, and be shaped by, social behavior. Legal drugs and alcohol are an important part of wellness culture today, and the ethics of selling and buying drugs is still in question. This book avoids teleology, however, and in fact it does not try to explain why the patterns of today are the same as four hundred years ago. Yet the patterns do persist.

Each chapter will focus on a separate theme that emerges from early modern European drug use, like the ethics of capitalism or changes in sociability. As a springboard for exploring that theme, the chapter will each foreground one of the seven drugs, though all of the drugs will appear in each chapter. Chapter 1 uses sugar as the focal point from which to approach stimulants and their engagement of the senses. Its use as a sweetener made the consumption of the bitter hot drinks of chocolate, coffee, and tea possible in Europe. Unlike the other rest of the new soft drugs, sugar was not controversial until the end of the eighteenth century, when it became the target of a boycott led by antislavery activists like Trotter hoping to end the transatlantic slave trade who believed that by eliminating the demand for sugar they would eliminate the need for enslaved labor in the Caribbean. The story of this boycott, which drew the participation of perhaps three hundred thousand families in Britain, is well known, as is the role it played in bringing women, who oversaw the use and purchase of sugar, into politics. But this chapter focuses on the sensory experience of ingesting sugar and its fellow soft drugs. Antislavery activists drew on a long tradition of excoriating the new psychoactive drugs for their filthiness and their offensive effect on the senses, beginning with chocolate and tobacco. At the same time the soft drugs extended an irresistible allure of pleasure that attracted consumers, and this tension between appeal and disgust characterized European's engagement with all the new exotic drugs.

Exotic drugs were also threatening because of their foreign origins. Chapter 2 uses chocolate as a starting point to explore the relationship between western European consumers and the rest of the world. A new commodity like chocolate was hard to categorize: Was it a drink, because it was consumed in liquid form? Or was it a solid, since it began as a cocoa paste to which water was added and incorporated many other ingredients? Could Christians safely use psychotropic drugs like chocolate that played such a prominent role in Native American religion—or, as it seemed to Europeans, the worship of demons? In the case of tobacco and chocolate in Spain, Marcy Norton has shown this to be a fundamental challenge for the incorporation of foreign drugs, and this chapter demonstrates that it was a problem for all the drugs throughout western Europe.[26] Would ingesting a drug like coffee make European men effeminate, as they imagined Turkish men to be, and make European women oversexed and infertile, as they imagined Turkish women to be? As the drugs became less expensive and more widely available, common people started to use them; would these drugs erase class distinctions? Each new foreign drug brought with it the cultural connotations of the peoples from which it came, and when it arrived in Europe it threatened to disrupt the racial, gender, class, and religious qualities of their users by disordering their users' bodies. At the same time, the exotic origin of the new drugs was a part of their appeal, and Europeans depended on the learning and experience provided by foreign countries to understand the medical effects and proper use of the new drugs. Yet they were also alarmed at how they threatened to reorganize European society. All of the stimulants carried with them racial, religious, gendered, and class-blurring dangers for their new users.

Chapter 3 investigates the addictive qualities of the new stimulants, starting with tobacco. The strange new sight of tobacco users inhaling and exhaling smoke gave rise to unfamiliar terminology: in England users were called "tobacconists" and the use of pipes "drinking" tobacco. It also led to attempts to understand the new drugs and their effects on the body. Europeans turned to medicine and botany to fit drugs like tobacco into frameworks that made sense to them, and Europeans justified the use of these drugs first as new forms of medicine, as opium already had been for centuries. Orthodox medical thinking rested on the inheritance of Galen and other physicians from antiquity, although medicine was changing due to the development of a new chemical-based understanding of the body and, later, the nerves. Physicians found it easy to understand the new intoxicants' effects on users' bodies and, through the humoral system, their minds. What medicine could not comprehend was why, once they had started, some consumers could not stop using the drugs. To address this new problem, observers reached for two traditional rhetorical strains for moralizing about people whose consumption was disordered, one that emphasized gluttony and debauchery and another that stressed luxury and custom. Critics also reached for another way of analyzing compulsive behavior that focused on the power of the drugs themselves, by employing the language of bewitchment and slavery. Historians of addiction have identified the origins of the modern idea of addiction with medical experts who were shocked by the compulsive drinking of gin in eighteenth-century England, but even before then observers of the new stimulants developed ways of talking about compulsive drug use, not just for distilled spirits but all the new drugs.[27]

Coffee, the point of departure for chapter 4, has drawn historians' attention mostly because of coffeehouses, which provided a location for the emergence of Habermas's public sphere; its effects on social life have seemed to be the most important aspect of its history. Yet early modern Europeans remained just as concerned about the substance of coffee. As the eighteenth century moved forward, and coffee and the other stimulants became an increasingly normal part of Europeans' diet, taken daily rather than as a medicine that targeted specific ailments, Western medicine shifted to a focus on the nerves. Trotter was not the only one to blame coffee and other drugs for a new epidemic of nervous disorders among the consuming elite of Europe. Supporters of exotic drugs like coffee, tea, and tobacco responded by claiming a role for their daily use as part of a new Western culture of wellness, where stimulants took their place besides diets, baths, mineral waters, exercise, and other new bodily practices that aimed to maintain the health of the body and, through the body, to regulate their emotional states. Critics countered that in truth the drugs caused the very same physical ailments and mental anxiety that they pretended to cure. Either way, governance over soft drugs was slipping away from the medical profession toward the power of the market.

Chapter 5 opens with tea as a way to explore the effects of the new drugs on sociability. Historians are most familiar with the rise of the coffeehouse as a new site for the public sphere and the fears raised by gin about the lawless disorder of the London poor, but all of the new drugs challenged the old social world of medieval Europe, which was centered on beer, wine, and the tavern. Tea became a symbol of domestic serenity by the nineteenth century, associated with genteel middle- and upper-class women. But tea originally appeared as a disruptive force, mistrusted for the way that it brought women together in new ways, crossing class boundaries in the densely crowded cities, leading them away from their domestic duties and into a new social space where they could exchange information—pejoratively called "gossip"—without the oversight of men. But while some observers feared the impact of the new drugs on social life, others found them liberating. Promoters of these drugs had to tame and domesticate them, depending on the users to behave themselves according to new standards of politeness in innovative rituals such as teatime. For tea and all the new soft drugs, their spread depended on social ties, as one person taught another how to use them, and, once begun, each new drug started to bend social life around its use.

Chapter 6 focuses on the ethics of the marketplace, using gin as a springboard. When studying morality and early capitalism, historians are most familiar with the way that the slave-sugar boycott emphasized the commodity chain that connected sugar consumption with the horrors of Caribbean slavery. According to the tenets of the Enlightenment, however, commerce was supposed to be civilizing, bringing people together from all over the world in a liberal exchange of goods, triumphing over the government-regulated mercantilist and absolutist policies that constrained trade, ideas, and people. But well before the sugar boycott, commentators were dismayed to find that the market brought enormous quantities of cheap gin into poor neighborhoods in London. Defenders of gin placed economic growth over the moral corruption of its consumers. Another avenue of criticism of the new psychotropic drugs claimed that use of the new drugs encouraged idleness, damaging the work discipline of the laboring poor and rendering them unable to help the nation's economy prosper. As Europeans found that psychotropic drugs were increasingly mediating their social relationships, they also saw that the market and its products were intruding not just into their consuming lives, but their moral lives as well.

The conclusion focuses on Thomas De Quincey, who wrote the first addiction memoir, *Confessions of an English opium-eater*, drawing attention to the problem of opium dependency and foreshadowing the modern drug epidemics that would arrive in the nineteenth and twentieth centuries. The early modern career of opium, known as a painkiller and sleep aid since ancient times, perfectly summarizes the history of early modern drugs, touching on all the themes of the previous six chapters. During the nineteenth century, beginning with De Quincey and his friend Samuel Taylor Coleridge, opium and its derivatives began to shift from a medicine to a recreational drug. Like other intoxicants, opium changed the social relations of its addicts, created concern over its bodily and mental effects, and, with its origins in Asia, brought fears of racial degeneration for its users in Europe. Opium would create a new moral problem thanks to the growing dependence of the East India Company on its sale, while helping usher in a new understanding of addiction that would form the basis for modern ideas of the problem. As such, opium proved to be an inflection point in the history of drugs and alcohol, summing up all the trends of the previous three hundred years and crystallizing them into the modern patterns that determined how we have used and thought about drugs and alcohol during the following two hundred years and more.

Chapter 1

Stained with Spots of Human Blood

Disgust, Pleasure, and the Senses

Humans first domesticated sugarcane in New Guinea, and the crop spread northwest from there, reaching the Mediterranean by the Middle Ages.[1] When the Portuguese and Spanish colonized the Atlantic islands of Madeira, the Azores, the Canaries, and Cape Verde in the fifteenth and sixteenth centuries, they realized that the climate was good for cane and quickly began transporting enslaved people from West Africa to work the fields. Sugarcane demanded an intensive year-round labor regime, including tasks like holing the ground, planting cane cuttings, harvesting the stalks, milling the cane, and boiling the juice into a syrup that then dried into sugar loafs. As Europeans began to colonize the New World, they brought sugar with them, along with the plantation slavery regime pioneered in the Atlantic Islands. As one imperial incursion followed another, sugar boomed in Brazil, Barbados, Jamaica, and Saint-Domingue, as well as on other smaller islands in the Caribbean. Increased production drove the price down, so sugar transformed from a luxury good that appeared as a medicine or in the form of sculptures gracing the tables of the European elite to an item that increasing numbers of people could use to make the bitterness of chocolate, coffee, and tea palatable. The boom also stimulated the Atlantic slave trade, and sugar became the primary commodity driving the forcible transportation of perhaps 12.5 million people, of whom 10.7 million survived the Middle Passage; half of those captives went to sugar plantations.[2] While the slave trade took place over three centuries, it accelerated over time, and the eighteenth century saw the largest numbers transported as the boom in sugar—as well as the chocolate, tea, and coffee it sweetened—took off. Sidney Mintz estimates that by 1800 the world was producing 245,000 tons of sugar per year, most of which was consumed in western Europe.[3]

Sugar did not become controversial in Europe until the late eighteenth century, when an organized antislavery movement began to coalesce in Britain. Led primarily by Quakers and evangelical Protestants, the activists formed the Society for the Abolition of the Slave Trade in 1783, seeking the legal abolition of the trade in the hope that, by cutting off the supply of new labor, slavery in the Caribbean would wither and disappear. As part of this effort William Fox proposed a boycott of sugar in 1791, which helped pressure Parliament into outlawing the transatlantic slave trade in 1807. Meanwhile the price of sugar was skyrocketing, thanks to the Haitian Revolution, beginning in 1791. Abolition of slavery itself would wait until 1833 in the British colonies, 1848 in French possessions, 1865 in the United States, and 1888 in Brazil. As part of their campaign, activists worked to call attention to the links between slaving ships, plantation slavery, and sugar. One tactic was to urge the women who oversaw the tea service in Europe to empathize with African women whose children were torn from them. Likewise, the Wedgewood motto "Am I Not a Man, and Your Brother" displayed on the china tea service reminded those who benefited from slavery of the common humanity of the enslaved, drawing connections between western Europeans sitting down at the tea table and Africans enduring the Middle Passage. This made the antislavery campaign arguably the first human rights movement in western European history, a landmark in liberal progress.

At the same time, a different, relatively unknown tactic of the antislave sugar argument emerged to remind users of the enduring physicality of the product they were ingesting, a tactic aimed at fostering disgust rather than empathy. In 1792 Andrew Burn published his *Second address to the people of Great Britain: containing a new, and most powerful argument to abstain from the use of West India sugar*, in which he explained that this new approach came to him while trying to persuade some friends not to purchase Caribbean sugar by using the method of urging sympathy for enslaved Africans. He was unsuccessful "'till one or two of the female part of the company, knowing he had been sometime resident on a Sugar Plantation in the West Indies, begged he would favour

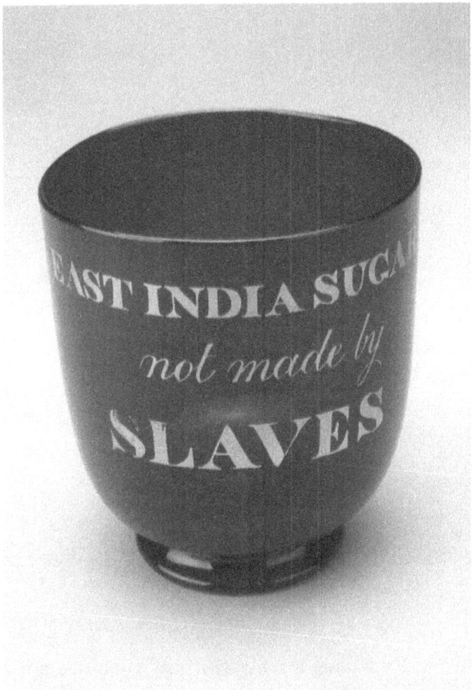

FIGURE 1.1. A sugar cup used during the English antislavery sugar boycott. The cup advertises that it contains sugar from India, which was used by some boycotters who did not wish to drink their tea straight as an ethical alternative to the less expensive sugar from Caribbean plantations. Reproduced courtesy of the British Museum.

them with a short account of the Process of making it?" He did so, and when "describing the manner in which the Negroes stamp it in the Hogshead, he could easily perceive an alteration in the complexion of one of his fair hearers; and as he proceeded, knit Brows, distorted Features, and disgustful Emotions, were visible in all their Countenances; till one unable to stand it out any-longer, exclaimed with the most determined resolution, 'Well! I'll never eat another bit of Sugar so long as I live.'"[4] Prompted by this reaction, Burn devoted much of his pamphlet to a physical description of the work of slavery. "The Consumers of Sugar and Rum, innocent or guilty," he wrote, "are actually the first and moving cause of all those torrents of Blood and Sweat, that annually flow from the body of the poor African. . . . Yet how difficult to persuade some, that when they eat Sugar, they figuratively eat the Blood of the Negro." They also literally did so, "as it flows copiously from the Body of the laborious Slave."[5]

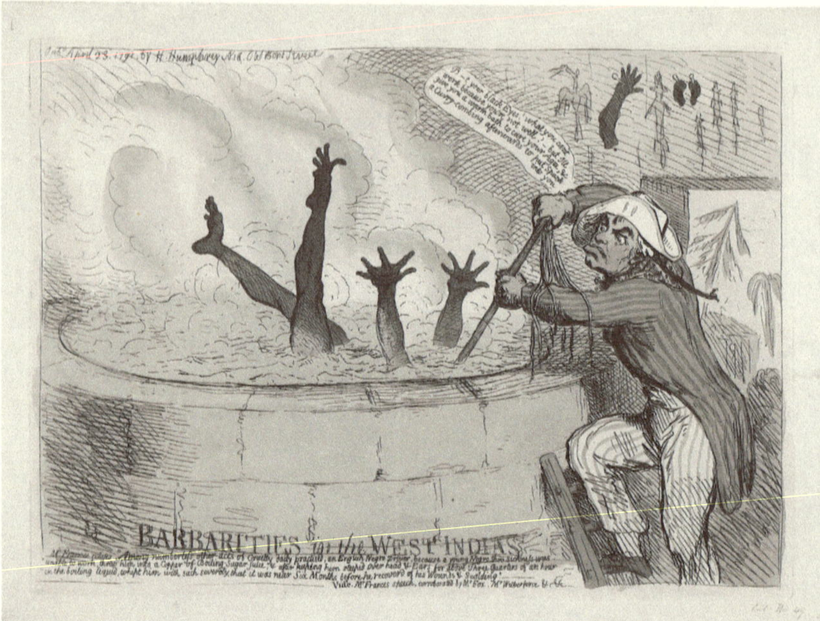

FIGURE 1.2. James Gillray, "Barbarities in the West Indias." Published by Hannah Humprey, 1791. This print depicts an anecdote told by antislavery campaigners of an overseer who, when confronted by an enslaved young man who was unable to work due to illness, threw him into a boiling sugar vat. This print makes the point that by consuming sugar, tea drinkers in England consumed the lives of the enslaved, both literally and metaphorically. Reproduced courtesy of the British Museum.

Burn went on to explain how sugar was packed, emptied out of draining molds into barrels and stamped down by two or three enslaved Africans. Touching the sugar with their bare feet, the men produced a foul odor, "nauseous effluvia emitted from them by excessive Perspiration." This was "absorbed among the Sugar; for nothing is more common than to observe little hard lumps among it, of a darker hew than the rest." Also to be found in the barrels of sugar were dead lice from the workers' hair, plus "a very disgusting fluid, of various colours" draining from sores in the workers' feet and legs caused by yaws, and, finally, pus that skin-burrowing insects known as "jiggers" produced in the stampers' feet.[6] Burn worried that he had not done justice to the full loathsomeness of sugar production and, were "all the filthiness of a Sugar House, laid open to public view, I believe it would be still more disgusting than the picture I have drawn."[7] Sugar was literally and metaphorically polluted, he argued, by the bodies of the enslaved Africans who created it.[8]

Although motivated by antislavery sentiment, Burn invoked racist beliefs about Black people, ascribing foul and repulsive qualities to their bodies that then spread to the sugar and rum they produced. Indeed his argument fit well with a new emphasis on bodies, and on the perceived uncleanliness of Africans, that helped shape ideas about race in the eighteenth century.[9] But the decision to emphasize the sensory details of sugar production to play on the "disgustful emotions" of his listeners had deep roots. All the new stimulants attracted attention for their bizarre new physical aspects as they were eaten, drunk, smoked. The mix of attraction and repulsion began with the Spaniards' ambivalent first reactions to chocolate and tobacco in Mesoamerica and continued with each new item that Europeans encountered.[10] Drugs and alcohol entered the body directly, which only made the concern about their physical aspects more intense, so the debates that arose were laden with the sensory language of filth, stink, and disgust. Although they seem natural and unchanging, to a large degree disgust and all sensory reactions are not objective but culturally and socially determined.[11] Norbert Elias has argued that the civilizing process that began in early modern Europe was marked by a recoil from the body and physicality as part of increasing self-discipline, and the attacks on the foulness of drugs conforms with that perspective.[12] In fact, the drugs' effects seemed to be readable on the users' bodies, befouling their faces while damaging the users' senses. The language of disgust and filth culminated in the attempt by Burn and other antislavery crusaders to transfer Europeans' feelings of repulsion from Black bodies to the sugar on their tables.

Defenders of the new drugs, however, countered with competing claims about senses and the exotic new substances: first, that they actually cleansed and preserved the body, and, second, that, far from being disgusting, the new drugs were pleasurable. These sentiments, which welcomed agreeable new bodily sensations, worked against the grain of Elias's civilizing process. Although arguments promoting the pleasurable sensations of sugar and its fellow new comestibles were less common than claims of foulness, the rapidly expanding production, import, and consumption of all the new exotic drugs certainly suggests that the critics' denunciations had little practical impact. If opponents of the new drugs were preaching bodily self-discipline, they were swimming against the tide—a tide of sugar, tobacco, tea, coffee, and distilled spirits rising and swelling into the cities, taverns, coffeehouses, homes, and bodies of early modern Europeans. Nevertheless, the fact that disgust remained a useful critique up through the early nineteenth century suggests that the physical attributes of early modern drugs and alcohol, and concerns about them entering the body, fueled a powerful ambivalence about alcohol and drugs.

Tobacco: Shocking Indelicacy and Nastiness

The idea, so dramatically employed by Burn, that exotic drugs were foul, began hundreds of years earlier, when Europeans first encountered tobacco and sugar in the New World. One hurdle preventing their immediate adoption by Spaniards who traveled there was their perceived loathsomeness. The success of these products today makes it seem like they would be naturally adopted by anyone who encountered them, but, as Marcy Norton relates, this was not the case. There was no natural, inherent appeal to chocolate, tobacco, and the rest of the new drugs, except sugar.[13] At first the Spanish associated tobacco with the diabolical Indian priests who used it, and they were repulsed by the smell of its smoke. Chocolate, with its frothy head on top of the drinking vessel, reminded Spaniards of feces. Chocolate also recalled human blood, which they associated with violent Mesoamerican religious rituals. Certainly chocolate and tobacco made the Spanish wary because they were symbols of racial and religious difference, but physical qualities themselves were repulsive as well.[14] Kristen G. Brookes notes that in England, too, fear of the exotic foreignness of tobacco was intertwined with a perception of its filthiness.[15] The 1602 *Work for chimney-sweepers*, published under the pseudonym "Philarates," lamented tobacco's ability to "pervert the natural use & offices of the parts of the bodie," where the mouth and throat, which nature intended as a receiving area for nourishment, "are made emunctuary clensing places and sincks . . . for the filth and superfluous excrements of the whole body," since it confused the face with the "most abject and basest part" of the body.[16] Moreover, "to this may bee added, his unpleasaunt and ungratefull smell . . . in their bodyes and breath, the loathsome Tabacco sent [scent]."[17] Other terms he used to describe tobacco included "noisome and irksome," "unpleasant," and "stench."[18] Here Philaretes established the pattern for those who disliked tobacco, framing its uncleanliness and odor as the two main objections.

A decade later the satirist Barnabe Rich noted that tobacco worked by making men salivate and spit and instead recommended: "Thou that so much desirest to drivell & to slaver, take but one dragme of the abstract that is drawne out of a Close-stoole," that is, a chamber pot.[19] A few years earlier the humorist Samuel Rowlands depicted an exasperated wife complaining about her husband, "'Tis the filthiest man":

Himselfe all day in Tavernes he bestowes,
And comes to bed at night in shooes and hose;
And there he lyes as cleanly as a Hog,
Perfum'd as sweet as any stinking Dog,
With filthy leaves he smoakes his head with all,
Such Weeds as Indians do Tobacco call:
But sure as Black-amores looke outward skin,
So Collier-like are English-men within,
That take such trash.[20]

The wife's solution was to throw the tobacco into the privy, symbolically putting it in the proper place for feces.

Equating tobacco with human waste was a common theme. The Castilian scholar Bartolomé Jiménez Patón asked in 1638, "Who sees the noses dirty with filth, and does not imagine a little child's buttocks full of crap?"[21] English humorist John Philips returned to the theme in several doggerel poems composed in the mid-seventeenth century. For example:

When I do smoak my nose with a pipe of Tobacco after a
 feast,
Then down let I my hose, and with paper do wipe mine [arse]
 like a beast . . . Tobacco's my delight,
So 'tis mine to sh[ite].[22]

In a different poem he gestured toward tobacco's humoral benefits:

Tobacco onely can draw the vapours down from my troubled
 brain;
And from the bashful Pan vapours rise 'twixt my thighs to my
 nose again.
Five Pipes I have devour'd,
Five pans I have deflow'r full of fume.

Another of his verses celebrated the friendship between the nose and the backside, while another mused on the fumes emitted from a smoker's pipe and his rear end and likened both to thunder and guns. Yet another played with social class and human waste:

> Tobacco is a dish for an Earl, for a Lord, for a Knight, for a
> Squire:
> Than shitting who can wish greater, if you please, or occasion
> require?
> Tobacco's a fine thing,
> But shitting's for a King; for the brains,
> For the pains of the belly.
> Tobacco who despise?
> Then shitting who denies?
> None, I think;
> though I stink, I tell ye.[23]

Perhaps Philips had tipped from a true concern for tobacco's smell into a Rabelaisian celebration of its foulness, playing around with the way that others perceived tobacco smoke in order to shock and satirize, using smoking and human waste as a social leveler connecting kings and noblemen with the common smoker. More earnestly, in 1797 Adam Clarke warned users who were not already put off by "its shocking indelicacy and nastiness" that tobacco sellers often moistened the leaves with urine.[24] The anonymous author of *Tobaco-mastix* in 1677 also dwelt on tobacco's connection to human waste, claiming that like the eel, thought to have only one orifice for its digestive tract, tobacco reversed the proper functions of the body, "immitting and emitting, eating and voiding, at once," feeding the nose and making "their mouth the tar-barrel."[25] The author also lamented the custom of using tobacco smoke as an enema, asking, "Doth it not cause the excrements of nose and mouth also to be as ugly and noisome of those of the anus to look upon?"[26] Tobacco here is linked to many types of uncleanliness befouling a clean space.

The most common objection to tobacco was its smell. The Cambridge "gentleman" complained of the breath of smokers in the late eighteenth century, and as early as 1595 Anthony Chute reported that when he lit a pipe bystanders would "crie fie, fie, how it stincks, smell you it not: or tell me he will hire an Irishman to chimney sweep my stomache."[27] Some of the early seventeenth-century complaints about its smell tied its odor to what they perceived as its exotic, pagan, and anti-Christian nature. Philaretes, who in 1602 dwelled on its odor, described it as "this hellish smoake, reeking foorth of Plutoes forge" when discussing its tendency to dry up men's seed.[28] The humorist Samuel Rowlands also traced tobacco's origins to Pluto, whom the gods then cast out of Olympus, owing to the stink, into the land of the "blackamoors," where the Spanish found it.[29] A poem by Ben Johnson published in 1669 placed tobacco "in the Devils Glister [enema]-pipe."[30]

Tabaco-mastix added that smoking was so foul that doing so near others "is a Treason and inexpiable breach against all the Royal Laws of Civility."[31] This touches on another theme introduced by Philaretes, that tobacco was so nasty that it destroyed normal sociability. He told a story of a man who stopped smoking thanks in part to how his breath made him "loathsome to eat or sleep with, or even to speak to."[32] Barnabe Rich addressed this theme in 1616, chiding smokers for their "rude incivility," as their spitting and slavering was so "loathsome and unmannerly" that it would make their companions sick, "especially if they were such as had beene trained up in civility, or had any regard of cleanliness."[33] Snuff made its users beastly, depriving them of their humanity. Francisco de Leiva y Aguilar also complained that tobacco destroyed sociability while likening snuff to human waste: "What kind of ornament is it to bring into the nostrils tobacco powder that seems like it was taken from urine? Is all of this not disgusting? Not vile? Not annoying to one's companions?"[34] William Tullett has observed that as tobacco became popular its supporters claimed it as a respectable, genteel comfort, but the lingering complaints about its offensive smell indicate that not everyone agreed.[35] As late as 1725 Francesco Arisi related an anecdote of a woman who divorced her husband over the bad odor and filthy handkerchiefs of her tobacco-using husband.[36] Snuff brought along its own catalog of filthiness, as did chewing tobacco. The anonymous author of 1722's *Of the use of tobacco, tea, coffee, chocolate, and drams* warned that smokers were better off than chewers of tobacco, whose teeth were "Foul and Black" and whose breath and spitting were also obnoxious.[37] The satirical *Whipping-Tom* wrote about "the Foppish Mode of taking Snuff, which of late Years is become so ridiculous in England" that one time "meeting a Fop in the Strand, besmear'd from nasty Nostrils to the very Ears," he mistook him for the chimpanzee that had recently been displayed at Moncrief's Coffeehouse.[38] These insults were particularly damning because one reason why snuff gained popularity in the eighteenth century was that it was supposedly less objectionable than smoking in the presence of women.

Coffee and Tea: A Turdy Turk

Coffee was an early target for satirists, especially in England, where there was an outpouring of scornful ephemeral literature when it first arrived. One broadsheet, *A cup of coffee, or coffee in its colours*, printed anonymously in 1663, called coffee "Sulphur," "Liquid fire," a "loathsome Potion, "Syrrop of Soot," and "essence of old Shooes." It claimed that coffee caused "Christians to turn Turks," thus proving that "Coffee's extraction has its heats from Hell." The poet drew attention to the Turkish origin of the drink, calling coffee sellers "Friends to the gross Turky-shore" and, taking the position of a coffee drinker, portraying himself "in the power of this Turkish Spell / I'm faithless as a Jew or Infidel." The author tied coffee's religious danger to its disagreeable physical nature, wondering if coffee was concocted from "the Devils [turd]" and urging people to profit from its popularity by turning their close stools into coffee pots, filling them up from their "Backsides," and then advertising their feces as coffee with "Strange Hebrew-English" to lure in credulous customers attracted to foreign fashions. "'T shall ne'er be said, a Turdy Turk could do / More . . . then you."[39] Sensory historians have been exploring early modern soundscapes for a generation, but few have tackled the emerging scent-scape of the early modern city.[40] Tullett points out that the distinct odor of brewing coffee, along with the tobacco smoking that so often accompanied the beverage, helped mark off the coffeehouse as a distinct space, an innovative and masculine site in the urban scent-scape.[41] Like the critics of tobacco, however, the author of this pamphlet thought coffee's proper place was in the close stool.

Another attack from 1663, *The maidens complaint against coffee*, also linked the exotic nature of coffee to sensory revulsion. *The maidens complaint* featured Snapshort, a servant who journeyed to the Royal Exchange in London to collect a debt for his employer. Finding himself bewildered by the foreign languages spoken among the merchants there, he entered a coffeehouse and ordered "a dish of that Hell-burn'd Liquor," hoping to settle his wits. Instead, the "ratling noise of Kettles, Skimers, and Ladles" made his "brains run round so swift as a Windmill" until he fled to Moorfields and drank some ale, which restored his mind.[42] At the Royal Exchange, the disorienting sounds of brewing coffee mirrored the foreign speech of visiting merchants, both symbolizing the confusion of modern, cosmopolitan life in London. "Don Bollicosgo Armuhaz," the pseudonymous author of yet another 1663 satire, also emphasized the physical nature of coffee, "that black, nasty, Hel-burnt Liquor."[43] Many observers drew attention to the bitter taste of coffee, like Isidro Fernández Matienzo, physician to the cathedral of Palencia in Castile, who used it to help determine coffee's humoral properties.[44] Also noteworthy was coffee's heat, which Edward Ward described as "a Liquor of infernal Race, / Black, scalding, and of most offensive smell," using touch as well as sight and smell to link coffee to exotic foreigners.[45] As late as 1792, Spanish writer Alexandro de Moya linked what to him was the unpleasant sensation of drinking coffee and its baleful effects on health: "I dislike that black and bitter drink, and what is more it is very dangerous and prejudicial, according to what I have heard from the most able experts: it attacks the nerves, producing pains and convulsions, it is very hot, and it inflames the blood."[46] Critics could use blood to associate coffee, like sugar, with slavery; the Jacobin politician and abolitionist Joseph M. Lequinio decried coffee as a crop, "watered with the blood of our brothers."[47]

The debauched and enchanted coffee and tea world, published in the Netherlands in 1701, also associated coffee and tea with disgust, labeling coffeehouses "filthy" because, there, men pretended to better themselves at penny universities but actually met with prostitutes.[48] The anonymous author added that despite the lofty claims made for them, all coffee and tea did was make their users urinate frequently after exchanging their "piss-gossip."[49] Another Dutch writer supported Norton's claim that Europeans had no natural desire for the new stimulants, wondering how tea or coffee could become so popular, given that the first taste of either was bad—tea tastes like soapy water at first.[50] In 1733's *A satyr against tea,* John Waldron he compared tea to hay for livestock and to a laxative that "make costive Ladies sh[i]te."[51] For Waldron, the claims that tea was a good medicine were false: "It cures the Megrim of the Head? / It rather helps to—p[i]ss the Bed."[52]

Spirits: What Is More Filthy than a Drunken Man?

The literature excoriating gin grew out of the much longer history of anti-drunkenness rhetoric. In 1596, before any of the new drugs became common in western Europe, Thomas Lodge wrote that "of all detestable sinnes dronkenness is most vilest, for it bréedeth lothsomenesse in those that most delight in it." "What is more filthie than a droncken man," Lodge asked, "who hath stench in his mouth[?]"[53] In 1727 the anonymous author of *A dissertation upon drunkenness* focused on the debased status, as he saw it, of those who frequented alehouses, calling them "the Scum of the Town and Country." He added that "the vile obscene Talk, Noise, Nonsense, and Ribaldry Discourses, together with the fumes of Tobacco, Belchings, and other foul Breakings of Wind" of taverns repelled the polite and attracted the low. The author related a misogynistic anecdote of a London miser who, whenever he felt the need for an emetic, instead of calling the apothecary sent for "an Alehouse Servant in the Neighbourhood, fam'd for her Nastiness. The Wench would no sooner appear before him in a Morning in her Dishabilee, but her Presence procur'd his Stomach an entire Discharge of the Load that oppress'd it." The author of the *Dissertation* next turned his gaze to gin and rum, portraying dram shops as vile, disordered spaces much the same as alehouses.[54]

In his attempt to turn his polite listeners away from the products of slavery, Andrew Burn followed his portrayal of sugar-making with a portrait of rum distillation. The waste product from the harvested sugarcane that went into its production was "abominably filthy and disgusting," with no guarantee that the impurities would be distilled out of the final product. Burn included a cautionary vignette of a merchant who ordered rum from Jamaica and found one cask to be bad and one good. Curious as to why that was so, he opened up the good cask and found "the whole Body of a roasted Negro." It was said that the burnt bodies of animals, including humans, made rum better, so, perhaps, Burn suspected, the corpse was included intentionally.[55] As a byproduct of sugar refining, rum, too, was both literally and figuratively "polluted" and "defiled with blood."[56] But even gin and Irish whisky, made in Europe, were susceptible to similar attacks, as William Henry related in 1753: "I have been informed by Officers in the Excise, that some Distillers distill human Excrement, to heighten the Spirit in their Whisky. . . . One has been caught with a Corpse dug out of the Church-yard in his Still," just like the rum casks hiding the body of an enslaved person.[57]

Sugar: Stained with Spots of Human Blood

As these vignettes demonstrate, when William Fox launched the campaign to boycott slave sugar in 1791 with the pamphlet *An address to the people of Great Britain on the propriety of abstaining from West India sugar and rum*, there was already a long-standing tradition of employing the rhetoric of disgust to criticize the new soft drugs. Emphasizing the bodily practice of ingesting sugar, Fox excoriated the British

Parliament for continuing to allow the slave trade, writing that the government "may hold [sugar] to our lips, steeped in the blood of our fellow-creatures; but they cannot compel us to accept this loathsome potion."[58] He calculated that for each English family who abstained from sugar for twenty-one months, one African would avoid enslavement and murder. "Nay, so necessarily connected are our consumption of the commodity," he contended, "and the misery resulting from it, that in every pound of sugar used . . . we may be considered as consuming two ounces of human flesh. . . . A French writer observes, 'That he cannot look on a piece of sugar, without conceiving it stained with spots of human blood.' "[59] When describing the enslaving of Africans, Fox described how slaves were whipped, emphasizing for his readers that, unlike flogging in the British Navy, enslavers and overseers ripped flesh from of the enslaved; again and again he repeated the image of lacerating enslaved people's bodies.[60] Britain was not the only place where antislavery writers connected sugar on the table with the bodily practices of Caribbean slavery. In 1775 the Dutch periodical the *Patriot* featured "Alintera," a young Dutch woman with her lover drinking coffee and sugar, holding a cup filled by the tears of the enslaved. It was no longer water in the cup, he claimed, but the blood and sweat of the wretched. "Drink that sweat my friend! Drink that blood, drink those tears, and then you can never be called a friend of the human race, of those who like you had the same God for their Creator. . . . Drink such blood that cries out for revenge and then do not call yourself a civilized European."[61] And in America, decades before Fox launched his campaign, the radical Quaker Benjamin Lay threw fake blood on his fellow Quakers to underscore the connection between sugar—which, in the 1730s, Lay was already refusing to eat—and slavery.[62] As Julie L. Holcomb and others have pointed out, Fox's metaphor of blood-stained sugar immediately became popular among antislavery writers.[63] Charlotte Sussman observes that by doing so Fox inverted the traditional European idea that other races were savages and cannibals, and, in a 1795 lecture, no less an influential figure than the poet Samuel Taylor Coleridge directly called sugar-eating cannibalism, a trope that Robert Southey and others picked up.[64]

When, in 1807, Parliament finally banned British participation in the slave trade, the antislavery movement turned to focus on ending slavery itself, and once again urged a boycott. In 1828 English abolitionist William Naish was still emphasizing the sensory experience of sugar, first repeating Fox's imagery about the government holding bloodstained sugar to the consumers' lips, then adding his own, focusing on feeling, hearing, and emotions:

> May every man, before he indulges his appetite with the blood-bought luxury, reflect upon the price it cost. Not eightpence . . . but groans, and wounds, and death. As he sweetens his tea, let him reflect on the bitterness at the bottom of the cup. Let him bring the subject home to his heart, and say, as he truly may, this lump cost the poor slave a groan,—and this, a bloody stroke of the cart-whip;—and this, perhaps, worn down by fatigue and wretchedness and despair, he sunk under his misery and died! And then let him swallow his beverage with what appetite he may.[65]

Here Naish united the sensory bitterness of coffee with the metaphorical bitterness of slavery.

These metaphors of bloody sugar represent the culmination of a long tradition of using sensory and bodily imagery to attack alcohol and the new drugs. Liquor, tea, chocolate, and especially tobacco and coffee drew attention from critics for their supposedly repulsive smell, sight, and taste. Their opponents associated these substances with filth, feces, urine, vomit, saliva, corpses, and blood and claimed that they perverted the natural functions of the body. Michel Foucault has ranked vision above all other senses as a tool for discipline in the eighteenth century, using the panopticon—a prison set up with a watchtower surrounded by a circle of cells, so that the inmates were always subject to observation—as the ultimate symbol of physical punishment giving way to the disciplining process.[66] The writers surveyed in this chapter demonstrate how smell, taste, touch, and even sound could also act as tools for discipline. These attempts at urging consumers to exercise self-discipline in avoiding the bodily practice of consuming drugs and alcohol were grounded in the physicality of the drugs, but their intention was to police moral boundaries as well.

A Trifling, Vain, Weak, and Contemptible Figure: Drugs Visible on the Body

As these examples have demonstrated, early modern Europeans believed that the use of the new intoxicants were readable on the face and body. Even before sugar became controversial for its connection to the slave trade, critics warned that it disfigured its users. In 1630, "Gallobelgicus" cautioned that sugar rotted out the teeth of women who consumed it, and the English dietician James Hart likewise claimed a few years later that "although Sugar in it selfe be opening and cleansing" of the body's humors, "yet being much used . . . rotteth the teeth, maketh them looke black; and withal, causeth many times a loathsome stinking-breath."[67] While defending tea against the claim that it destroyed the beauty and spoiled the breath of the young people who drank it, Bontekoe cast the blame on the added sugar instead.[68] Black, rotten teeth, stinking breath, and ugliness were the marks of those who consumed sugar. Likewise, Daniel Sennert and Abdiah Cole claimed that taking opium not only induced sleep but, after awakening, "there is a strong scent over all the body like Opium, the lips swell, there is hickets [hiccups], little breathing, the eyes are dim, the nose is awry, & there are Convulsions."[69] Not only were these stimulants disgusting in themselves but they made the faces and bodies of their users disgusting.

Gin, and drunkenness in general, left its foul marks on drinkers' physical appearance as well. In 1683, before the Gin Craze, Thomas Willis told a cautionary tale about a gentleman who gave himself up to drinking as he aged, "became dull and stupid, and also Dropsical, with a great paunch, and his thighs and legs swelled," and he was beset with a powerful drowsiness. These symptoms would disappear whenever he was able to stay sober.[70] As distilled spirits became more common, critics pointed out their physical consequences. Edward Whitaker's "Satyr upon brandy" in 1700 described a gin-soaked sot,

> His greasie Eye-lids shoar'd above their pitch,
> His Face with Carbuncles, and Rubies rich,
> His Scull instead of Brains supply'd with Cinder,
> His Nose turns all his Handkerchiefs to Tinder;
> He breaths like a Smiths Forge, and wets the fire
> Not to allay the flame but raise it higher.[71]

Similarly, *A dissertation upon drunkenness* explained that drunkenness was easily legible in one's appearance: "Look upon the Drunkard, when his Eyes stare, his Mouth drivels, his Tongue falters, and his Feet reel; how ugly, how loathsome, how monstrous does he seem?" Its author wondered why, "seeing what a trifling, vain, weak, and contemptible Figure he makes," his visage did not deter more people from drinking.[72]

Women were especially susceptible to the visible marks of gin. *An epistle to the fair-sex on the subject of drinking* warned that alcohol destroyed women's complexions.[73] In 1726 Saynought Slyboots wrote a dialogue in which a brewer and a distiller articulated opposing stances about the effects of beer and gin on the body. The distiller claimed that gin was good for the appearance of basket-women, while ale made its drinkers fat and "their Eyes stare out of their Heads."[74] The brewer countered that gin gave women "filthy diseases," hinting at sexually transmitted infections that marked gin drinkers with pox and sores.[75] Other supposed physical effects of gin drinking included making hair harsh and dry (thanks to the Gin Craze, English hair dealers in the wig trade allegedly were forced to import hair from France), trembling hands, bad skin, and bad teeth, and making the legs of hard drinkers swarthy and covered with purple spots, or "as smooth as polished ivory, and the soles of the feet even glassy and shining."[76] The most famous portrayal of a female gin drinker, of course, was in William Hogarth's *Gin Lane*, the centerpiece of which was a negligent, drunken mother whose legs are riddled with ulcers.[77]

The three hot drinks threatened the face and body as well, with Daniel Duncan cautioning in the early eighteenth century that the abuse of coffee, tea, and chocolate blackened the teeth.[78] According to *The women's petition against coffee* in 1671, coffee, along with tobacco, dried out men's bodies, and when women turned to their coffee-drinking lovers they "only meet A Bedful of Bones, and hug a meager useless Corpse."[79] This was a dig specifically at the way coffee enfeebled men's sexual prowess, but note how the enfeeblement was tangible. The physician Nicolas François Joseph Éloy lamented that Flanders and Holland were full of women who, thanks to tea, had become "living specters thanks to the pallor that reigns over their faces."[80] The satirical author of *Whipping-Tom* in the early eighteenth century poured scorn on tea drinking for distorting the way people carried themselves. Upon observing people drinking tea for the first time, he noted "some holding the Rim at the bottom of the Dish, betwixt their Thumb and the first, second, and third Fingers; others holding the Top and Bottom of the Dish, betwixt the Thumb and middle Finger only, with the Palm of the Hand outwards, so that one skill'd in Chiromancy, may easily tell their Fortunes."[81]

Moreover, the countenances and bodies of smokers were susceptible to permanent damage. In 1621 the Bath physician Tobias Venner noted that smokers could be identified by their "smokie faces" due to tobacco, and swollen and flatulent bellies due to the drinking that followed.[82] Thomas Short observed that "Habitual Smoakers have a foul squalid Tongue, a white Mouth, their Senses of Smell and Taste are impaired and sometimes lost, the Smell of their Breath is more nauseous than that of a Boghouse [outhouse]. . . . Their Complexion (if not red or carbuncled with drinking) is pale or bad. . . . They are always dribbling at their Mouth, and Spitting."[83] One anonymous writer noted that snuff caused polyps to appear inside the nose, sometimes filling the nostrils and growing outward into plain view, as well as damaging the nerves of the face, leaving the muscles "flaccid, and to give the visage a furrowed, wrinkled appearance, causing the complexion to have a sallow, cadaverous colour."[84] In his medical guide for families, Hugh Smythson warned that smoking tobacco would blacken and decay the teeth, while snuff would destroy the sense of smell in addition to fostering nasal polyps, sometimes even extending into the mouth, threatening suffocation unless a surgeon could remove them.[85] Another, less immediately visible effect of tobacco could be found inside users' bodies: in 1635 Tomás Ramón wrote that when a smoker's cadaver was opened, it revealed that tobacco had turned the interior of its head black.[86] Tobacco was also said to blacken the entrails or, as Joshua Sylvester put it, to shrink the entire body like a smoked herring.[87] Truly, tobacco insulted all the senses, as Sylvester wrote:

> Offend the Eyes, with foule and loathsome Spawlings:
> Offend the Nose, with filthy Fumes exhalings:
> Offend the Eares, with loud lewd Execrations:
> Offend the Mouth, with ougly Excreations:
> Offend the Sense, with stupefying Sense."[88]

Not only did tobacco offend the senses; it also damaged them, especially tobacco. In 1634 Francisco de Leiva y Aguilar complained that tobacco impaired sight, thanks to the ill effects of its heat and dryness on the humor of the eyes.[89] The anonymous author of *Tobaco-mastix* in 1677 accused tobacco smoke from tobacco of ruining the taste of tobacco as well as damaging hearing and smell through its ill effects on the brain.[90] The most common complaint was tobacco's ruinous effect on taste and smell, with snuff in particular dangerous to the sense of smell.[91] And, while not one of the five senses, speech, too, could be ruined by tobacco; as the anonymous author of *A dissertation on the use and abuses of tobacco* observed in 1720, smokers were marked by a speech impediment, "commonly called Snuffling."[92] On the other hand, Antonio Lavedán countered that tobacco lent agility to the tongue and made them more fluid speakers.[93] The wearing away of the senses helped promote the use of tobacco itself, as Tobias

Venner argued, since long, immoderate use of the weed made users "Insensiles, without sense." Here he meant both the bodily senses and common sense, as smokers became immune to tobacco's bad effects, "because that by long use and custome, it becommeth familiar to their bodies."[94] Although English dietician Henry Butts warned that it dulled the senses, he claimed that tobacco, taken moderately, could in fact sharpen them.[95] Certainly, either way, tobacco affected the workings of the body's five senses. Nor was it just tobacco that had these effects: J. B. Sassenus, an Antwerp physician, recommended tea to the elderly as restorative of eyesight, hearing, and the sharpness of mind.[96] Duncan, who warned against hot drinks harming teeth, cautioned that coffee led to poor vision and hearing; its drinkers would have earlier recourse than others "to make use of Spectacles and a Horn."[97] If one found one's senses debilitated from the abuse of coffee and tobacco, however, the English physician and natural scientist Frederick Slare had, in 1715, an antidote: sugar. Spread on the hands, administered to the tongue, or even blown into the eyes as a salve, sugar healed and soothed the sense organs.[98]

Cleansing and Preserving the Body: Sweet Ointment for Sour Teeth

While antislavery activists were emphasizing sugar's immoral and disfiguring aspects, others maintained that it was unproblematically sweet and that it purified the body. The anonymous author of *An essay on sugar* claimed in 1752 that it was tea that rotted the teeth and gums, and that sugar actually whitened teeth.[99] In 1599 the dietician Henry Butts contended that sugar was a healthy alternative to honey and that it cleansed the body, especially the kidneys.[100] This was the case for other drugs, too. A judge in England named Walter Rumsey praised tobacco and coffee both for their ability to scour the body of corruption (and worms), and, indeed, the expulsion of corrupted humors was key to their usefulness as medicines (Rumsey had invented a instrument made from whalebone that could induce vomiting without the bad taste of tobacco- and coffee-based medicines).[101] Cornelis Bontekoe urged the use of coffee and tea to clean the mouth and sweeten breath, making the saliva "lovely" and "fragrant" and strengthening the teeth. Coffee, meanwhile, was a good counteragent for bad breath as well.[102] One Spanish observer reported that young women drank coffee because it made their faces prettier, and an English advertisement from 1660 claimed that chocolate would whiten the skin of "The Nut-Brown Lasses of the Land," tanned from working outside in the sun, erasing their low status.[103] Many English observers argued that far from blackening the teeth, tobacco was a cleaning agent, including Thomas Tomkis, who wrote in 1607 that it made a "sweete ointment for sowre teeth."[104] Some defenders of tobacco, like Richard West, even defied the common trope of "stinking tobacco" to claim that tobacco was "stinking breaths perfumer."[105]

As Edmund Gardiner pointed out, many medicines had terrible odors, many of them worse than tobacco, so its stink was not a sign of anything unhealthy.[106] He also praised the healing and cleansing abilities of tobacco in the form of unburnt leaves, which, he asserted, cured ulcers and sores, as well as killing the "crawling wormes" in the wound. He continued: "I know a certain man that had an ulcer in his nose out of which there issues forth a virtulent or filthy matter . . . who by mine advise dropped in som of the juyce of the leaves of Tabacco, and when hee had done so twise together, a great many worms first came forth, and . . . after a fewe days the sore was absolutely cured."[107] Gardiner also recommended tobacco powder for healing "stinking and rotten gums" caused by scurvy."[108] And, of course, the normal medicinal use for tobacco was as a cleansing purge, expelling phlegmatic humors from the stomach, lungs, and head, drawing "slimie and pituitous humours from the mouth and nostrels."[109]

Gardiner's praise was part of a deep undercurrent that welcomed tobacco for its sweet smell and cleansing qualities. Nicolás Monardes, one of the first observers to describe tobacco to western Europeans, explained in 1574 how Native Americans used tobacco to cleanse wounds, purge the stomach, and expel worms.[110] One early, nearly universal recommendation for tobacco was to burn it during plague epidemics in order to dispel the contagion and keep people healthy. Even in the second half of the eighteenth century there were proponents of tobacco as a cleanser. Thomas Short conceded that "Habitual Smoakers have a foul squalid Tongue, a white Mouth," that "the Smell of their Breath is more nauseous than that of a Boghouse, or of Wind broken downward after taking Flower or Milk of Brimstone," and that the smell of the smoke in an enclosed space was enough to make non-smokers vomit.[111] Nevertheless, he recommended tobacco ashes as a teeth cleaner and asserted that tobacco juice could expel worms from the rectum.[112] Antonio Lavedán also believed that tobacco could whiten and clean the teeth.[113] Juan de Castro y Medinilla recommended tobacco for clearing sickness from diseased organs, and for dispelling bad odors emanating from the body.[114] Cornelis Bontekoe argued that tobacco did not stink, that in fact its users had sweeter breath than drinkers of wine or beer.[115] Perhaps John Taylor summed up the ambivalence about tobacco's sensory effects best when he called it "stinking sweet Tobacco."[116]

Pleasure: Better to Be Tasted than Described

No matter how often critics deployed the language of filth, disgust, and stink to warn people away, they could not change the fact that, for so many consumers, sugar and its fellow stimulants brought physical pleasure. As the anonymous author of *An essay on sugar* put it in 1752, even infants knew it was good. When milk was unavailable, nurses gave babies sugar, which was perhaps even better for them than breast milk. Insects and animals, like ants or sugar-mill horses, were also drawn to eating sugar, proving that "Nature itself" wisely chooses "this excellent and pleasing Sweet."[117] As Kim Hall points out, by 1700 sugar had captured the imagination of the English that for them the sensation of sweetness had become almost exclusively associated with white crystals produced from Caribbean sugarcane.[118] How could something that tasted so good be unhealthy or immoral? Michael Kwass notes that one defense of luxury goods put forward in eighteenth-century France was simply that they were pleasurable. The "new luxuries" of the day were no longer adopted for display and status like the furs, jewels, and spices favored by the nobility during the Middle Ages. Now the luxury market aimed for bodily comfort and physical pleasure. Comfortable carriages, down bedclothes, well-constructed housing, and white bread were all aimed at pleasing the senses.[119] So were sugar and all the new drugs.

As Kwass suggests, exotic drugs arrived in Europe just as thinking about pleasure and the senses was shifting. The seventeenth and eighteenth centuries witnessed a changing assessment of pleasure and the five senses, inspired in part by an increased attention to ancient Greek and Roman epicureanism. The theorists behind the Scientific Revolution, for example, with their new regard for empirical evidence, developed an appreciation for the information that the senses provided for the mind.[120] Defenders of the new intoxicants supported them in ways that fit nicely into these trends, articulating a language of bodily pleasure that helped justify their use. Emboldened by new respect for the senses and for exotic physical pleasures, promoters of sugar and its fellow drugs leaned into the same sensory language used by critics such as Burn. Like these critics, they used their assessment of the drugs' physical qualities to make moral points about their users.

Early modern writers were more comfortable giving voice to their emotions in verse than in prose, and it was often poems that expressed the pleasure of using the new soft drugs—the flip side of the mocking doggerel verse that they used to express disgust. In one eighteenth-century poem, Girolamo Giuntini praised the smell and taste of chocolate, expressing the wish that his throat could be a long well, or a crane's neck, to make the sensation of drinking it last longer.[121] In 1789, Italian clergyman Giambattista Sbalbi published a poem in praise of chocolate (or perhaps translated it from Latin into Tuscan) in which he described his anticipation before drinking it, and how refreshed he felt just thinking about it.[122] Sometimes the language of pleasure snuck into prose, though. The celebrated Neapolitan chef Vincenzo Corrado explained that "people educated in the comforts and pleasures of life" drank chocolate hot in the morning and cold during the day.[123] Giacomo Sanvitale argued that, like wine, the main reason people drank chocolate was for the taste. It delighted the palate and appealed to different people for various qualities of its taste: sweetness, bitterness, spiciness, or sourness.[124] Gregorio Mayáns, a Valencian jurist and man of letters, lauded chocolate in the eighteenth century as an invigorating force, "similar to divine nectar and ambrosia." He wrote: "Oh sweet drink, even more pleasant than wine mixed with honey!" He liked it so much he sometimes took It twice a day.[125]

As early as 1620, Castro y Medinilla dwelled on the pleasing smells of tobacco and the comfortable rituals of smoking that Native American elites employed. They stored their tobacco carefully, and at mealtimes they combined tobacco leaves with scented ingredients and shaped them into a thin cigar, mingling their smoking and eating just as Europeans combined wine with meals.[126] Francesco Maria della Volpe also praised the sensory pleasures of snuff and chocolate in two neo-Latin poems published in Rome in 1722.[127] The Elizabethan playwright Francis Beaumont claimed in a poem that neither beer nor wine could compare with tobacco "for taste, and for smell."[128] The praise could also come in a simple description of how it felt to sneeze after taking snuff; as Luigi Zorzi Prete put it, "A torrent flows through me, which unloads my head and refreshes me, and fills me with sweetness and contentment."[129] Writing in 1819, the Genoese physician Michele Nicolò Chiazzari attributed the rapid spread of tobacco throughout Europe not to fashion, vice, or compulsion, but to its flavor and "narcotic odor,"

Which people liked. After wondering whether snuff was truly a necessity, he countered that "perhaps the nose has its own needs, as do the other bodily senses, needs truly founded on the deprivation of a pleasure which could be satisfied with so little expense?"[130] A century earlier the Ferrarese Jesuit and man of letters Girolamo Baruffaldi had declared in his ode to tobacco that every sense has its delight, and the delight of smell was tobacco.[131]

The sensations of drinking coffee and tea also spurred praise, as in 1750, when the Bergamasque priest and satirical poet Anton-Maria Borga da Rasa published a poem in praise of the pipe, and of the "gentle idleness and delicate sloth" that one experienced while alternating sips of coffee and puffs on the pipe.[132] Irish dramatist Nahum Tate published a poem about tea, "Panacea," in 1700, describing "the warm Nectar's pleasing Force," which set spirits dancing around the heart and the brain. This feeling was so different from the "woeful mirth" that came from drinking wine.[133] In a classicizing poem printed in the *Spectator* placing tea among the nymphs and groves of ancient Greece, Peter Motteux reveled in the sensory pleasures of the tea table, singing that "the lovely Colour courts, / The Flavour charms us, but the Taste transports."[134] Repeatedly calling tea a nectar, Motteux expressed his enjoyment of its ability to refresh the mind and spirits. Cornelis Bontekoe wrote that the judgment of what is good or bad for health and life belongs to the tongue, and the tongue judged tea to be "pleasant, delicate, and refined." "But . . . the pleasant flavour of tea is better to be tasted than described, even if one if insensible to this delicate flavour, which far surpasses all that passes for sweet and delicious."[135] The mere anticipation of drinking tea could cause pleasure, as one poet described the sounds of the boiling kettle and the sight of the clean and shining saucers bringing comfort to a student in a dark November season.[136] While less common, there were those who praised the scent and taste of coffee as well.[137]

Gin was more difficult to find pleasurable. Alexander Blunt praised its scent in a backhanded fashion, as a way to ward off all of the evil smells of London, drawing on the connection made by contemporary medical thought between foul odors and contagious disease. He portrayed juniper as heroically staving off the stench from jails, outhouses, sewers, and slaughterhouses, as well as the dead animals lying in the streets of the monstrously expanding city.[138] The naturalist and man of letters Pierre Jean-Baptist Legrand d'Aussy speculated that people given to coarse diets might find their taste so blunted that only the strongest flavors could please them, which might account for why some people found brandy delicious. Apparently it took either a depraved diet or depraved surroundings to make distilled liquor palatable.

Opium was easier to find enjoyable. The anonymous Dutch author of *A brief on opium* explained that while opium relieves pain, it also "awakens to a certain extent the vital spirits, just like wine, and then beckons and invites nature to rest again."[139] In Turkey the recreational smoking of opium led to "joy and cheerfulness," and when mixed with spices like cinnamon and nutmeg, "a delight, yes, even a kind of ecstasy arises."[140] James Handley, in a 1721 work devoted to the new, post-Newton mechanical medicine, went out of his way to describe the "Relaxation" that opium's "Pleasure causes," likening it to listening to fine music or sitting indoors in comfort while hearing the wind blow outside.[141] However much critics emphasized the foul, nasty experience of using the new drugs and alcohol, defenders explained how the sensory pleasures of ingesting them acted as a powerful enticement for their use. Historians who have studied pleasure in the early modern period have focused almost exclusively on sexuality, but the acclaim that these commentators showered on the new soft drugs shows that Europeans of that period were sensitive to other types of physical sensations as well.

Senses and Knowledge

Bontekoe's insistence that the tongue could determine whether or not tea was wholesome pointed to another connection between the new soft drugs and the senses: the belief that the senses were the best judge of both healthfulness and moral character. Speaking of sugar, Frederick Slare's recommendation was to "appeal to this Organ [the tongue] as to the most accurate Judge" of what was good for the body. "Let this distinguishing Faculty speak out," he wrote, "and utter only the just Praises of Sugar."[142] This was a recent development, since it was only in the late seventeenth century that western Europeans stopped associating taste with material, edible things and began to think of it as a moral quality. The man of good taste was also an ethical man, and "taste" became a way to know the world, not just to experience food.[143] The rise of taste as a kind of knowledge coincided with the increasing trust that empirical evidence, experience, and the five senses could lead to knowledge about the physical world—in other words, the Scientific Revolution.

In the earliest years of tobacco's appearance in Europe, James I, the king of England, believed that tobacco's stench was a clear sign of its dangers, "the Nose being the proper Organ and convoy of the sense of smelling to the braines, which are the onely fountaine of that sense, doeth ever serve us for an infallible witnesse, whether that Odour which we smell, be healthful or hurtful to the braine."[144] Others, of course, thought that tobacco smelled good and was therefore healthy, but what about the artificial scents added to tobacco? Juan de Castro y Medinilla considered scented tobacco as a medicine, concluding that it was fine for the purpose and should be used if the patient finds it convenient.[145] In keeping with the new respect for pleasure and the role of the senses in natural sciences, Lorenzo Serafini opened his investigation of chocolate with a long disquisition that the senses, not reason, tells people what is good and bad to ingest.[146] French agronomist Antoine-Augustin Parmentier explained how the quality of raw chocolate could be determined by its taste, scent, and feel in the mouth.[147] Tea especially could be judged by its smell and taste, as Cornelis Bontekoe noted in 1678: "The more it smells of newly dried hay the fresher and better it is. The taste is the chief connoisseur of tea; to this it ought to appear to be bitter, strong, delicious, penetrating and somewhat astringent." Tea's color also told its quality. Further, he argued that the tongue would naturally approve of the "pleasant, delicate, and refined" taste of tea, signifying its healthiness, so long as its powers had not been eroded by luxurious eating and drinking. Nevertheless, stale tea could be deceiving, and weak tea might still taste and smell good even without doing anything to benefit the drinker's health.[148] Two decades later the English clergyman John Ovington distinguished between different types of tea, with their different effects on the body, through the senses. "The finest Sort" of bing, or imperial tea, "looks both green to the Eye, and is crisp in the Mouth, and the smell of it is very pleasant, which inhances the Price of it here in England, and 'tis highly esteem'd likewise in China."[149] Around the same time, *The debauched and enchanted coffee and tea world* ranked teas using sensory information, as did Thomas Short half a century later.[150] "Sometimes the fine Green Teas shall have a most fragrant, cordial, reviving Smell and Taste," Short explained, while "at other times (as is the present Mode) all good Tea shall smell so rank of Soap, that it would make any delicate Person's Stomach peuk."[151] The sensory features of the tea indicated their qualities: "What more wretched fainty Stuff, and miserable Tipple, even to the strong and healthy, far more hysteric and hip'd than Bing Tea? What most nasty and nauseous

Smell than Soap Sudds at your Nose? What more comfortable and cordial, than the natural Smell of the finest Green Teas?"[152]

Thomas Short went on to offer more detailed instructions for telling whether true brandy was of exceptionally high quality, and how to detect if Dutch swindlers had tried to pass off "Molossos Spirits" as true French brandy.[153] Thomas Dossie agreed that one could distinguish rum, brandy, molasses, and malt spirit from each other and also determine their quality by their taste and smell. In his mind, rum was superior to French brandy, which had a "very disgustful smell and taste."[154] Dossie explained that the more spirits are distilled, "they gain, by time . . . a grateful flavor and odour; and, in those, where volatile oil abounds, their seeming rankness of smell and taste . . . is converted, by degrees, into a species of perfumed odour."[155] Note how the plain judgment of the senses and the chemical analysis of "volatile oils" reinforced each other.[156] M. de Reynal also combined sensory and scientific knowledge when discussing coffee in 1813. "It is true that the tincture of roasted coffee does not strike the taste or smell except by a manifestly empyreumatic quality," he wrote, "for one drinks this liquor with pleasure. However, it is not possible that the degree of torrefaction that the beans have undergone . . . has not changed the character of their oil; indeed it could not rise and evaporate through heat . . . without losing the soft, creamy quality of the fatty oils; similar to butter . . . and just like butter . . . that on the organ of taste creates a sensation that one finds pleasant only because it is activated by an acrimonious principle."[157] Short believed that, like tea, the nature of distilled spirits revealed itself to the application of the nose, tongue, eyesight, and skin. To discern brandy from inferior stilled spirits, he recommended rubbing a little of the liquid between the hands and then smelling it; a more "vinous" and lingering smell indicated true brandy.[158]

Quality was something that taste could judge, but taste was a subjective form of evaluation that depended greatly on the person making the judgment, and one can see how a sense of connoisseurship could develop from the ever-increasing refinement of one's taste. These drugs, of course, had physical properties that did not change unless their composition altered. The three hot drinks were all bitter, while sugar was sweet. Tobacco's scent was distinctive, as was gin's. Nevertheless, individual appraisers judged those permanent qualities in variable ways, as good or bad, pleasing or foul. In her study of judging quality in the production of tea, Sarah Besky demonstrates that there is no natural good or bad quality inherent in any consumable substance;

instead critics assign quality to substances, making moral judgments about their value.[159] There is no doubt that inhaling smoke from a pipe was novel in early modern western Europe, but observers differed in their assessment of that smoke's value. Sweetness was intrinsic to the experience of eating sugar, but whether that sweetness created a pleasing sensation or choked the consumer with blood depended on the context in which the taster imagined the sugar to be.

Both Andrew Burn and Frederick Slare paid close attention to sugar's physical qualities. Slare claimed that sugar's appeal to the tongue spoke for itself, as did its pleasant sensation when applied to other parts of the body. Burn turned his readers' attention to African bodies and their alleged filthiness, which became inextricably linked to sugar's physical nature. Both men were making moral judgments about sugar through their consideration of its physical qualities. Slare gave sugar a clean bill of health, while Burn insinuated that the inhumane manner of producing slave sugar in the Caribbean contaminated its western European consumers. Both men inhabited a long tradition, beginning with the Spaniards' first encounter with chocolate and tobacco in the Americas, of linking the physical qualities of psychotropic drugs and alcohol to the moral impact of using them. Critics of the new drugs emphasized the foulness of the drugs, especially by comparing them with nasty things sloughed off or expelled from the human body. Tobacco, chocolate, and coffee were all comparable to feces, while alcohol was associated with vomit, tea with urine, and sugar with blood, sweat, and pus. They also perverted the functions of the body, acting as purgatives in the old Galenic tradition but in the wrong way, letting smoke out of the nose, making the mouth and face sewers and chimneys for filth. But, as viewed by their defenders, the new stimulants were cleansing. Sweetening the breath, cleaning the mouth, eyes, and teeth, healing and generally scouring corruption from the body. Either way, the effects of the new drugs were easily readable on the body. Legs, bellies, hands, hair, teeth, and especially faces announced to the world that a person was a drug user. They also allegedly damaged the senses themselves through their overuse, and, in doing so, they hurt the very tools by which western Europeans knew whether the drugs were good or bad, healthy or ill, high or poor quality. Another undercurrent of praise for stimulants was for their sensory effects on the body in the form of pleasure. Pleasure and cleanliness persisted despite the torrent of abuse poured on these drugs, highlighting the ambivalence with which observers measured their impact in early modern Europe. The intensity of commentators' focus on the senses emphasized their experience of these drugs as physical things, ingested into their bodies and affecting their bodies, as much or more than they did for their mental or social effects. The smells, taste, touch, and sight of the new drugs intertwined with all of the anxiety that they felt about the bodily consequences of using them.

This complicates the story that Norbert Elias has told about civilization and the body: that modernity rests in part on an increasing threshold of shame surrounding the body and bodily functions, like excretions, eating, and even cleansing actions like blowing one's nose. Historians have taken Elias's ideas and used them to suggest that early modern Europe saw elites drawing away from popular culture. This enabled them to make a moral distinction between their refined, rational behavior and the crude, Rabelaisian peasants and urban poor, with their childlike lack self-control or shame about their bodies. In keeping with Elias's thinking, critics harnessed the rhetoric of filth and disgust to try to restrain people from using the new psychotropic drugs. Self-discipline demanded that, to keep control over one's bodily autonomy and social status, European men and women keep away from these disgusting new comestibles. The writers who praised the pleasure derived from consuming the new drugs constituted the most dangerous threat to Elias's idea of the civilizing process—the seductive pleasure of consuming drugs, among other new luxury items like cotton clothing, white bread, and comfortable home furnishings—drew European consumers, rich and poor, away from bodily discipline toward sensory pleasure. The ambivalence about the bodily experience of using drugs was profound; there was great encouragement to move away from the body, but the counterpressure of pleasure persisted, enticing Europeans into ever-increasing amounts of drug and alcohol consumption.

CHAPTER 2

Chocolate, or an Indian Drink

The Cultural Geography of Drugs and Alcohol

In his 1682 work *The natural history of coffee, chocolate, thee, tobacco*, John Chamberlayne observed that "most Nations under the Sun ha[ve] their drunken Liquors and Compounds; the Turk his Maslack, the Persians their Bangue [bhang, a form of cannabis], the Indians their Fulo, their Rum, their Arak, and Punch. The Arabians, Turks, Chinese, Tartars, and other Eastern Countries do make inebriating Liquors out of their Corn, and Rice: some rather than not be Drunk will swallow Opium, Dutroy [datura], and Tobacco, or some other intoxicating thing, so great an inclination has Mankind to be exalted."[1] Chamberlayne mapped out a global cultural geography of intoxicants that by the late seventeenth century was becoming familiar to the literate elite of Europe. When Chamberlayne published his *Natural history*, two of the drugs he targeted, coffee and tea, were quite new to western Europeans, while tobacco and chocolate had been known for decades. Nevertheless he felt it necessary to describe the cacao tree and its "fruits" and "nut" to his readers, as well as the regions where it grew, the process of making chocolate, and chocolate's physical effects. He took pains to make his information intelligible to English readers, explaining that "the Tree is said to be as large as our English Plumb-trees," its leaves were similar to those of the chestnut, the nuts the size of large almonds. He also narrated some of the episodes of the history of the European encounter with chocolate, such as Moctezuma serving it to Hernando Cortés and his followers in the waning days of the Aztec empire.[2] One hundred and eighty years after Christopher Columbus encountered a canoe containing cacao among other trading goods off the coast of Honduras, and a century after Spanish natural scientists like Francisco Hernández began to make chocolate comprehensible to Europeans, Chamberlayne still had to describe its exotic origins to contextualize it for his readers.[3]

Chocolate's exoticism was not simply a matter of benign curiosity. Decades earlier Bartolomé Marradón, a medical professional from Andalusia who had traveled to New Spain, warned that Spanish immigrant women had learned from Native American women how to work sorcery through chocolate, harming their rivals through supernatural powers derived from the devil.[4] Marradón's words of caution about the connections between chocolate, Native Americans, and the devil were echoed in European thinking about all the early modern stimulants. As Marcy Norton has demonstrated for chocolate and tobacco, not only did western Europeans have to grapple with these psychotropic drugs as chemical agents with biological consequences, they also had to interpret them as cultural artifacts. During the centuries that Native Americans had been using these drugs, they developed ceremonies and rituals around their use. Mesoamericans infused chocolate and tobacco with religious meaning, consumed them in different settings and in different ways by different classes of people, and prepared and used them in gendered patterns. Western Europeans had to decide which of these meanings and practices to adopt and which to discard, and indeed whether it was possible to discard them at all. When incorporated into European consumption patterns, the American drugs began to stir up changes in European culture as well.[5] Chocolate and tobacco threatened to reshape aspects of gender, class, courtship, sex, and fertility in ways both subtle and profound when they arrived in western Europe, and this would repeat itself with coffee, tea, opium, and sugar.

The anxiety and fascination that Europeans harbored toward foreign peoples arrived in Europe along with the drugs, even as they were learning about the exotic drugs from those same people. The first chapter of this book introduced this anxiety, showing that western Europeans associated sugar with the supposedly filthy bodies of enslaved Africans, for example, or coffee with the Muslim Middle East. Commentators mapped the disgust and pleasure that they experienced onto the exotic foreigners from whom the new drugs originated.

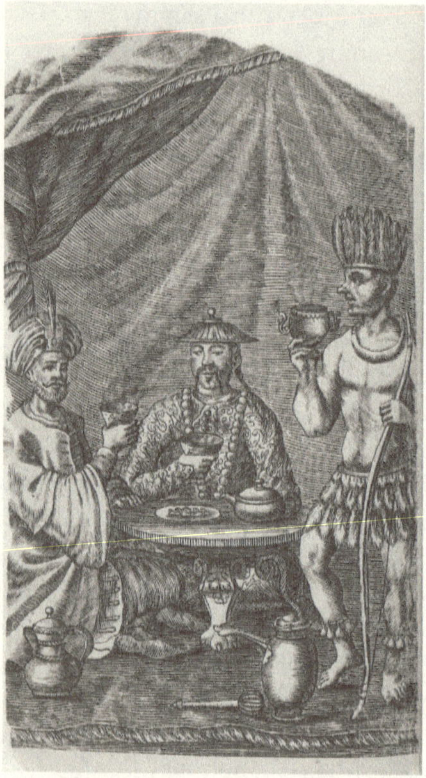

FIGURE 2.1. Philippe Sylvestre Dufour, *Tractatus novi de potu caphé, de Chinensium thé, et de chocolata* (Paris: Pierre Muguet, 1685), frontispiece. This engraving links the three hot drinks, coffee, tea, and chocolate, with caricatures of the peoples from whom Europeans obtained them: the Turks, the Chinese, and Native Americans. Reproduced courtesy of the British Library.

All of the stimulants carried with them racial, religious, gendered, and class-blurring dangers for their new users, threatening to loosen control over their behavior and modify the composition of their bodies. So much of the discipline that theorists like Weber, Elias, Oestreich, and Foucault tell us was intensifying during the early modern period focused on increasingly self-aware control over the body and on the efforts of church and state to enforce morality, especially sexual morality. Yet chocolate and its fellow stimulants threatened to erode that self-discipline and even erode the bodily integrity of European consumers by imprinting the cultural markers of the societies from which they came. At a time when Protestant and Catholic clergy both worked to shape their parishioners into members of religious communities bounded by sharply defined ethics, theology, and practice, these stimulants offered to seduce Europeans away from Christianity altogether. However much historians who have examined drugs and alcohol from the viewpoint of the consumer revolution want to write a triumphant narrative of chocolate and its sister intoxicants, quickly brushing away the initial hesitation at incorporating the new foreign substances into western Europe, a thick strain of ambivalence remained through the seventeenth and eighteenth centuries about the threats these exotic goods posed to their self-conception. As Irene Fattacciu observes, chocolate's exoticism was both an obstacle to adoption and part of its allure, and the same was true for all of these drugs.[6] Even as they imported and ingested increasing amounts of them, Europeans searched for ways to make them safe.

Chocolate, or an Indian Drink

Although sailors and other travelers during the sixteenth century brought small quantities of cacao back to Seville for their own use, it was not until the 1590s that Spanish merchants began to import it for sale.[7] It remained a rarity until midway through the seventeenth century, when chocolate began to be prepared and sold in English coffeehouses, where the diarist Samuel Pepys tried some.[8] Initially, Castile held a monopoly on all of the cacao imported into Europe, since the Spanish crown controlled the territory where it grew, and the Spaniards spread its cultivation from Mesoamerica to New Granada.[9] The Dutch began cultivating it in Curaçao and the Dutch East Indies, and by the 1630s the international market had shifted from Seville to Amsterdam. The English began planting cacao in newly seized Jamaica after 1655, bringing in enough of the commodity for Parliament to impose an excise tax in 1660, while the Spanish imported a half million pounds during the decade of the 1650s, rising to two million in the 1660s.[10] Irene Fattacciu estimates that by 1700 one million pounds per year entered Europe through Seville and Amsterdam, rising to fifteen million per year by 1800, with an untold amount smuggled in unrecorded.[11] By this time chocolate had shifted from an American drink to a European beverage, and producers dropped hard-to-find American ingredients like achiote from the recipe and added sugar. In the eighteenth century, chocolate became commodified as a preground, premixed paste of cacao, sugar, and cinnamon, ready for drinkers to just add water and consume.[12] Drinking chocolate was associated with Italy and even more so with Spain, with foreign travelers noting the drabness of the diet there except for the remarkable amount of chocolate consumed. The moneyed elite in Madrid took chocolate every morning for breakfast and then drank more during the day and at night during social events, as well as in coffeehouses, from stalls along the Paseo de Prado, and in the park of the Retiro. Chocolate's relatively high price kept it largely out of the hands of the nonelite until the end of the century, but Fattacciu reports that while in 1727 Madrid consumed 70 percent of all the chocolate in Spain, it share had fallen to 30 percent by the 1790s as the rise in imports and the fall in price made it more accessible to consumers beyond the capital.[13] Outside of southern Europe, chocolate consumption largely remained an urban phenomenon until the nineteenth century.[14]

Chocolate provides a good entry point for exploring Europeans' concerns about the threatening nature of the new drugs. Norton has shown that chocolate's deep enmeshment with Native American religion was especially troubling. Mesoamerican religion symbolically linked chocolate to blood, and it became a surrogate for blood in religious rituals, especially after Catholic authorities put a stop to bloodletting and human sacrifice. Moreover, anxiety grew about the influence of Native American customs and habits on the Spanish living among them, the more so as Spanish authorities began to realize that the conversion of the Native Americans to Christianity often resembled a thin veneer that did little to suppress traditional forms of worship and belief. If Native Americans continued to use chocolate to gain access to their gods—or, as the missionaries believed, devils—and creoles were adopting Mesoamerican behavior, did this mean that drinking chocolate turned Christians into devil-worshiping pagans? This possibility is what had Marradón alarmed when he warned that chocolate served as a conduit for superstition, idolatry, and the demonic to enter into Christian society in America, and perhaps Europe, too. These fears only grew as Spanish authorities periodically uncovered groups of Native Americans clandestinely trying to keep their ancient faith alive, substituting chocolate for blood in their makeshift rituals of religious resistance.[15]

Chocolate's natural properties could be troubling as well. William Hughes, a physician who had traveled to the Caribbean, published a treatise in 1672 on the various exotic plants grown on English plantations there, drawing on humoral theory to discern who should drink chocolate and where. He recommended it for sailors who arrived in the islands ravenous for fresh food after their long journey. After overeating, they developed skin problems, for which, Hughes advised, chocolate served very hot "is excellent to drive forth such offensive humours, opening the pores, and causing moderate sweats." But because of its heat, consumers in England should not indulge in chocolate often, since their stomachs were already hot and needed colder food, and young people especially were prone to stomach problems if they drank too much.[16] The Scots-French Huguenot refugee physician Daniel Duncan also wrote about hot drinks—chocolate, coffee, and tea—in 1706, warning about the problems that drinkers of chocolate brought on themselves by introducing so much excess heat into their bodies, especially in their blood. Differences within Europe informed Duncan's thinking, as chocolate was especially dangerous for Italians and Spaniards, who were already too hot.[17] On the other hand, Duncan noted that "the Inhabitants of the cold and moist North excuse their Intemperance in Coffee, Chocolate, Tea, Strong-Waters, Salts, Spices and Tobacco, by the necessity there is of it to avoid an intemperate Coldness and Moisture," but they used this medical excuse to overindulge.[18] The English physician Martin Lister also believed that chocolate-drinking residents of Paris risked harming themselves. "The Wild Indians . . . no doubt digest it," he wrote, "but our Pampered Bodies can make little of it."[19] This American drink was meant to be consumed in America.

The unease many felt at Christians sampling Indian chocolate was founded in part on the belief that one's bodily identity was changeable. Ideas about race and ethnicity were looser and more varied in early modern Europe, before the pseudoscientific racism of the nineteenth century assigned a biological essence to race, marked by skin color and physiognomy.[20] One early modern strand of thinking about racial difference connected directly to religion: the Iberian idea of *limpieza de sangre*, or "purity of blood," held that the alienation of Jews and Muslims from Christianity was somehow embodied, and that even if they received the sacrament of baptism they could never become truly Christian. Throughout Europe the salient markers of difference between the various races not only included skin color but also manners, dress, climate, and religion. Altering one or more of these elements could alter an individual's place among the peoples of the world.[21] Moreover, medical advice warned of the susceptibility of the body to change. According to humoral theory drawn from Galen and other ancient physicians, the balance of humors in each individual's body gave them a unique complexion, but that complexion was heavily dependent on the climate, food, and drink of one's original home. Changing those factors, either through travel or the introduction of foreign food and drink, could disturb that equipoise and cause illness.[22] Furthermore, in the late seventeenth and eighteenth centuries, the English physician Thomas Sydenham and his Dutch follower Herman Boerhaave took inspiration from Hippocrates's *On airs, waters, and places*, launching a neo-Hippocratic revival. Their ideas reinforced the sense that the body was shaped by its environmental surroundings, and they refocused medical attention on environmental influences to explain health and disease during a time when their countrymen were increasingly journeying around the globe. Everything about the New World environment threatened Europeans, as the air, stars, and food could all supposedly alter their humors and shift their bodies to become like those of the Native Americans, whom Europeans viewed as fragile and distressingly prone to disease and death as they observed wave after wave of epidemics crash into American societies. As soon as they could, Spaniards tried to establish European agriculture to nurture the Europeans who made America their home and to keep their bodies healthy, providing familiar provisions like wheat and wine. Inducing Native Americans to switch to European foods was also part of the reforming project to civilize and Christianize them—there could be no Eucharist without wheat and grapes.[23] Hughes, Duncan, and Lister drew on an emerging body of scholarship that aimed to explain the dangers of foreign areas to travelers, to explain how the local people's bodies were adapted to their climates, and to help preserve Europeans' health in the tropics.[24]

Although by the seventeenth century chocolate-drinking was common even on the lowest rungs of Mexican society, the earliest Spanish observers noticed that chocolate was a luxury good used more frequently by the elite merchants and nobles of Mesoamerica.[25] This pattern replicated itself in Europe, as the Andalusian surgeon and physician Antonio Colmenero de Ledesma pointed out when commenting on how popular it had become among aristocrats in Spain, Italy, and Flanders.[26] In fact, until the second half of the century, chocolate and cacao probably circulated in Spain less as a commodity on the market and more through gift exchange between noble households, and, together with the porcelain serving cups, pots, and other utensils associated with it, chocolate became an important aspect of fashionable display to demonstrate a host's taste and class.[27] In 1690 a London satirist mocked the "modish town-sparks, drinking Chocolate" in coffeehouses as even more socially pretentious than the other customers there.[28] François-Guislier du Verger, a master distiller from Paris living in Brussels, noted that after thirty years of chocolate's presence in the Francophone world it had become customary to offer chocolate to guests twice a day, at morning and at dinner, "among people of quality and even among the distinguished and well-off bourgeoisie." This would be understandable in Spain, Italy, and the Indies, he continued, because one should drink hot things where it is hot, but it hurt the digestion of those living in colder climates.[29] In 1753 the Carmelite friar and later bishop of Durango in New Spain José Vicente Díaz Bravo observed that, while previously "only Kings, princes, and other grand lords" drank chocolate, "today its use is so common, that even the poor yearn and go around begging for it."[30] The moralizing friar may have exaggerated how widespread chocolate drinking had become, but certainly he shared a preoccupation with other social observers about chocolate's interaction with social status.

Among chocolate lovers, Díaz Bravo singled out women for abandoning their families, failing to cook for them, all in search of cups of chocolate.[31] This kind of scolding exemplified another way that chocolate confused and threatened stable patterns of western European life. Associated with sex, courtship, and fertility in Mesoamerica, chocolate brought those associations with it when it traveled across the Atlantic.[32] In a "Panegyric for Chocolate" written in 1640, among the wonders that chocolate performed was its ability to make lovers beautiful, bringing a flush to their faces and the vigor of youth to the old.[33] On the other hand, thirteen years previously the Castilian converso Fernando Cardoso, writing as a physician in Madrid (although he later moved to Verona, Italy, where he changed his name to "Isaac Cardoso" and lived as a Jew), recommended keeping chocolate away from boys, "because it effeminizes them."[34] By disordering gender roles and sexualizing both men and women, chocolate threatened bodily integrity and moral discipline. Chocolate could also affect fertility, as suggested by an English broadside from 1660 titled *The vertues of chocolate East-India drink*. Among the benefits of drinking chocolate was that it would beautify women by whitening them, increase their ability to conceive, and prevent miscarriages.[35] The Dutch physician Stephen Blankaart claimed that it would increase male virility, asserting that chocolate was good for newlyweds because it improved the blood "and in consequences increases the seed."[36] Even as it became increasingly familiar in western European cities, chocolate's sensuality compromised the religion, civilization, and bodies of Europeans who were tempted to drink it.[37] This pattern repeated itself with the other new drugs, especially tobacco, coffee, tea, and opium. As David Courtwright has commented, "What we think about and how we regulate [modern drugs] depends very much upon the characteristics of those who consume them."[38]

The Mighty Emperor Tobacco, King of Trinidado

Tobacco entered western Europe around the same time as chocolate, and it carried with it the same troubling connections to indigenous Americans. As early as 1567 the French physicians Charles Estienne and Jean Liebault reported in their household advice and medical book that Native American priests used tobacco to divine the future, employing it to access "diabolical and terrible visions."[39] Five years later the Spanish royal surgeon Juan de Fragoso published a catalog of medicinal drugs imported from the rest of the world to Seville, where he had practiced medicine. "In many parts of our Indies," he wrote, distinguishing Spanish America from Asia, there existed a plant called "tobacco" that a priest would use for divinations, putting the leaves in a pipe and sucking the smoke into his mouth until he appeared to be dead. "And either by the power of the herb, or maybe the devil was doing it, he imagined a thousand phantasms and strange visions" in which he received answers to questions put to him by his followers.[40]

In England commentators picked up on the warnings about tobacco's demonic powers, beginning with the minister and future vice-chancellor of the University of Cambridge, Henry Butts. Butts included tobacco in a cookbook he published in 1599 where as an aside he repeated Estienne and Liebault's story of Native American priests receiving prophetic "phantasms and visions" after knocking themselves out "dead-drunke" on tobacco smoke.[41] As Kristen G. Brookes argues, this fed into a more general fear of the foreign food, manners, clothing, and luxury goods that were entering England and eroding national and racial integrity.[42] Three years later an English physician who adopted the pen name "Philaretes" prefaced his anti-tobacco pamphlet by putting Estienne and Liebault's vignette about tobacco-intoxicated Indian priests into verse. He repeated one of the main objections to tobacco, "that the author and finder hereof was the Divell, and the first practisers of the same were the Divells Priests, and therefore not to be used of us Christians."[43] The Elizabethan soldier, poet, and moralist Barnabe Rich decried the growing popularity in England of tobacco in *My ladies looking glasse*, also objecting to its use by devil worshippers.[44] As the use of tobacco spread, fear of religious contagion grew to include other non-Christian groups. The English translator and poet Joshua Sylvester based some of his suspicion about tobacco on its popularity among "Moores, Turks, Tartars, Persians," and other heathens, in addition to Catholic Spain, archenemy of Protestant England in the 1610s, when he published *Tobacco battered; & the pipes shattered.*[45] In 1614 the famous London boatman and "water poet" John Taylor decried its popularity among "Moores and Pagans," and "Jewes and Turks."[46] Italian authors also emphasized the anti-Christian properties of tobacco, with Pier Luigi Origoni and Matteo Pinelli both recalling its diabolical origins to their readers in the middle of the seventeenth century.[47]

At the same time there was an effort to extract tobacco from its connections with the heathen, devil-worshipping religion of the Americans, denying that it had any supernatural power that could spread to Europe's shores. Roger Marbeck, physician to Elizabeth I, published *A defence of tabacco* as a rebuttal to Philaretes in 1602. He parried the objection that tobacco was used by the devil's priests to gain supernatural powers by denying that Native Americans were devil worshippers at all; as Cicero wrote, there was no group of people that had no "feeling of God." But even if they were the devil's servants, Marbeck continued, "shall it therefore be thought either impious or inconvenient, or unlawfull, for Christians to use it? For my part I am not of that mind." After all, consider the Turks, "the professed enemies, of Christ, and of his sacred Gospell: and yet, I am sure there are many things both invented and devised by them . . . which are held in great price, and estimation, with all Christians." To condemn tobacco would be to condemn all things and practices that originated with infidels.[48] The Castilian physician Francisco de Leiva y Aguilar believed that Native American priests were actually victims of the devil, who always used the good to pursue his evil designs. In a book published to defend tobacco in 1634, Leiva y Aguilar argued that Satan tricked the Indians into using tobacco for their rituals, just as he tricked Adam into eating the forbidden fruit.[49]

Both attitudes toward tobacco—that it had diabolical powers, or that pagan priests simply used its natural powers—had appeared in the work of an important early popularizer of tobacco in 1571, the Seville physician Nicolás Monardes.[50] Even as tobacco became more commonly used in western Europe, it could never quite shed its association with the devil, as the English Catholic controversialist Thomas White showed in a 1659 story about a young man he knew who had been saved from a life of "debauchery with Drink and Tobacco." This man experienced a vision of "a lively portraiture of the Devil drinking to him, and puffing Tobacco by his side," the memory of which helped keep him on the straight and narrow.[51] Throughout the seventeenth and eighteenth centuries, the anti-Christian associations of tobacco lingered, and, of course, the mere fact of blowing smoke out of the mouth and nose—startlingly new at first—could always conjure images of Satan.

Even setting religious questions aside, should western Europeans adopt cultural practices of these supposedly savage races? James I, the king of England and Scotland, did not think so. He penned an attack in 1604, *A counterblaste to tobacco*, focused on tobacco's origins with Native Americans: "Good Countrey men let us . . . consider, what honour or policie can moove us to imitate the barbarous and beastly manners of the wilde, godlesse, and slavish Indians . . . aliens from the holy Covenant of God?"[52] Three years later Thomas Tomkis wrote a comedy for the students at the University of Cambridge called *Lingua: or The combat of the tongue, and the five senses for superiority*. In it he depicted the character "Tobacco" with bare brown arms, feathers around his neck, painted face, pig's tusks through his nose, and "on his head a painted wicker crowne, with Tobacco pipes set in it, plumes of Tobacco leaves, lead by two Indian boyes naked, with tapers in their hands, Tobacco boxes and pipes lighted." The character was called "the mighty Emperour Tobacco, King of Trinidado, that in being conquered, conquered all Europe, in making them pay tribute for their smoake." The Emperor Tobacco embodied both tobacco and Indians, conflating the physical qualities of the tobacco leaf with the physical appearance attributed to Native Americans, as well as speaking a made-up "Indian" language: "Ladoch guevarroah pufur shelvaro baggon."[53] Coincidentally, Tomkis had composed a comedy several years earlier for Cambridge students to perform before James I during a royal visit to the university. Combined, the playwright and the king pointed to the exotic barbarity of tobacco's original users and posed a question about tobacco in England: Would users take on the attributes of the people who first discovered how to smoke it? Could smoking tobacco make an Englishman uncivilized, slavish, exotic, and brown?

Lauren Working has explored the tensions between the supposed savagery of Native Americans and the civility that befit the elite young English men who enjoyed smoking.[54] James I and others feared a degeneration of the English to barbarism, both in Virginia where tobacco was beginning to take off as a cash crop, and in England, where smoking was growing in popularity. "Why doe we not as well imitate them in walking naked as they do?" asked the king. "Yea why do we not denie God and adore the Devill, as they doe?"[55] Others took up the warning call, including the minister John Deacon in his 1616 anti-tobacco tract, where he complained that in general the minds of English travelers abroad were too easily swayed by the customs of foreign lands, from Scotland to Turkey, including being "Indianized with the intoxicating filthy fumes of Tobacco."[56] Eventually the urgency of saving the Chesapeake colony, bolstering English customs revenue, and depriving revenue from the Spanish, who had been supplying England with tobacco, led English elites to deemphasize its Indian origins and anglicize tobacco. Masques performed at James's court in the 1610s, in particular, helped change tobacco from an exotic good with the potential to turn its users savage and heathen, as in Tomkis's play, into a celebration of the loyal English planters who provided it.[57]

Yet the focus on tobacco's production in English American colonies further racialized tobacco. The English began to associate tobacco with the enslaved Africans who grew it and, as slaves in America or servants in England, served it.[58] As early as 1617, Richard Braithwaite, in a satirical attack, claimed that the god Pluto had created tobacco, depicting him instructing a personified Tobacco how to promote its sale by setting up booths decorated with "the picture of some sallow-faced Blackamoore, or a Virginia-man."[59] Humorist Samuel Rowlands likewise associated tobacco with Africans in several poems, one of which featured a wife complaining that when her husband returned from smoking his skin was black, and another claiming that Pluto created tobacco and then, thanks to its stinking odor, cast it out of Olympus to the land of the "blackamoors," where it was found by the Spanish.[60] Spanish writers also associated tobacco with Africans, beginning with Monardes who reported that enslaved Africans in the Americas quickly adopted tobacco. The friar Tomás Ramón described slave owners trying to keep tobacco away from Africans because they smoked it "until they are like drunkards" in secret rituals where they worshiped the devil.[61] Even in Spain itself in the late eighteenth century, the Spanish physician and military surgeon Antonio Lavedán claimed that in Andalusia Moriscos owned establishments that featured hookahs.[62] Even as tobacco became associated with African slavery, the fear of Native American influence on the bodies of Europeans remained, as Brookes points out: Philaretes worried about a "swartie Indian" corrupting "faire Albion."[63] Brown, Black, Muslim, and barbarous: western Europeans who ingested tobacco risked changes to their bodies and their religious selves.

Henry Butts registered another objection to tobacco: its effect on public manners and social rank. He began his discussion of tobacco with a satiric poem where the author objected to a "Lock-Tabacco-Chevalier" clouding the air of a theater with smoke.[64] Even without alluding to American barbarity, critics of tobacco might ask whether it fostered or corroded civility, and who should be allowed to smoke it. While young elite men quickly adopted tobacco as it arrived in western Europe, so did nonelite men, and low-class Spanish sailors were among the pioneers who spread its use in port cities along the Atlantic coast.[65] England was no different than Spain, as the water poet Taylor observed: Pluto commanded his devils to spread tobacco among all the Christian lands, to be used by everyone, "rich and poore," and "Let every Cobbler with his durty fist,/ Take pride to be a blacke Tobaconist" (meaning a smoker, not a seller of tobacco).[66] The poet Richard West also noted tobacco's ability to cross class boundaries in 1608: "Yet Countries cloth breech, and Court velvet hose, / Puffe both a like Tobacco through their nose."[67] Working argues that the English government hated the idea of the poor using tobacco, so, while gentlemen might smoke in their homes or other privileged sites like the Inns of Court, poor men smoking in public signaled disorder.[68]

As West's verse suggests, one distressing aspect of tobacco was that it obscured differences of rank. If apprentices, who were notorious for dressing above their station, could get hold of tobacco, who, then, could tell if a smoker in a tavern was a gentleman or an idle young apprentice? Rowlands played on this theme in two poems in his 1604 publication *Looke to it: for, ile stabbe ye*, which featured a disreputable figure using tobacco to help adopt a false higher-ranking social persona: in one was a "Swaggering Ruffian," a highwayman who adopted tobacco as well as a fancy hat, boots, and hairstyle to make him appear as a gentleman, while in the other was a "Filthy Pander," whose sinful profession is betrayed by his own body, "in-side all Tabacco, and the Poxe."[69] The following year Rowlands published an epigram mocking a boisterous young man who displayed numerous badges of aggressive masculinity:

> What gallant's that whose oaths flie through mine eares?
> How like a lord of Plutoes court he sweares:
> How brave in such a bawdiehouse he fought;
> How rich his empty purse is outside wrought;
> How Dutch-man-like he swallows down his drink,
> How sweete he takes Tabacco till he stinke:
> How loftie sprited he disdaines a Boore,
> How faithfull hearted he is to a [whore]

How cocke: taile proud he doth himselfe advance,
How rare his spurres doe ring the Morice-daunce.
Now I protest by Mistris Susans fan.
He and his boy, will make a proper man.[70]

Like Butts, Taylor, and Sharpe, Rowlands disliked the disorder that tobacco caused, mixing gentlemen, apprentices, ruffians, artisans, and servants all together in taverns, brothels, and theaters. Tobacco also became a symbol of an assertive, boisterous masculinity that moralists disapproved of as a false virtue, signifying not a true virility but an ostentatious and ultimately empty masculinity marked by vanities such as drinking to excess, wearing flashy clothing, gambling, and smoking tobacco.[71]

These concerns about masculinity show that, like chocolate, tobacco threatened to disorder gender, sex, and fertility. James I warned that tobacco would prevent the English from making war, as soldiers would linger at their pipes, growing soft, rather than attack the enemy. "Mollicies and delicacie," he wrote, "were the wracke and overthrow, first of the Persian, and next of the Roman Empire." Tobacco, he continued, "is even at this day accounted so effeminate among the Indians themselves" that they would not purchase a slave who smokes tobacco.[72] The king's objections leaned on the idea that any foreign luxury would weaken England and its men, which was a long-standing trope in moral thought dating back to Livy. John Deacon, the minister who warned that tobacco would "Indianize" the English and who dedicated his anti-tobacco jeremiad to James I, urging him to extirpate the weed from England, also worried about foreign luxury, finding that it distracted Englishmen's minds from true Christianity "and their bodies withal, very monstrously transformed from their former ancient simplicity."[73] He contrasted the contemporary English with the brave and simple Germanic tribes whom Julius Caesar encountered in his wars in Gaul and Germany, unsullied by foreign trade and customs. Deacon's concerns about religious waywardness mixed with worries about bodily change and luxurious softness. He specifically warned against the feminizing powers of tobacco, upbraiding the English by asking what caused them to become "such cavallering Carpet Knights, such fantasticall effeminate fellows," unfit for military service, if not drinking and smoking, "and our contagious conversing with the vicious customes of forreigne countries?"[74] His rhetoric was shot through with images of tobacco entering English bodies, in phrases like "insatiably swalloweth the filthie fume of Tobacco" "so wildly do use the inward taking of filthie Tobacco fumes," "the venomous and deadly contagion," "taken such deepe roote in those our besotted Tobacconists minds," an "inordinate sucking up of filthie Tobacco Smoke," and an "insatiable swilling in of filthie Tobacco fumes," all of which portrayed a violent, self-willed invasion of the body by pollution.[75]

The attention to bodies and gender led to an intense concern about tobacco's effects on sex and courtship. The poet and controversialist John Phillips published a collection of licentious, humorous poems in 1656 that included a song featuring an extended metaphor featuring tobacco and pipes, reading in part:

> She will be ready at your call,
> And take Tobacco, Pipe, and all,
> So ready will she be to fall
> To tast your good Tobacco.
> Your Stopper must be stiff and strong,
> It must be large and long,
> Or else she sweares you do her wrong.
> She scorns your weak Tobacco.[76]

Snuff, however, could be a part of an acceptable, or semi-acceptable, romantic courtship, such as in a collection of poems by the Castilian writer Luis Antonio. One poem featured snuff while describing playful flirtation between aristocratic men and women, while another depicted the offering of snuff as the beginning of a romantic relationship, and yet another related how a man, blind with love and reaching over to kiss his lover, bit her nose instead and ended up with a mouth full of snuff.[77] The anonymous English author of a treatise on tobacco noted that snuff helped amorous men and women engage with one another by giving them an excuse "to prattle the Praises of their different Kinds of Snuff and Snuff-boxes, and give Directions where to buy the best." Moreover, taking snuff allowed women to show off "their handsome Hands, and well shap'd and snowy Arms."[78] But just as often tobacco was associated bluntly and crudely with an increased sex drive. In 1669 the London printer John Playford published a collection of songs that included "The Tobacco-Takers Song," in which a man called for tobacco while singing its praises, including its ability to make him too "Valiant" for his wife's liking.[79] Another English writer featured a newlywed man whose strength began to fail from too much sex, and whose friends jokingly tell him to avoid his wife and tobacco (and drink chocolate instead).[80] Tobacco was further associated with promoting disordered, illicit sex. Humphrey Mill created a scene in his 1646 poem where a man accosts a prostitute in a smoky tavern, his moral judgment clouded by wine and tobacco.[81] *Whipping-Tom* mentioned snuff boxes painted with sexual scenes, "more obscene and lascivious Pieces than can be shewn in Aretine's Postures," a notorious work of Renaissance pornography.[82]

Other writers, however, took the view that tobacco discouraged sex, like the Flemish Huguenot refugee physician Raphael Thorius, whose *Hymnus tabaci*, first published in 1625, was translated into English in 1650. Thorius portrayed the discovery of tobacco as a scene from the mythology of the ancient Roman gods, and tobacco angered Venus because it bridled lust—not extinguishing it, but setting it within its proper bounds and preventing the poor from having more children than they could support.[83] The satirical novelist Richard Head mocked contemporary young men as given over to luxury, claiming that their mistresses had to forbid them to use tobacco since it dried up "their radical moisture."[84] Head was joking, but his reasoning followed more serious warnings of men like the Huguenot physician Duncan, who asserted that tobacco "takes away virility."[85] Thorius and Duncan were among a group of writers who warned about tobacco's impact on the fertility of both men and women. Philaretes advised that tobacco's head would dry up the "sperme & seed of man," Sylvester cautioned that it decreased virility, and the London physician Everard Maynwaring claimed that the Turkish sultan banned tobacco because it made people infertile.[86] The Spanish physician Lavedán agreed that tobacco caused sterility in both men and women, but the Italian physicians Giovanni Piccino and Sebastiano Laghi disagreed.[87] Like chocolate, tobacco threatened to complicate one's control over bodily integrity and appearance, not only racially but also socially.

Coffee: The Marriage of the Turk

Ephemeral pamphlets from late seventeenth-century England are a good place to start looking at coffee's reception because it was in this time and place that coffee made its first sustained mark in print. Take, for example, *A broadside against coffee; or the marriage of the Turk*, published anonymously in 1672, during the early years of coffee adoption in England. The pamphlet depicted coffee as a Turk who had come to London to marry the Thames, personified as a nymph, and it employed a series of visual puns to mock the misalliance and the problems that troubled their union. Arriving on England's shores, the Turk was "brown as a [coffee] berry" and "Too swarthy for a Nymph so fair, so clear." As the courtship found itself in trouble, the poet admonished coffee, the "Bold Asian brat," to leave England. The poet played with the contrasting humoral properties of water (wet) and coffee (dry), and claimed that much of the trouble between the two was sexual: while the Thames was willing, "the Slave Coffee must be beaten to't." Nevertheless the Thames had the upper hand: Coffee lost the breeches when he found that "she's above and he lies undermost." Then, in a nod to Shakespeare, coffee "shuns her as a Whore, / And loves, and kills, like the Venetian Moor," and toward the end the poem compared coffee to prostitution. The poet also warned "Christian water" that "Coffee, a kind of Turkish Renegade," or a convert from Islam, could not be trusted: "No faith is to be kept with Infidels." And "Water, though common, is too good for thee," the poem added, fretting about the mix of "clean and the unclean."[88]

Note the emphasis on the body in this satire, which racialized and sexualized foreign coffee and domestic water. The disordered sex featured so prominently in the poem aligned well with western Europeans' obsession with Turkish sexuality, including eunuchs and the homosexuality that they imagined to be common Ottoman practice, both of which signified emasculated men, and the harem signifying oversexed women.[89] The poet underscored the physicality of the Anglo-Turkish marriage with the constant references to sex and the many references to the mixing of roast grounds and water that created coffee. The poem also evoked the then-novel sensual experience of preparing and drinking coffee, describing "Coffee a crust is charkt into a coal" and tongues burning when they touched the hot liquid. Despite all the ways that Turkish coffee seemed to be inappropriate for the English, coffee was apparently there to stay, "both the Water and the Men bewitcht" by the new drink. Indeed, people could not stay away from it, caught between "Dread and desire" and drawn to coffee like "hungry Dogs" to "scalding porridge."[90]

Other satirical writing likewise emphasized the foreign origin and unpleasant sensation of drinking coffee, such an anonymous pamphlet from 1673, *The character of a coffee-house with the symptomes of a town-wit,* which painted a picture of a coffeehouse proprietor as a "Stygian-Puddle-seller" who wore a turban that, together with "his Antichristian face, made him appear perfect Turk." Alluding to the Gunpowder Plot to destroy Parliament in 1605, the poet asserted that the coffee vendor's drink would scald one's throat like "Gunpowder-Treason," and that he substituted freshly ground coffee with the soot scraped off his unwashed coffee pots to sell a counterfeit drink. As he served his "hot Hell-broth," he gossiped with his customers "that the Great Turk is a very good Christian, and of the Reformed Church, because he drinks Coffee."[91] One broadsheet from 1674 simply described coffee as "The Sweat of Negroes, Blood of Moores."[92] These pamphlets combined the novel sensory experience of drinking coffee with its foreign origin, concluding that coffee was disgusting, hellish, Turkish, and anti-English.

Other satirical attacks ominously linked the foul underworldly qualities of coffee with the way it blurred its aficionados' religious identities between Christian, Muslim, and Jew. *The maidens complaint against coffee* employed a racial slur to associate coffee with yet another group of non-Europeans in 1663, claiming that

> It makes a Christian blacker far within
> Then ever was the Negars outward skin:
> Its of a Berry, men, this liquor make,
> Which is transported from a Stygian Lake[93]

Mercurius Democritus, the pseudonymous author of *The maidens complaint* (probably the bookseller John Crouch), also voiced sexual anxiety about coffee. Cast as a satirical dialogue, at one point *The maidens complaint* featured a conversation between two servants, Snapshort and Toby. Snapshort describes the giddy confusion he felt after drinking coffee in Lothbury, a street in London near the Royal Exchange, that he cured by drinking good English ale. Toby responds that he was not surprised by Snapshort's misadventure drinking "that cursed Indian liquor," as he himself tried some recently and afterward tried to seduce the maid Joan but failed. After drinking ale, he had great success with another young woman. For their part, the two servants' companions, Joan and Dorothy, complain about their beaux, with Joan lamenting that "I believe I shall never enjoy any comfort from our man Snapshort since he went, with my Master to the Coffee-house, he is so dry as a kix." Dorothy replies that "truly our Toby is come to the same passe; for since he drank Coffee, he is no more like the man he was then an apple's like an Oyster." Joan says that the devil invented coffee to plague women, and the two women agree that they will no longer entertain the courtship of coffee-drinking men. "And for my part," declares Joan, "I'le hang my Maiden-head on a Wind-mill to be bated to death by the four Winds, rather then be poyson'd with the scent of old crusts, and shreads of Leather burn'd and beaten to powder, of which I believe this cursed Coffee is made."[94] Here the new sensory aspects of coffee were linked to its malign influence on sexual ability. Again, suspicion of coffee's novel sensations was joined with fears of racial and religious impurity and sexual deficiency; such a mysterious, exotic, and harmful drink could only displace traditional English ale thanks to its supernatural charms.

Outside England, commentators on coffee joined in the debate on its effects on sexual ability. In 1671 Philippe Sylvestre Dufour, a Lyonnais apothecary, asserted that it "effeminizes the body, and the mind," due to the sulfur inherent in coffee.[95] Angelo Rambaldi explained that while some believed that such a hot and dry drink "dulls the senses of Venus," and that the Turks drink it as a method of birth control, this could not be true—first, because the Turks had large families, and, second, because Rambaldi himself drank coffee and yet, even as a man in his seventies, his wife was expecting a child.[96] One hundred years later, Francesco Merli, the royal physician for the army and hospitals of the Kingdom of Naples, took a commonsense empirical approach, explaining that while it was once believed that coffee caused sterility, experience taught that it could not be the case.[97] Thus, while some observers defended coffee against the suspicions of its exotic foreign nature, the more common vein of writing linked its origins in the Turkish and Arab lands to racial mixing and change, with European drinkers wearing turbans and "turning Turk." Becoming Turkish also meant becoming a religious renegade, and the religious taint of coffee was also strong, associating it with hell or the Greco-Roman underworld for its hot, black, bitter sensual experience and also with faithless infidelity to Christianity. More than anything, however, coffee was viewed as connected with a physical change in the gender and sexual performance of its drinkers, effeminizing the men who drank it, making them impotent or at best unable to produce children. In all these respects, coffee followed the pattern established beforehand by chocolate and tobacco, although connected to effeminate Turks and Arabs rather than savage Indians.

Like American drugs, coffee caused a disturbing mixing of different classes of men. While the coffeehouse is usually seen as a site of polite conversation among well-behaved elite men, there was an undercurrent of concern and disdain for the place as a site of disordered, unpoliced talk, bringing together men from different classes and stages of life in a way that no one could be sure of who was sitting next to him.[98] *The character of a coffee-house with the symptomes of a town-wit*, published in

1673, carried over concerns from the social upheavals of the English Civil War when criticizing the coffeehouse: "As you have a hodge-podge of Drinks, such too is your Company, for each man seems a Leveller, and ranks and files himself as he lists, without regard to degrees or order; so that oft you may see a silly Fop, and a worshipful Justice, a griping Rock, and a grave Citizen, a worthy Lawyer, and an errant Pickpocket, a Reverend Nonconformist, and a Canting Mountebank; all blended together, to compose an Oglio [a type of stew] of Impertinence."[99] Edward Ward similarly sneered at coffeehouses, since "the place no manner of distinction knew, / 'Twixt Christian, heathen, Turk, or Jew." Fools, philosophers, knights, sailors, soldiers, courtiers, tailors, tradesmen, clergymen, quacks, and

> Lawyers and Clients, Sharpers and their Cullies,
> Quakers, Pimps, Atheists, Mountebanks and Bullies,
> Clean or unclean, if here they call,
> The place, like Noah's Ark, receives 'em all.[100]

As with chocolate and tobacco, coffee promoted a leveling of social rank and a blending of religions. It changed the bodies of its drinkers, making women barren and enfeebling men. And although coffee became engrained into everyday life in western Europe over the course of the eighteenth century, in the minds of its users it never did lose its connections to the Middle East. As late as 1796, the Spanish physician Lavedán opened his discussion of coffee by explaining that coffee is most common "in Turkey and Arabia, and other Eastern areas where wine is prohibited."[101]

Tea: The Chinese Drink

Lavedán also wrote about tea. More common in England and Holland than in Spain, tea, he wrote, was even more ubiquitous in the places whence it came: China and Japan. While discussing tea's effects on the drinker, Lavedán commented on the physical and moral character of the Chinese. A people of medium build and strength, they were "incapable of great labor and weaker than all the other nations," and "we see them as cowards, dissolute, cunning, furtive, conceited, effeminate, vindictive, and duplicitous." He went on to wonder how much of this was attributable to the Chinese way of life, especially tea drinking.[102] Lavedán wrote in the 1790s, over a century after tea first arrived in western Europe—evidence of tea's enduring association with east Asia and the characteristics that Europeans imagined its people to possess. Historians portray the adoption of tea in western Europe as a smooth process, eased by the respect that Europeans had for the sophistication of Chinese culture and society. It is true that western Europeans admired the vast wealth and size of the Chinese empire, coupled with the sophistication of the mandarins who administered it, steeped as they were in a centuries-old tradition of learning.[103] Of course, the Chinese were also viewed as heathen, but at least they were not Muslim like the Turks and Arabs, or devil worshippers like the Native Americans. Still, testimonies like Lavedán's reveal that the translation of Chinese tea into European culture was not entirely without friction. As with chocolate, tobacco, and coffee, tea brought with it worries about race and religion, and, as Erika Rappaport points out, concern about its potential to disorder gender roles, sex, and fertility.[104]

The Danish physician Simon Paulli believed that, like coffee, tea emasculated its users. "The present Europeans," he wrote in 1661, "are vastly different from what they were before the Asiatic Effeminacy was known among us." Paulli thought that tea was good for the climate and manners of east Asians, but not for Europeans. "Thus Tea seems by Nature adapted to the Inhabitants of China, Coffee to those of Persia, Chocolate to those of America, and Ale and Wine to those the different parts of Europe," he wrote.[105] A century later, the London merchant, traveler, and philanthropist Jonas Hanway published his "Essay on Tea," in which he expressed astonishment that the English would imitate "the most effeminate people on the face of the whole earth."[106] He excoriated the men of England for squandering the masculine prowess they inherited from their forebears, who had defeated the French in the glorious battles of the Hundred Years' War and again against Louis XIV. "Were they the sons of TEA-SIPPERS, who won the fields of CRESSY and AGINCOURT, or dyed the DANUBE's streams with GALLIC BLOOD? What will be the end of such EFFEMINATE customs extended to those persons, who must get their bread by the labors of the field!"[107] Even the reforming Quaker physician John Coakley Lettsom, who was not wholly against drinking tea, wondered, like Lavedán, whether tea was responsible for the effeminacy of Chinese men.[108]

Tea's racializing power had religious connotations as well. John Waldron's 1733 satirical attack on the pro-tea John Ovington mocked the English ladies who insisted on having their tea served by Black servants, whose appearance should put them in mind of the devil while they drank their "Stygian evil."[109] As late as 1787, the critic Godfrey

McCalman observed that "a vein of idolatry seems to be congenial with the culture, importation and consumption of tea. The ancient, and so far as we know, the modern Chinese worship material objects; the Japanese, at the same time are represented the grossest of all idolaters." Dutch traders, McCalman went on, were forced to abjure Christianity while residing in Japan, "and tea, in its last and consumptive stage, is regarded by ourselves to a violent pitch of fancy, that borders on idolizment."[110] Even as tea became engrained in English manners and foodways, its links to nonwhite non-Christians remained a liability.

But the most troubling aspect of tea remained its perceived effects on gender roles and sex. As with snuff, tea was associated with false, unmasculine men. Simon Mason believed that teatime was especially dangerous when the talk there drifted to commenting on the sexual morals of female neighbors and praising neighborhood men who let their wives dominate them. The husband who bought luxuries for his wife, or handed over the family finances to her and avoided spending money in the alehouse, or the man who "tamely submits to all his Dame directs" won praise, while the husband who tried to command his wife earned disapproval.[111] Tea created hollow men undeserving of respect while encouraging women to gather and conspire to rule the household and the community. Commenters further debated tea's effect on sex and fertility. The anonymous author (perhaps the Dublin physician, mathematician, and natural scientist Richard Helsham) of *An essay on the nature, use, and abuse, of tea* warned in 1722 of tea's effect on women's bodies. A ruinous luxury that weakened the blood and spirits of its drinkers, in women specifically it caused hypochondriacal disorders, reduced the energy necessary for sex, induced miscarriages, and prevented mothers from nourishing their babies—both as a fetus and a nursing infant.[112] Two tea sellers based in Rome, Giovanni Agostino and Morison Scozzese, claimed the opposite effect two years earlier in their advertisement for "the Chinese drink"; not only did it make both men and women more likely to produce offspring, but "for wet-nurses it is the most excellent drink in the world for purifying the blood and rendering the milk healthy and very nutritious for the infant."[113] Effeminizing men and putting women in control while rendering them unfit for motherhood, tea could not shake its association with the Chinese and western Europeans' ambivalence about East Asian civilization. Like the other exotic imported drugs, tea embodied the ability of a foreign civilization to enter into and change the bodies and manners of western Europeans.

Sugar, Distilled Spirits, and Opium

Sugar did not usually carry with it the baggage of an alien culture, despite the fact that it came to western Europe from the Muslim Mediterranean during the Middle Ages and, later, from Brazil and the Caribbean. Nevertheless the merchant, vegetarian, mystic, and reformer Thomas Tryon did protest: "What agreement or affinity is there between our Fruits, Grains, Herbs and Seeds" in England, with those from tropical lands? "Not so much as that between the complexion of a . . . Blackamore, or swarthy Bantamen," and the faces of the English women who put sugar into their tea.[114] Distilled spirits were indigenous to Europe, but they did raise some of the same anxieties as the drugs that arrived from abroad. Tryon also attacked "Brandy, Rumm, Rack, and other Distilled Spirits" in 1682, arguing that, when distilling begins, "this dark Fiery Brimstonie Spirit appears in its own form, and becomes like a Mad furious Devil in Nature."[115] Besides this association with anti-Christian devilry, brandy caused confusion about social rank, as expressed in Edward Whitaker's "A satyr upon brandy" from 1700. Whitaker deployed an extended conceit about the fiery effects of the "damn'd Stygian Juyce" and claimed that it "doth bewitch" everyone across the ranks of English life. Although it had its origins among the dregs of society, brandy now gained popularity in high society, mingling among and spilling on "Gold Chains and Fur."[116]

Another characteristic of distilled spirits was its promotion of disordered sex. The satirical attack on gin by "Saynought Slyboots," published at the height of the Gin Craze, featured the character Swell-Gut, representing the brewers' interest, who lamented that gin made young people debauch themselves: "They commit Lewdness in the open Streets; . . . Girls of 12 and 13 Year of Age . . . this damn'd bewitching Liquor makes them Shameless, and they talk enough to make a Man shudder again . . . this fills our common Fellows with lewd Notions, and filthy Diseases."[117] Ten years later, *The deposing and death of Queen Gin* connected gin with visiting brothels.[118] And, of course, the Gin Craze of early eighteenth-century London was based on intense anxieties about class, focused as it was on the poor who drank gin in the streets rather than the wealthy who drank madeira in their townhouses. As Samuel Johnson pointedly remarked, when he was a boy "all the decent people of Lichfield"—his hometown—"got drunk every night, and were not thought the worse of."[119]

Despite its long history of use in Europe, opium was imported from the Middle East and India and brought with it many of the same connotations as coffee. The recreational use of opium was strongly associated with Turks and Arabs, as opposed to western Europeans, who supposedly used it only as a medicine. Turks took opium to "make themselves drunk without wine," reported Nicolas de Nicolay after his sixteenth-century visit to the Ottoman Empire; it made them "loose both their wits and understanding, for they go reeling about the streetes, holding one of another, as the other Drunkardes doe, foming out of the mouth like unto chafed boares, making fierce and terrible cries and howlings like unto dogs."[120] The idea that they resorted to opium for intoxication because wine was forbidden was a common trope about Muslims. A century later an English physician scolded a fellow practitioner for giving patients too much opium and for too long, wondering, "I cannot imagine from whom he should learn it, unless from the Turks, when he was at Constantinople; and they, you know, make Opium . . . their daily bread."[121] Accusing Europeans who used too much opium of behaving like Turks became a stereotype, such as when a Tuscan physician in 1807 lamented the shortage of opium for medical use, owing, he believed, to the fact that the new practice that has "seduced, little by little, the Europeans to make use of opium in place of wine, just like the habit of the Orientals."[122] Opium could also be associated with Africans, as in the case of one anonymous Dutch writer who claimed that opium was banned in the Caribbean "because of the abuse that the Blacks make of it, since they thereby work themselves up to a murder-lust."[123] Some observers believed that opium as a daily habit, while not appropriate for western Europeans, was fine for inhabitants of the Middle East. In 1580 Timothy Bright argued that opium was more fit for Turks, Moors, and Persians than not for Europeans, and that it would not work as well as it did in its land of origin.[124] Partly this fit into a European medical tradition that medicines drawn from plants were suited for the diseases and people of the same locality.

Because opium was associated with the East, it invoked connotations of irregular sexual practice and infertility. In 1664 the London-based Huguenot chemist Nicaise Le Fèvre claimed that in India men took opium before sex to "to be more enabled to satisfie longer the lust and luxurious inclination of the Indian women."[125] The English physician Henry Stubbe likened chocolate to opium, claiming that both help men "yield a more vigorous Seed" and assisted ejaculation, just like the "amorous and Martial Turk drinks Opium, and Shirbet, to continue his lust."[126] In 1700 the English physician John Jones published a study of opium that asserted its ability to encourage sex when applied, either internally or externally, "to the Perinaeum." In fact opium produced more "seed" and "cause[d] a great promptitude to Venery, Erections, &c." which explained why men used it so much in the Middle East, where polygamy was legal.[127] He also believed that it helped women during labor. Indeed an English traveler named Brooke attending medical lectures in Italy wrote of meeting a Turk in Viterbo who explained to him how opium was used in the Ottoman Empire; because it increased fertility in women, "opium is administered to favourite wives if they should not prove pregnant."[128]

Learning from Others

Despite western Europeans' disdain for the peoples from whom they obtained the exotic drugs, observers like Brooke had been translating foreign knowledge about them into European ways of thinking since Bartolomé Marradón and other Spaniards in Mesoamerica derived their understanding of chocolate and its properties from Native Americans.[129] For example, in the seventeenth century, a controversy erupted about whether drinking chocolate broke a religious fast, a dispute complicated by the split between the Dominican order, who tended to hold that drinking chocolate was impermissible during fast days, and the Jesuits, who disagreed, perhaps because they had invested in cacao plantations.[130] The Spanish attorney and historian Antonio de León Pinelo intervened in this debate by reaching for examples of how Native Americans used it, sometimes sucking pellets of chocolate as though smoking tobacco.[131] In order to discern the nature of chocolate in the very European ritual of religious fasting, he relied on Mesoamerican practice. In other examples, one of the early broadsheets published to introduce English consumers to coffee, *The nature of the drink kauhi, or coffe, and the berry of which it is made described by an Arabian phisitian*, was simply a translation of a description of coffee written by the Cairo medical man Dawud ibn Umar al-Antaki.[132] The Bolognese naturalist Luigi Ferdinando Marsili published a tract in 1685 in which he made a bid for authority by explaining that he was translating Ottoman knowledge about coffee for Italians.[133] Quinto Alcaldolana, who published a collection of pro-coffee writings in 1691, quoted Italian travelers to Arab, Turkish, and Persian cities who learned described all about the good qualities of coffee from physicians and other coffee drinkers they met there. Even the coffeehouse itself was modeled after the institution that travelers found in the Middle East. While western Europeans worried about chocolate turning its drinkers into heathen and coffee introducing disordered sex in Europe, writers continued to cloak themselves in the authority and wisdom of Indians, Turks, and Arabs. Perhaps this should come as no surprise, since Stephen Blankaart opened his discussion of coffee by announcing that "those great nations, like the Turkish realm, the Chinese, Japanese, and all those whom we have considered as the greatest barbarians, have in all things (aside from knowledge of the Gospel) much more subtler minds than us."[134]

While most western Europeans writers would hesitate to extend this courtesy to the Turks, they certainly believed that the Chinese were civilized and worth emulating. In his 1665 account of his mission to China, the adventurer and diplomat Johan Nieuhof carefully described how various classes of Chinese and Manchus drank tea, including the types of utensils they used and other minutiae, to instruct his Dutch readership at home.[135] In 1700 the Irish-born poet laureate of England Nahum Tate wrote a classicizing poem on tea that combined Roman mythology with a story about a hermit who traveled to China and brought back tea to a grateful Europe. According to Tate, tea is what made China superior to Europe: "Tea came to rescue China from ills of western civilization: / While the Chinese remain'd a Virtuous Breed, / From Western Vices and Distempers Freed."[136] Tea, Tate stated, had helped restore ancient Chinese virtues after a descent into tyranny and vice, and it could do the same for England. Even as late as 1772, John Coakley Lettsom drew heavily on Chinese and Japanese authorities to explain the natural history of the tea shrub and its medical properties.[137]

Surprisingly, given that opium was a staple of the classical Greek pharmacopeia, western Europeans continued to draw on foreign expertise to help them understand it. Angelo Sala's *Opiologia*, first published in 1614, argued that opium was still very poorly understood by physicians, and he drew on accounts of its use in the Ottoman Empire to discuss its medical properties and the effects of heavy daily usage.[138] This borrowing habit continued, with the English physician John Jones and the Scots physician George Young both incorporating knowledge derived from Turks and Arabs in their treatises on opium, published in 1700 and 1753, respectively.[139] Despite western Europeans' apprehension about Turks, Arabs, Chinese, Japanese, Africans, and Native Americans, they were dependent on them for learning about the exotica that they imported. As the next chapter will show, the awareness they gained about the medicinal properties of chocolate and its sister drugs helped domesticate them and make them safe for western European consumption.

Exotic goods called consumers' attention to exotic people. None of these drugs were neutral objects, affecting their users merely because of their chemical properties and the way they hit the senses as either foul or pleasing. None of them could be severed from their cultures of origin, not least of all because it was from these cultures that western Europeans first learned about these drugs: how to consume them, and what potential they possessed to delight or to heal. They understood chocolate and the other new drugs by borrowing knowledge from the people who used them, but they also applied all their stereotypes of exotic foreigners to the exotic foreign drugs. For example, Julie Landweber explains that even when coffee had been thoroughly assimilated into French cultural life, sold at Parisian coffeehouses by French vendors importing it from French colonies, it retained its association with the Middle East.[140] Incorporating these stimulants into European practice was fraught with anxiety; all the certainties of masculinity, femininity, Christianity, class, and race were cast into doubt as consumers of chocolate and its sister drugs risked the erosion of control over bodily autonomy and self-discipline. Or perhaps they were not certainties at all, and the new products simply reminded Europeans of their anxieties about gender, class, race, and religion.

Why was that so? Why were chocolate and tobacco thought to be demonic and barbarous? Why were coffee and opium considered feminizing and anti-Christian? Why was tea feared for emasculating men and coarsening women, and gin for disordering social rank? Today we think of drugs mostly as intoxicants, possessing psychotropic powers that primarily affect the mental states of their users and, through their behavior, their social position. In the early modern period, observers acknowledged this aspect of drugs, but they focused more intensely on the fact that drugs and alcohol were ingested into the body. They also conceived of their bodies as less stable and more malleable than we do today. Drinking chocolate meant drinking in all the things associated with Native Americans as an embodied experience. The new stimulants arrived at a time when western Europeans understood race, religion, gender, and class as aspects of their bodies and behavior, influenced by places, airs, and waters. What did it mean to be Christian, Muslim, or pagan? Spanish, Indian, or African? A woman or a man? Elite or common? How much of these aspects of their selves depended on maintaining control over their bodies, and how much of that control did Europeans jeopardize by incorporating new drugs into their routines? Early modern bodies were unstable, and perhaps the most surprising aspect of the uncertainty introduced into western European identity by the new drugs was how religion formed a part of that bodily instability, how much even one's status as a Christian was compromised by the ingestion of chocolate, tobacco, tea, coffee, and gin. How could one distance oneself from bodily functions, as Norbert Elias believed elite Europeans strived to do, if their bodies were under threat from seductive new drugs? How could the emergence of capitalism depend on a religiously motivated work ethic, as Max Weber asserted, if exotic drugs were threatening the religious integrity of their users? Whatever the causes, western Europeans had reason to be concerned as the entire geography of drugs that Chamberlayne described was rushing into western Europe throughout the early modern period, directly into the bodies of his readers.

Chapter 3

Who from Excess Is Free?

Medicine and Addiction

Western Europeans first experienced the curative effects of tobacco in Lisbon around 1560. Jean Nicot, the French ambassador to Portugal, had been cultivating some specimens of this herb, newly brought over from the New World, when one of his pages reported that a young boy had applied tobacco leaves to an ulcer growing on his nose and achieved a miraculous cure. Nicot consulted with the Portuguese royal physician, who confirmed that the lesion had indeed healed, and the two of them spread the word throughout the city about tobacco's virtues. Others afflicted with skin lesions came to Nicot's garden and they too recovered. The ambassador reported back to France where the physicians Charles Estienne and Jean Liebault included this story in subsequent editions of their household advice and medical book, *Country house and husbandry*.[1] Eventually the name of the discoverer of tobacco's healing properties found commemoration in its scientific name, *Nicotiana tabacum*, and its most important alkaloid, nicotine.

A century and a half later an Englishman named Lawrence Spooner penned a warning against tobacco, drawing from his long experience of smoking, quitting, and smoking again. *A looking-glass for smoakers*, published in 1703, described how he was lured to tobacco as a young man, smoking up to twenty pipes a day, but found tobacco to be "accurst" because it tempted him into idleness and drinking. Then he experienced "a mighty Gale of Grace," which showed him how sinful his behavior was, and he managed to quit. Twenty years later he took up tobacco again, because friends advised him that it would help him recover from a serious illness. Soon he fell into a habit of smoking one or two pipes a day. Reflecting on his relapse, he composed a confessional poem:

> The Herb is good for Medicine and Use:
> Fear not to use it, only fear Abuse . . .
> Yet prithee who from Excess is free?

He lamented, "Then Tobacco laid on me its Chains," inducing him again to waste his days smoking and drinking with others; "it made me such a Slave" that he could barely find time to pray. Yet, once more,

> God did me restore
> Out of the House of Bondage, where I lay
> To Satan and my own Heart's Lusts a Prey.[2]

Groping for words to explain his feelings, Spooner filled the poem with an array of metaphors to describe his experience of what we today would call "addiction": prison, death, bewitchment, warfare, poison, sin, disease, "this Indian witch," and, again and again, slavery.[3] How could tobacco encompass the experiences of both Nicot and Spooner? How was it possible that tobacco represented both a miraculous cure and a bondage that only God could break?

Responding to the ways in which tobacco, as well as all the other early modern drugs, threatened to alter stable categories of religion, gender, class, and race, Europeans scrambled to understand how their bodies reacted to these substances. In doing so they reached for tools they already possessed in their conceptual toolbox, beginning with botany and medicine. The solution that emerged was to label the new drugs as medicines, just as sugar, distilled spirits, and opium already had been for centuries.[4] European medical thinking rested on the humoral system of Galen and other classical physicians, although this was changing thanks to the development of a new chemical-based understanding of the body. Physicians found it easy to comprehend the new intoxicants' effects on users' bodies and minds through Galenic humoral theory, as well as the ideas of chemical and nervous medicine that followed. However, it soon became clear that once consumers grew accustomed to these substances, it became difficult or even impossible to stop using them. Traditional medical learning could not explain why some consumers found themselves compulsively taking the new soft drugs; instead, they pivoted to other models in their culture, especially to moral rhetoric like Spooner's, to develop an early notion of addiction.[5]

The origin of the modern idea of addiction as a disease has been traced to the Philadelphia physician and signer of the Declaration of Independence Benjamin Rush, who published *An inquiry into the effects of ardent spirits upon the human body and mind* in 1784.[6] More recently, Roy Porter and Jessica Warner have pointed out that Rush's British contemporary Thomas Trotter developed much the same idea, and indeed that Rush's thoughts on drunkenness were similar to those of ministers and physicians stretching back to the seventeenth century.[7] These moralizing observers asserted that distilled spirits—newly available as consumer goods—were much more dangerous than the traditional alcoholic drinks of beer and wine, that the loss of control over drinking was the key to this new problem, that it was as much a disease as it was a moral failing, and that its only cure was abstinence.[8] A few even used the term "addicted" to refer to people given over to habitual drunkenness, although it had a broader meaning than it would take later; throughout the eighteenth century "addiction" simply denoted a devotion to any sort of activity, such as studying.[9]

Even in the seventeenth century, gin was not the only new substance that attracted attention for inducing compulsive behavior. Commentators on tobacco and other new drugs were struck by their habit-forming properties and, independent of those like Trotter who focused on alcohol, began to articulate an understanding of what we today call "addiction." Tobacco, chocolate, coffee, tea, and opium forced observers to find a way to describe involuntary overconsumption. One way they did so was with traditional moral categories like gluttony and luxury that located the blame in human frailty or social decline. They also identified seductive qualities of the drugs themselves, noting their ability to bewitch, enchant, and enslave. These models could be applied to a broad array of stimulants, not just alcohol, and they provided explanations of compulsive behavior that did not rely on the "modern" idea of addiction as a disease. At the same time, the addictive behavior that users of these drugs displayed posed a counterpoint to the overarching theme of increasing self-discipline that is supposed to have been taking hold in the early modern period, whether it is Weberian self-denial, Oestreich's Neostoicism, or Foucauldian self-discipline. In an age when western Europeans were supposed to be exercising more self-mastery, drugs played an ambivalent role. Used as medicines, they might help their users gain more control over the body and its maladies, but simultaneously they eroded the ability of the will to moderate the consumption of those same substances. As the first exotic drug to generate substantial medical commentary in western Europe, tobacco makes an excellent place to start an examination of medicine and addiction in the early modern period.

Tobacco: It Cureth Any Grief

Tobacco entered western Europe as a commodity for sale in Seville at the very end of the sixteenth century. Over 400,000 pounds of tobacco were recorded entering the port per year by 1616, as Spanish colonists planted tobacco for export in Cuba, Santo Domingo, Central America, Trinidad, and especially New Granada, or modern Venezuela.[10] A group of Portuguese merchants gained control of the shipping of tobacco from Spanish America and quickly began cooperating with the Dutch and English to smuggle tobacco to northern Europe. By 1620, around 150,000 pounds of tobacco entered London per year, either legally through Seville or illegally from the Caribbean.[11] By the late seventeenth century, the holders of the tobacco monopoly in Spain estimated that about 1 million pounds was consumed per year there, both from the Caribbean and from the Chesapeake, and by 1739 over 3 million pounds, or over one-third of a pound per capita, were sold in Spain, not counting smuggled tobacco.[12] The monopoly was so successful that taxes on tobacco sales provided more revenue for the Spanish Crown than American gold and silver.[13] In 1612 English colonists began raising tobacco, exporting 370,000 pounds by 1628, while an additional 800,000 pounds were coming to England from English and Dutch colonies in Guiana and Brazil. Tobacco cultivation spread throughout the Americas from the Amazon to New France, and Europeans began to grow the crop at home as well. The Netherlands was the largest European procurer of tobacco, peaking at up to 28 million pounds by the early 1700s. During the eighteenth century cultivation became concentrated in the Netherlands, Brazil, and especially the Chesapeake, which alone was producing over 100 million pounds of tobacco per year by the 1770s, crowding out production in the Caribbean islands and elsewhere.[14] London and Amsterdam became the entrepôts for the international tobacco trade, both licit and illicit, but the production and consumption of tobacco quickly spread throughout the world, reaching Russia and alarming Muscovite authorities so much that they banned it in 1627.[15] Brought by European sailors, tobacco became a commercial crop in southern China and a robust pattern of cultivation and consumption was rooted in East Asia from Java to Japan by the early seventeenth century.[16]

As Marcy Norton has shown, the earliest writer to explore the medical potential of tobacco systematically was Nicolás Monardes. A physician steeped in the classical humanist training of Renaissance Castile, Monardes lived in Seville, which, in the sixteenth century, was, along with Nicot's Lisbon, the most important port for the transmission of people, goods, and ideas between Europe and the Americas. He supplemented his medical work with trade, investing in the export of enslaved Africans to the Caribbean and all manner of things from America to Castile. Among his imports were plants with a reputation as medicines, some of which, like Nicot, he began to grow in his botanical garden. Combining his medical training, experience in trade, and curiosity about the New World, in 1565 Monardes published a volume in which he tried to reconcile the discovery of new medicinal plants from America with the classical inheritance from Greece and Rome, especially Galen's medical theories and Dioscorides's *De materia medica*, the pharmacopeia from antiquity that early modern Europeans relied on to understand plants and their effects on the human body.[17] Subsequently he issued new editions of his work, including in 1571, when, perhaps prompted by Estienne and Liebault, he included tobacco in *The second part of the book, treating all the things brought from our West Indies that can be useful to medicine*.[18] In this text he included knowledge, gained from Native Americans, about tobacco's curative properties, such as the ability of the leaves to clean any dirty wound and heal it.[19]

This topical use of tobacco was similar to Nicot's practices in Lisbon. From Mesoamericans, though, Monardes learned about lighting the dried leaves on fire and breathing in the smoke in through the nose or mouth, which helped asthmatics by expelling rotten material from the lungs. Smoking the tobacco also helped users go for long periods without eating or drinking.[20] In all, Monardes found twenty ailments that tobacco would cure, including parasites, stomach complaints, and problems with the uterus. He also determined that the humoral properties of tobacco were hot and dry in the second degree.[21] Drawing from classical medicine, medieval and early modern medicine held that each ingestible substance must possess two qualities out of four possible: hot or cold, and wet or dry. Bodily health depended on balancing those qualities according to four bodily fluids, or "humors": blood, phlegm, yellow bile, and black bile. Each humor had a unique combination of qualities, as black bile was hot and dry, for example, while phlegm was wet and cold. Additionally, each individual had their own complexion that skewed toward one or two of the humoral properties, and organs within the body did so as well—the brain, for example, was cold and wet. Other paradigms of health and sickness were beginning to challenge humoral theory during the sixteenth century, but it still provided an important way for physicians and patients to understand health, illness, and the effects of ingesting food or medicine, which introduced their own humoral properties and thus effected the balance of the humors inside the body. Identifying tobacco as hot and dry meant that it would serve best as a corrective for diseases and symptoms caused by

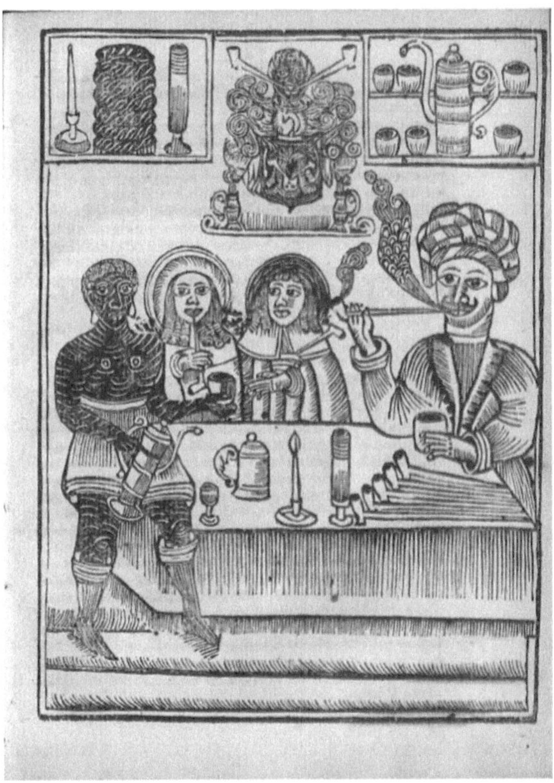

FIGURE 3.1. *Two broad-sides against tobacco* (London: John Hancock, 1672), 63. A Turk smokes and drinks coffee with two English patrons of a coffeehouse, attended by an African servant. Both coffee and tobacco remained strongly associated with the exoticism of non-Europeans, even as western Europeans learned from them about the new drugs. J147, image 7081, used by permission of the Folger Shakespeare Library.

an excess of cold and wet humors in the body, and it would exacerbate illnesses caused by excessive heat and dryness.[22]

In England observers began writing about tobacco even before it became the dominant crop in the Chesapeake, analyzing the new plant in ways similar to Monardes in Spain. In 1595 Anthony Chute, a tobacco user himself and a self-described poor gentleman and scholar, published a collection of opinions by physicians on tobacco, including Nicot and Monardes. He considered tobacco as applied as a green leaf to the skin as well as according to the new method of smoking its dried leaves in a pipe, which he and others called "drincking" tobacco.[23] Chute concluded that smoking was a good remedy for coughing, for treating a "rheume" in the stomach, and for clearing the head and eyes.[24] The best time to use tobacco, he believed, was in the morning before breakfast, and it was also useful for staying awake.[25] Chute concluded by suggesting that tobacco could cure just about any medical problem in the chest or head.[26] Here he leaned on Iberian precedents to identify tobacco's humoral properties, cures, and methods of usage, and he was not the only early English writer on tobacco to do so.[27]

In 1599, the minister and future vice-chancellor of the University of Cambridge Henry Butts published a cookbook that aimed to correct what he saw as his contemporaries' increasing tendency to eat for pleasure instead of health.[28] In it he included tobacco as part of a healthy daily regimen, describing the plant, its preparation, and its benefits for its users. It could be taken in the nose as "snuffe" and also served as a broth: "It cureth any grief, dolour, opilation, impostume, or obstruction, proceeding of cold or winde: especially in the head or breast: the leaves are good against the Migram [low spirits], cold stomacks, sick kidnies, tooth-age, fits of the moother, naughty breath, scaldings or burnings," and also agues.[29] Hot and dry in its humoral properties, it served "against Rumes, Catarrhs, hoarsenesse, ache in the head, stomacke, lungs, breast: also in want of meat, drinke, sleepe, or rest" when smoked in a pipe. Advertising tobacco as a cure for almost all ills was common, especially in this early period. The Scots humanist and physician William Barclay opened his panegyric to tobacco by boasting that as Hercules slayed monsters with his bag and club, so Barclay would slay disease with his tobacco and pipe.[30] He listed many of the same illnesses as Butts, Chute, and Monardes, as well as the French Pox (syphilis), which was relatively new to Europe. He added the observation that ever since Hippocrates there had been only five ways "to voyd this our body of filthy corruption": bloodletting, vomiting, purging by the stool, urinating, and sweating, but now there was a sixth, using tobacco.[31] Purging the body was crucial in Galenic medical practice, devoted as it was to expelling excesses or corruptions of humors, so discovering a new purge was an important achievement. Smoking was not the only method of purging that tobacco could achieve: "Take of leafe Tabacco as much as being folded together, may make a round ball of such bignesse that it may fill the patients mouth, and inclyne his face downward towards the ground, keeping the mouth open . . . there shall flow such a flood of water from his brain and his stomacke, and from all the parts of his body that it shall be a wonder." At the same time, Barclay puzzled over the humoral properties of tobacco, listing the reasons why it might be hot ("it hath acrimonie") or cold ("because it is narcoticke and stupefactive, it maketh drunken, and refresheth, it maketh hungry and filleth, it maketh thirstie, and quencheth thirst").[32] Barclay serves as a good example of early attempts by physicians and natural scientists to understand tobacco. They were excited about the physical maladies it might address, experimenting with different ways to incorporate tobacco into the body and attempting to fix the humoral properties of the new American herb in order to explain precisely how it affected its users' bodies and how it might help cure illnesses.

As the seventeenth century wore on, observers throughout western Europe continued to consider the nature of tobacco, all the while referring to previous writers like Monardes. Although a consensus emerged that tobacco was hot and dry, there were still some doubters, like the Northampton physician James Hart, who suspected that it might be cold, due to its "narcoticke or stupifying nature," which was what made it such a good painkiller.[33] Sebastiano Laghi, a physician from Porlezza, north of Milan, working in Lugano was convinced that it was hot and dry and therefore warned that tobacco might be damaging to the brain, which needed to be wet and cold, and to the reproductive organs.[34] Another Italian physician, Giovanni Piccino, from Orte near Viterbo, cast aside the usual practice of targeting medicines to specific humoral imbalances in individuals and argued that tobacco was useful for everyone, regardless of their humoral complexion. Only tobacco was suited to every age, every season, each sex, and each status of person: poor, rich, base, illustrious, artisan, peasant, layman, the cloistered, and so on.[35] The Spanish moralist Bartolomé Jiménez Patón disagreed, countering that tobacco should be used as Monardes prescribed, and if it were taken indiscriminately it could only do harm, especially to the brains.[36] The Cordovan pharmacist Juan de Castro y Medinilla recommended tobacco as a purge for cleansing the kidneys, curing "the French disease," and inducing menstruation in women.[37] The Spanish friar Tomás Ramón had a different take on tobacco, judging that it made a poor medicine because a purge should encompass the whole body, not just the head.[38] Other authors continued to experiment with its use as a medicine beyond pipe smoking and snuff, including as an emetic to induce vomiting, as a salve to heal sore or decaying eyes, as a dewormer for small children, as a remedy for lice, as a lambitive (a medicine ingested by licking), and as a smoke enema to cure wind and colic.[39] In 1671 the entrepreneurial English royal physician John Archer included an entry on tobacco in his medical guide for laypeople, *Every man his own doctor*, which provided a summary of the conventional wisdom about tobacco that had coalesced by the late seventeenth century. Good for cleaning and curing wounds, when smoked in a pipe "it makes a pump of the mouth," drawing moist and wet phlegm out of the head and stomach, which was good for people of a wet and cold complexion but dangerous for people who were hot and dry.[40] Regardless of the details, many experts throughout Europe agreed with Dutch physician J. I. W. Beintema van Peima that "smoking is one of the foremost means of preserving health and long life."[41]

Not everyone agreed that tobacco belonged in the European pharmacopeia. In 1634 the Castilian physician Francisco de Leiva Aguilar denied that it was a medicine at all, because people used it without reference to the principles of Galenic medicine, not accounting for the time of dose; region of the earth; or humoral complexion, age, weight, or habits of the user.[42] He had physicians like Piccino in mind, prescribing tobacco to all and sundry, contrary to sound medical practice. In 1604 James I took up his own pen and wrote a *Counterblaste to tobacco*, in which, like some of the more cautious physicians, he expressed the belief that tobacco threatened to dry out and overheat the brain. Arguing against its use as a purgative, the king claimed that it purged nothing but itself—tobacco smoke went into the nose only to be distilled into moist and watery phlegm by the brains and then drained again.[43] By the late eighteenth century, physicians were warning that snuff caused the growth of polyps inside the nose and throat.[44] Critics sometimes used stronger language, calling tobacco a poison. In 1602 the English physician "Philaretes" warned that it was such a violent purge that it should be considered toxic, causing "violent vomits, many and infinite stooles, great gnawings and torments in the guts and inward parts. Coldnesse in the outward and externall members, Crampes, Convultions, cold sweats, ill colour, and wannesse of skin . . . giddinesse of the head and braine, profound and deep sleepe, faintnesse, soundings, and to some hastie and untimely death."[45] Another problem was adulteration, as a Dutch writer known only as "van R." pointed out, cautioning that merchants mixed tobacco with other leaves, and that when he spoke of the medical properties of tobacco he meant only the best from Virginia and the Spanish Caribbean.[46] So, despite the great enthusiasm that many physicians expressed for tobacco, a vigorous discourse of opposition emerged as well. Nevertheless the debate and experimentation circulated within well-established parameters of botanical, pharmaceutical, and medical discourse, and well-defined lines of argument developed in a cosmopolitan and homogeneous conversation that crossed the boundaries of nation and language. While they disagreed about the details, all of the observers conducted their discussions within the shared vocabulary of medicine.

Everyone Seems to Have a Darling Liquor

As each of the new drugs arrived in Europe, a similar debate took place among scholars of medicine, pharmacy, and botany. Norton identifies Francisco Hernández as the first physician to incorporate chocolate into Western medicine, playing the same role that Nicolás Monardes played for tobacco, although, while Monardes stayed in Seville, Hernández traveled to New Spain to investigate American natural history for himself. Sent by Philip II of Spain, whom he served as a royal physician, Hernández used Mexico City as his base to explore Mesoamerica between 1571 and 1574 and returned with thirty-eight volumes of written reports, which remained unpublished during his lifetime. Other scholars consulted his manuscripts to learn about the cacao plant, the preparation of the chocolate drink, and the medicinal effects of chocolate, which could be consumed either cold or hot, since the roasted cacao seeds were always served mixed with other ingredients that had their own humoral properties.[47] Bartolomé Marradón, another Castilian with a medical background who traveled to New Spain, reported that chocolate helped with digestion; everywhere he went Native Americans and Africans were making it and selling it to each other to treat colic. He described how it was made and warned that, although it was an energy-boosting drink, thanks to its cold and dry qualities it was probably also the cause for so much of the constipation and hydropsy seen among Spanish women in New Spain.[48] The Sevillian medical professor

Santiago Valverde Turices demurred, protesting that people prepared chocolate in so many different ways, mixing it with so many different ingredients, that it was difficult to tell just what the health benefits or dangers might be.[49] Italian observers, too, worked to fit chocolate into the understanding of Galenic medicine, and the Florentine physician Giovanni Batista Felici warned in 1728 that too much chocolate led to heart palpitations, intermittent pulse, and convulsions and had killed many users through apoplexy.[50] As with tobacco, early adapters experimented with methods of using chocolate that may seem odd today; the English promoter of hot drinks John Chamberlayne suggested that, to increase male libido, chocolate be applied to "the Testicles with a Balsam, or a Sap."[51] Be that as it may, as Irene Fattacciu has explained, by folding the new drink into the discourse and rituals of medicine, physicians blunted the fears of chocolate's exoticism and taught Spaniards how to properly consume it in ways that were physically and morally safe.[52] All of the early modern soft drugs underwent the same process.

When they appeared in western Europe in the middle of the seventeenth century, coffee and tea underwent a similar process, including experimentation with consuming the products in ways that now seem bizarre.[53] Two tea sellers in Rome, Giovanni Agostino and Morison Scozzese, suggested that the health-conscious should either eat its leaves in a salad with oil and vinegar or smoke them like tobacco.[54] Most tea enthusiasts, however, followed the Chinese example of drinking an infusion of tea leaves in a broth, including the most influential early booster of tea's health benefits, the Dutch physician Cornelis Bontekoe, who published his *Treatise on the most excellent herb tea* in 1678.[55] Bontekoe was a champion of iatrochemistry, or chemical medicine, which physicians like the idiosyncratic German Paracelsus and the Flemish Joan Baptista van Helmont proposed as an alternative to galenic humors in the sixteenth and early seventeenth centuries. They believed that salts, acids, and alkalines, not humors, were the important components of food that influenced health and sickness, although in practice the iatrochemistry and humoral medicine coexisted in the thinking and treatment of most seventeenth-century physicians.[56] Nicolas de Blégny's book on hot drinks went into great detail about coffee acting as a medicine that was good for almost everyone. To Blégny, humoral complexion did not matter; one should assume that coffee would promote the health of all—bilious, sanguine, phlegmatic, and melancholy alike—unless individual experience proved otherwise.[57] The Palermo physician and poet Giuseppe Galeano had heard from some Jesuit priests that coffee dispelled crudities from the stomach, and decided to investigate it himself. He found that it invigorated him because of its hot and dry humoral properties, and published a treatise about it in 1674.[58] An anonymous "Declaration of the virtue of the coffee drink" printed in Rome in 1683 also listed several health benefits, including improving digestion and vision.[59]

Under the labels "aqua vitae" or cordials, distilled spirits had a long history as medicines in western Europe, as did sugar and opium. The alchemist Isaac Hollandus had recommended aqua vitae mixed with sugar, and various early modern forms of alcohol continued to draw praise for their health benefits.[60] William Hughes, who had traveled to the Caribbean, noted that Europeans there drink "Rum, Brandy, and other strong and hot Spirits; which . . . are best in summer, when the weather is most hot"; along with chocolate, distilled spirits helped people sweat out the local fumes and ill humors that troubled them.[61] Hughes was adhering to neo-Hippocratic ideas that held that what one should consume depended on where one lived. Although the weight of medical and public opinion increasingly disapproved of distilled spirits, the memory of them as effective medicine lingered on. As the medical essayist Thomas Short lamented, while advising that Britons should forego wine and spirits for beer: "Every one seems to have a darling Liquor, which he is disposed to commend and celebrate at the Expence of all the rest."[62]

Like cordials and aqua vitae, sugar had a long history in the European pharmacopeia, appearing mostly as a sweetener for repellent boluses and syrups. But there were those who claimed that sugar itself had a healthful influence, including Thomas Newton, who in 1580 suggested sugar for lung problems and for the stomach, as long as the patient was not already hot and choleric.[63] As late as 1800 the physician Benjamin Moseley, who had spent years practicing in Jamaica, touted sugar for remedying coughing, for assisting in generating healthy blood, and for helping the lungs, kidneys, bowels, and bladder.[64] Opium was well known since antiquity as a sleep-inducer—for which Estienne and Liebault recommended it—and as a painkiller and a remedy for fevers and diarrhea.[65] Well into the early modern period, practitioners frequently recommended opium, as they had in the Middle Ages, as part of a mix of different drugs, such as lettuce, henbane, purslane, endive, dragons' blood, camphor, basil seeds, hemlock, adamant stone, among other herbs and medicines that the Swiss naturalist and philologist Conrad Gesner endorsed for his readers.[66] Not always internally, either—Gesner suggested applying a paste of opium mixed with garlic to the temples, forehead, and wrists to induce sleep.[67] Beginning in the sixteenth century, Paracelsus popularized laudanum, a tincture of opium in distilled alcohol, as a common way to administer opium.

Taken into their bodies, tobacco and the rest of the new drugs augured a loss of autonomy. Bodies—and selves—threatened to slip free of the boundaries of race, gender, religion, and class. But reconceived as medicines, the soft drugs promised mastery over the body. Enthusiasts touted them for purging, killing pain, helping wounds heal, alleviating symptoms like fever and rheums, and improving specific organs like the lungs and kidneys. Promoters promised a more general control over the body as well. Monardes, for example, emphasized how Native Americans used tobacco to ward off hunger and thirst, which he likened to the way that the Portuguese and Indians used opium and cannabis to refresh themselves in the East Indies.[68] Similarly, Thomas Willis explained that opium worked the same way for the Turks, enabling them to "do or suffer any thing . . . without any great sense of pain or weariness."[69] Even gin, according to the satirist "Saynought Slyboots," helped the poor ignore cold and hunger.[70]

Natural Melancholy Be Converted to Unnatural

While physicians, natural scientists, and other observers engaged in a debate about the effects of early modern stimulants on the body, they used a shared language about medicine, more or less in agreement about how to assess bodily health and disease and physical facts about plants and medicine. Whether the drugs were ancient like opium or new like tobacco, physicians and botanists pinned down the ways they could heal the body and experimented with different methods of employing them, some familiar like smoking tobacco leaves and others less so, such as smoking tea leaves. In so doing, they categorized the drugs by their humoral properties, or, as the paradigm shifted to chemical medicine, their salts and alkaloids. All the while some observers cautioned against the drugs' ill effects when applied in a manner inappropriate for the humoral (or chemical) conditions of their patients. As opium's ability to cause sleep suggests, the workings of drugs and alcohol on the mind was integral to this conversation: all of these comestibles affected it, which would come as no surprise to early modern observers, since their medical theories applied to minds just as much as to bodies. As much as the heart or the stomach, emotions, moods, and mental dispositions were governed by the humors, and the humoral properties brought by consuming drugs would realign the mental states of the users just like their physical states.[71]

Of all the subjects touching on tobacco and the brain, observers placed the most importance on melancholy. This disease occupied the forefront of the sixteenth-century imagination when considering mental illness, much as hysteria did in the late nineteenth century or schizophrenia in the mid-twentieth century.[72] Although recognized as a category of mental illness since the days of Hippocrates, in the early modern period melancholy remained an ambiguous disease without a clear definition. As its name suggests, melancholy (Greek: *melas*, "black," and *chole*, "bile") was caused by an overabundance of black bile, one of the four humors. As it took up an increasing amount of space in the Renaissance repertoire of diagnoses, it encompassed a broad range of symptoms including lethargy, obtrusive and depressing thoughts, capricious decision-making, sadness, rage, and psychotic breaks with reality. There were also moral and religious components to melancholy, and it was sometimes associated with genius and creative insight.[73]

English commentators like Philarates warned about smoking and melancholy. He believed that tobacco worked through the blood to eventually increase the amount of black bile in the body and should under no circumstance be used by those with a melancholy disposition, lest "naturall melancholy be converted to unnaturall."[74] According to the converso physician Fernando Cardoso, chocolate, too, caused melancholy and should therefore be used only as a medicine, not as a refreshment, as many people did in Madrid, especially elite women, who drank chocolate three or four times a day.[75] Others believed that tea and coffee were antidotes to melancholy, like Bontekoe, who defended tea against the accusation that it caused bile and anger and asserted that it was a powerful cure for melancholy.[76] Leonard Biet, a French apothecary devoted to chemical medicine, wrote that the nature of the alkaloids and salts in coffee "strengthens the memory and judgment, and gives the will complete freedom to direct all voluntary actions, by rectifying all melancholy and taciturn dispositions."[77] The Huguenot physician Daniel Duncan split the difference when he explained that coffee "occasions a Gayetie at first, which very soon determines a Melancholy."[78] Beer and wine had long been known for changing the mood and mental abilities of their drinkers, but distilled spirits were something new to early modern observers, and as the Gin Craze reached its height, they continued to attract the opprobrium of moralists concerned in part for their impact on the mind. Thomas Wilson, attacking rum and brandy along with gin, called attention to liquor's effects on the body and mind. In particular he warned about the damage done to the memory "by hardening and spoiling" the brain. Continued drinking would cause "Dispiritedness," and long years of immoderate drinking of spirits led to ill health, financial ruin, and "Melancholy and Despair, which ends in a Pistol or a Dose of some quicker Poison."[79]

Of the traditional drugs that Europeans had at their disposal, sugar was not touted as much for its effects on the mind, while opium attracted more attention. In his pioneering 1547 guidebook to health, the English intelligence agent and physician Andrew Boorde did recommend sugar to help against melancholy.[80] The English surgeon Thomas Brugis suggested laudanum for curing melancholy, and also "in phrensies, and madness." The French Protestant apothecary Nicaise Le Fèvre, who served Charles II of England, reported that in India opium was consumed to "prevent melancholly from seizing upon them."[81] The Welsh physician John Jones delivered a measured warning about opium's effects on the mind in *The mysteries of opium reveal'd*, published in 1700. When first administered, opium soothed the mind, "pleasing and comforting the sensitive soul," but after the dose wore off, "Melancholy does often (if not always) happen in some degree," and "the Sense of Pleasure, newly lost, aggravates the Sorrow."[82] Just as they did when talking about the body, medical experts had a shared language for discussing the effects of tobacco and its sister drugs on the mind.

However, medical discourse had no way of explaining these drugs' curious hold on one particular aspect of the mind: the will. In 1620, when tobacco was first gaining popularity in western Europe, the Córdoba apothecary Juan de Castro y Medinilla described the rise of tobacco's status as a commodity, originally something used by "slaves and tavern-drinkers" but cherished by all grades of society in his day, and "people with means enclose a great quantity of tobacco, and put it in good-smelling places and keep it there, just as in Spain with fine wine."[83] Further, Castro y Medinilla's smoking friends "have sworn to me with powerful oaths that many times they have resolved to cast it off, tobacco-users throwing it away with the intention of never returning to it; but it has such a hook in their hearts that they return after a while, as if seeking pardon."[84] Once people became used to smoking tobacco, they could not stop.

A Miserable Captivity, from Which They Can Scarcely Be Free

But why? Lacking any precedent in humoral theory or chemical medicine, observers grabbed a cluster of metaphors as they groped toward an explanation for tobacco's hold on its users. The English translator and poet Joshua Sylvester published a doggerel verse in the 1610s, soon after tobacco's introduction to England, titled *Tobacco battered; & the pipes shattered*, full of the kind of language that Spooner would employ a century later. Sylvester dedicated the poem to the Earl of Buckingham, James I's favorite, reasoning that since the earl was a staunch defender of Christendom he should call on him "against the proud Oppression / of . . . That Indian Tyrant . . . Thousands of Ours here hath He Captive taken . . . kept under slavish Yoak . . . To follow Follie and to feed on Smoake."[85] Tobacco was a despot "Greater than Great Can [Khan], / Great Turk, Great Tartar, or Great Tamberlan!"[86] Tobacco worsened all other vices, Sylvester continued, magnifying the cursing, swaggering, drinking, gambling, and adultery of smokers, making any place where smoking occurred a place fit only for blasphemers, atheists, and libertines, even devils and Jews.[87] Like firearms, pipes were a smoky engine invented by Satan. Sylvester accused tobacco of causing melancholy, "Sathan's fit Saddle," which allowed the devil "To ride . . . his wretched slaves to Hell" with two spurs: excess and despair.[88] In Sylvester's telling, smokers were idolaters, living in a "New Babylon," all the more because tobacco was so popular among the enemies of true Christianity: "Moores, Turks, Tartars, Persians," and Catholics in Spain.[89] Smoking was a habit that made custom into a second nature, with its users unable to live without it, even as they feared that it was causing them more harm than good, and so they lived in bondage to tobacco.[90] Sylvester also likened smokers to blind mill horses walking in the same fruitless circle every day, and he likened smoking to being ensnared in a cobweb.[91]

The language Sylvester employed, invoking custom, slavery, bondage, vice, and sin, was repeated again and again when writers tried to explain the hold of tobacco over its users. The Spanish clergyman Tomás Hurtado wrote a tract in 1645 aimed at determining whether chocolate and tobacco were foods and whether consuming them would therefore constitute breaking ecclesiastical fasts. Hurtado tried to explain the compelling qualities of tobacco while dismissing the idea that the devil had imbued them with supernatural powers. "And so that inner force that tobacconists feel that impels them to take it is not the force of some pact [with the devil], but rather that of evil custom. . . . That anxiety, or inner force that take those who are accustomed to smoke tobacco, that hastens them along to it when they lack it," he wagered, came from "the wretched habit, engendered by repeated acts that create a taste, and the delight that is already in the smell, already in the value that this herb possesses."[92] Once started, Hurtado explained, the habit of smoking was one with "such a great force that compels, and attracts one to need to use it even against one's will, and against the command of reason."[93] Tobacco users "have a miserable captivity, from which they can scarcely be free," he elaborated. "Good judgment is lacking in those who have become slaves of Tobacco."[94]

From early on, commentors saw that people could become habituated to tobacco, and that leaving it off might need to occur gradually. The physician Edmund Gardiner, writing in 1610, noticed that people unaccustomed to smoking felt dizziness, vertigo, headache, and other ill effects at first. In this aspect, Gardiner observed, smoking was just like drinking beer, ale, or wine, where new users needed to get used to the new intoxicant, but, once they had, "hee must not sodainely leave it, but by degrees."[95] In his family medical handbook, published in 1650, the physician and Leveller Humphrey Brooke took up the subject of custom in general, describing the way people could become accustomed to new commodities or habits by gradually building up a tolerance through repeated exposure. "She gains footing upon us by degrees, and must therefore gradually be removed, they therefore err, who advise the sudden abolition thereof," he wrote. "This Rule must carefully be observed by such as having long accustomed themselves to that which is hurtful and prejudicial to their Healths, have acquired thereby an Evil Habit and Constitution of Body; whether it be by too much use of Wine, Tobacco, Carnall Coition, Exercise . . . or whatsoever else either in Sickness or Health."[96] The English physician James Primrose similarly warned against quitting tobacco abruptly, lest all the humors that the tobacco was purging from the body rush back at once.[97] Another English physician, Richard Carr, allowed that snuff was an effective purgative but advised that a patient wait for natural sneezes instead because snuff would gradually lose its power, just as "Opium by frequent Repetition ceases to procure Sleep, altho' given in a prodigious Dose."[98] Steven Shapin has demonstrated that this was a principle of early modern medicine—that custom was a second nature, and physicians should tell their patients that suddenly quitting something to which they had become accustomed was dangerous, even if that practice was itself unhealthy.[99]

Observers noticed habituation for all the early modern soft drugs. N. F. J. Éloy, a physician in what was then the Austrian Netherlands, warned that those who drank coffee became habituated and required more until they were slaves to it, needing it daily.[100] Gin and opium attracted more attention, as when Edward Chandler, then the bishop of Lichfield and Coventry, gave a sermon against gin to the Society for the Reformation of Manners in London in 1724, where he warned that first-time gin drinkers "feel a loweness of spirits afterwards, which eggs them on to repeat the potion, and increase it's quantity."[101] Carr cautioned that "the more we accustom our selves to spirituous Liquors, the more we want Spirits," and advised that spirituous liquor was best given up gradually, both in quantity and in kind, from gin to wine to ale.[102] Habituation to and tolerance for drugs was most noticeable in opium, and European observers took it for granted that Turks consumed an amount as part of a daily habit that would kill a western European.[103]

At stake was mastery over oneself. If the new exotic drugs promised control over the body and mind in the form of medicine, they also threatened an erosion of the will. Bodily autonomy and the collapse of self-control vied for prominence in discourse about stimulants. With their long discussions of the subject, Sylvester and Hurtado provide good examples of the three main tropes that observers engaged to explain what we would now consider addiction. Two of them had existed for centuries, long before the new psychotropic drugs became so readily available to western Europeans, and one was new. The first was vice, the tendency of humans to behave in ways they knew to be wrong because they were pleasurable. Vice encompassed a rhetoric of debauchery and voluptuousness that evoked sensual, illicit pleasure, these themes that stretched back to the philosophy and literature of ancient Greece and Rome. The second was luxury, the idea that once users started they fell unthinkingly into durable habit. Luxury came from a tradition of discourse about fashion and custom to explain why people indulged in habits that were unhealthy and immoral, especially when imported from abroad, that also drew on Christian thought and classical Roman and Greek philosophy. While vice emphasized the depraved will of individuals, luxury pointed to problems gripping an entire society. The third, however, did not have such long roots, and this was spiritual language, one that invoked individual sinfulness, bewitchment, and the bondage of the will. This is not to say that each writer chose only one of these three rhetorical strategies when discussing one of the new soft drugs, since they were similar concepts that overlapped and shaded into one another, all attempts to explain how people could feel forced to do something like smoke tobacco seemingly against their will.

His Sensual Appetite: Gluttony, Vice, and Debauchery

When considering beer and wine, medieval European moralists folded drunkenness into the sin of gluttony, due to their disinclination to separate drinking from eating—excesses in both were considered equally sinful elements of gluttony. Beer and wine led to sinful behavior like violence and illicit sex, but gluttony was bad enough, because it took food away from the starving and drew humans into beastliness as drinkers lost the use of their reason, fell to the ground, and soiled themselves.[104] Drinking began to separate from eating in the seventeenth century thanks in part to the impulse—found most famously among English Puritans, but truly throughout western Europe—to reform the manners of the common people. The change in attitude mirrored a change in drinking habits. Beer and wine consumption had been a part of everyday life, with families drinking at home from breakfast and into the night, but now it was beginning to become a separate, recreational activity, with men imbibing in alehouses and taverns away from women and children. Drunkenness began to peel away from gluttony into its own sphere of sinful behavior worthy of moralists' attention even before the advent of cheap, mass-produced distilled spirits.[105]

As demonstrated in chapter 1, all of these drugs possessed a strong pull because of the sensual pleasures they led to, pleasures that could slide from benign physical contentment into seductive debauchery. When it arrived in Europe, tobacco fit nicely into preconceived ideas of drunkenness and gluttony. As early as 1604 James I noted that so many Englishmen had begun to smoke continually "as now they are not able to forbeare the same, no more than an olde drunkard can abide to be long sober." The king charged tobacco with leading to "sinnes and vanities," especially lust, since it was "a branche of the sinne of drunkennesse, which is the root of all sinnes."[106] In 1616 John Deacon, in a treatise dedicated to James I, chose to make tobacco a symbol of all the "carowsing and quaffing, all gulling [gluttony] and gormandizing, all excessive and riotous banqueting" taking place in England and blamed the tobacco's dryness for motivating men to drink too much.[107] The Dutch authors of *Bacchus' miracles* and the Italian physician Benedetto Stella explicitly likened tobacco smoke's effects on the brain to drunkenness.[108] Another seventeenth-century Dutch compilation, *The treasure of sobriety*, was careful to provide a broad definition of sobriety, including moderation in eating, not just in drinking, and generally preserving good health.[109] Even Beintema van Peima, just two years after claiming that tobacco was a sure road to health, warned in another publication that "tobacco-smoking makes men drunk, and all drunkenness is sin."[110] While debating whether consuming chocolate broke a fast, the Castilian jurist Antonio de León Pinelo differentiated chocolate, which sustained the body, from tobacco, which was simply a vice or sin like drinking.[111] In a posthumously published 1639 spiritual tract, the London Puritan minister Henry Ramsden addressed the glutton, whom he described as one who "gives too much way to his sensuall appetite," and cautioned that those who were so devoted to a certain food or tobacco that they could not live without it risked becoming slaves to what St. Paul called "the power of a thing" (1 Cor. 6:12).[112] An anonymous French author writing on snuff in 1700 counseled the elite to avoid tobacco, but he recognized that for those who indulged in the seductive pleasures of tobacco the habit changed into a necessity, because "voluptuousness, the enemy of reason, prevents us from following good advice and closes the eyes to the enormity of vice."[113] Even someone who "has thrown down his pipe, he who has resolved not to take tobacco in the future, and to avoid the contagious company of those who use it, it does not take long. . . to deceive himself, and to take back his snuff or pipe in secret."[114] Reason fell to self-deception, as the sensual vice of tobacco was too much to resist.

The other drugs fit the same profile of seductive debauchery, using pleasure to lure users into a trap from which they could scarcely escape. While visiting the Canary Islands, the French Jesuit traveler André Thevet lamented that, while the sugar grown there was once used only in medicines, nowadays "voluptuousnesse is so increased, specially in our Europe . . . but that every sause must be sugered, and also our meates and drinkes."[115] Cornelius Bontekoe believed that people who disliked tea only did so because their sense of taste had been corrupted by "wine, beer, and other unclean drinks," so he advised his readers to stop imitating "the irregular desires of sensual people, who constantly destroy themselves in those things that God has given for their sustenance."[116] The Huguenot physician Daniel Duncan, in his book about hot drinks, lamented that "the World grows daily more Voluptuous and by that means more unfortunate. Every Age opens a new Source of Pleasures, which produces abundance of new Diseases."[117] He observed that drinkers of coffee, chocolate, and tea did not drink because they were thirsty, but solely for pleasure.[118] The Napoleonic military physician M. de Reynal warned against letting a young man drink coffee, since his inexperience "only makes him all too easily a slave to the senses."[119] And, of course, the age-old concerns about beer and wine transferred easily to distilled spirits, which quickly became associated with debauchery and vice. The Scots minister James Yates was concerned in the 1810s that habitual drunkards would promote the abuse of ardent spirits, among other substances, in order to take away the disgrace of being alone in "that vice, to which they are themselves addicted."[120] This strain of thinking emphasized individual behavior. Debauchery, voluptuousness, and vice were all choices that people made when they indulged too much in the pleasures of the new stimulants, which would then ensnare them.

Our Strange and New Fangled Fashions: Custom, Fashion, and Luxury

"How great the force & power of this cruell tyrant Custome is, that creepeth in by little & little, insinuating and conveighing himself slily into our natures, so that at length he will [have] the whole rule and government of our bodies, prescribing and limiting new lawes . . . and abrogating olde ancient orders, constitutions, and fashions." Thus mused Edmund Gardiner about the power of custom, noticing tobacco's hold over its users.[121] The Bath physician Tobias Venner admitted that tobacco could be a good medicine, but believed that most people smoked not for health reasons, but as a "vicious custome."[122] In dietetic writing custom could mean a corruption of the diet, the rejection of what was natural to eat and drink and the consumption of what was unhealthy instead, or an excess of healthy things. Just as good habits led to virtue, bad habits led to vice. Customs changed with fashion and in pursuit of luxury, and, like gluttony, luxury had a long history in European moral thought.[123] The ancient Romans worried about it, believing that riches and imported luxury goods from the East corrupted both Roman morals and the Roman state. The historian Livy thought that luxury softened Roman soldiers, debased Roman statesmen, and corroded the Roman Constitution. Imported goods and foods formed an important component of luxury both in antiquity and later. Maxine Berg argues that early modern moralists saw tobacco and its fellow imported drugs chocolate, tea, coffee, sugar, and opium as part of an influx of luxury items that were washing over western Europe and threatening its social structure and moral fiber. Other foreign luxuries included textiles like silk, cotton, and tapestries, coveted woods like mahogany, Italian marble, and porcelain serving dishes for chocolate, coffee, and tea.[124] Whereas vice and debauchery were individual choices, luxury, fashion, and custom were trends that swept through entire societies.

James I leaned on this premise in his *Counterblaste to tobacco*, blaming the popularity of what was after all "a common herbe" on "an inconsiderate and childish affectation of Noveltie."[125] The English poet George Wither wrote a satire of tobacco, wondering why so many people wanted to smoke:

> What's their reason? . . .
> they have seene some doe
> Forsooth, and therefore they must use it too.
> Nay, wonder not; The Sunne lights not a Nation
> That more addicteth Apish imitation
> Then doe we English.[126]

Barnabe Rich, an English soldier and a writer, introduced his attack on tobacco by invoking "our strange and new fangled fashions" that brought such an unnecessary item into English usage.[127] In a reforming tract published during the Restoration, Edward Chamberlayne proposed a tax on "all such Commodities as occasion either Excess or Luxury, Wantonness, Idleness, Pride, or Corruption of Manners," including distilled spirits, coffee, chocolate, sugar, and tobacco.[128] Outside Britain tobacco had the same reputation. In a satirical poem about tobacco published in 1643, the Catalan satirist Burlot de Campaña labeled it a vice, but he also described its users as "accustoming" themselves to tobacco, which was a "luxury."[129] An anonymous Dutch moralist scolded men for acting like sheep, "where one walks through, there are more, and without any reason to see they ape each other." Whether or not tobacco was healthy did not matter, the writer thought, so long as tobacco was fashionable.[130]

The other psychotropic drugs received the same analysis as tobacco, as the physician and natural scientist Martin Lister observed. Writing about a visit to Paris in 1698, Lister noted something new since the last time he was there: that distilled spirits flowed freely at the conclusion of dinners. "Add to these Drinks the daily use of Coffee with Sugar, Tea and Chocolate, which now is as much in use in Private Houses in Paris, as with us in London," not to mention the increasing number of Parisian coffeehouses, all of which he attributed to changes in fashion. "I wonder at the great change of this Sober Nation," Lister reflected, "but Luxury like a Whirlpool draws into it the Extravagances of other people."[131] In 1662 the radical Protestant and English polymath Henry Stubbe published a tract in which he tried to defend the value of chocolate. He argued that it was pure and healthy in its simple, original form, the way the Indians made it; it became suspect only when "Spanish luxury" led to it being mixed with a variety of exotic things.[132] In the early eighteenth century, Joseph Browne, a physician who urged his readers to take cold baths for their health, lamented that bathing had fallen out of fashion since antiquity "with the Luxury and Delicacy of the present Age, which may be attributed, in a great measure, to . . . the Interest of Foreign Trade, which has introduc'd Tobacco, Tea, and Coffee, with all the Brandy, Spirits, and Spices."[133]

John Chamberlayne bemoaned the fact that while junipers and elderberries, native to northern Europe, could make an infusion that was healthier than coffee and tea, fashionable young men and women disdained anything that "comes not from France, or the Indies."[134] Although not a foreign import, gin, too, was associated with luxury; one anonymous moralist during England's Gin Craze wrote disapprovingly of English farmers who grew prosperous by providing grain for the distilleries. They began to "consult their Ease and Luxury at such a Rate" that they would no longer drink good English beer and were not content unless they had their daily doses of tea, coffee, and gin.[135] The Capuchin friar Gaetano Maria da Bergamo wrote a spiritual exercise in the early eighteenth century aimed at helping the reader determine if he was addicted to the habit of drinking in taverns. "Would you currently find it difficult to abstain entirely from the tavern, with a strong resolve never to go there again?" he asked. If abstention seemed impossible, then "it is a sign that the vice has become strong in you, and has dominion over you."[136] Even opium, entrenched as a part of the pharmacopeia since antiquity, attracted the attention of moralists by the eighteenth century. In London in 1785, Hugh Smythson published his *Compleat family physician*, in which he cited common knowledge that opium was abused in Muslim countries, where alcohol was prohibited. Smythson reported with alarm that European travelers to these places had begun using opium in the same way to lift their spirits, dampened by the hot climates; later, when they returned home, they continued with "this pernicious custom." Even worse than tea, tobacco, and stuff, opium was dangerous except used strictly as a medicine, "as an article of luxury or indulgence, bring on a species of present intemperance, and is pregnant with future mischief."[137]

As an interesting counterpoint to these admonitions, some British writers in the 1790s described sugar, once a luxury, as a new necessity. These arguments came out of the context of the enormous opportunities for profit by the British West Indian sugar islands after the collapse of French sugar production thanks to the Haitian Revolution on the one hand, and the growing strength of the antislavery movement in Britain on the other. One anonymous defender of slavery announced that medical authority and common sense made it clear that "sugar is not a luxury; but has become, by constant use, a necessary of life." He asked: "Is rum a luxury? Is cotton a luxury? Is ginger a luxury?" Banning sugar made as much sense as banning those other items, once luxurious but now entrenched in Europeans' daily practice.[138] Another anonymous defender of slavery concurred, arguing that once sugar was "a superfluity" but "the constitution, from long habits of luxury, becomes so much changed as to render that at last necessary, which originally owed its introduction to caprice and effeminacy," and returning to a state of nature would mean abandoning many other commodities besides sugar.[139] Perhaps this line of reasoning persuaded readers in the 1790s, but a moralist proposing higher taxes on sugar thirty years earlier had an answer: "If the Universality of any customary Luxury was to make us consider such Luxury as a Necessary of Life, why not admit Dram-drinking, Gaming, and other Debaucheries by the same Rule?—But Tea and Sugar are Luxuries, not Necessaries, and it is, perhaps, a Misfortune to Society, that they are so cheap as to make them universal."[140]

Bewitched Blindness: Sin, Enchantment, and Slavery

However well the ancient categories of luxury, fashion, vice, and gluttony described the grip that early modern stimulants had on their users, they were not enough. They did not capture the full power of these drugs, or the astonishment of observers of their effects. Take, for example, the testimony of a certain Dr. Bellamy, from the earliest days of tobacco's use in England. The doctor described himself as having been "leane, feeble, full of defects and infirmities full of fleame and rheumaticke humidities" as a young man. Urged by a friend to take tobacco as a medicine, he refused, behaving like a "Madde Dogge . . . whose propertie is, to shunne, flee, and refuse, the fresh running waters, his principall and chiefest comfort." Bellamy's afflictions made him barely able to eat or drink without retching and left him exhausted at the slightest exertion. He woke up every night with coughing, sweating, and bleeding from the nose, "in such sort, that I did seeme unto most men, destitute, and deprived of all earthly comfort," until finally he did try tobacco, as his friend suggested. "I felt myselfe at large happily redeemed from captivity to liberty, from sickenesse to health, from paines to delight, from continuall discouragement, to comfort and consolation," and he praised God for the transformation of his health through tobacco.[141]

Bellamy's tale of captivity and redemption serves as a mirror opposite of Spooner's, from the beginning of this chapter. While Spooner felt that freeing himself from the habit of smoking was a release from bondage, Bellamy hailed tobacco itself as freedom from bondage and the limitations of the flesh. Spooner was dismayed to see tobacco taking over his life, where Bellamy gained a new purchase on life thanks to tobacco's curative powers. A friend gave Bellamy the healing gift of tobacco, while Spooner's friends helped bind him with the chains of smoking. Putting the two vignettes together reveals a profound ambivalence about tobacco in western European experience, but, despite their different experiences, both men reached for spiritual language to describe their deep emotions. The rhetoric they employed—starting with a life incapacitated by enfeeblement and malaise, refusing at first the thing that will lead to freedom and then finally embracing it, with relief and transcendence—reads like nothing so much as a religious conversion.[142] The spiritual nature of Bellamy's tobacco tale recalls Nicot's first discoveries of the healing properties of tobacco in Lisbon, similar to a saint's miracle tales: with one ill person after another learning of the powers of Nicot's holy weed, coming to be healed, then spreading tobacco's fame further, first throughout Lisbon and then throughout Europe. Just as it is difficult to describe changes to the will, it is difficult to describe the connections between the will and the physical world. The new soft drugs appeared at a time when western Europeans had been reexamining their understanding of free will and human agency in the wake of Martin Luther's insistence on the depravity of the will—of the individual Christian's inability to stop sinning despite a desire to do so.[143] Religious language, with its rich vocabulary of miracles, ecstasies, mysticism, bodily transformation, witchcraft, conversion, and rebirth, offered an intimately familiar language for early modern Europeans to understand and describe the will. Where the language of medicine, pharmaceutics, and natural science failed, spiritual language rushed into the gap to help understand and describe the experience of using drugs and being transformed by that use.

One way to understand how religious language could be so useful for explaining the effects of drugs and alcohol is to examine how English writers also used drugs and alcohol as a metaphor to explain sin. Clergymen and moralists enlisted drugs and alcohol to describe the ways that sin could catch and hold Christians. For example, a collection of the sayings of James I published in 1643 featured the king making an elaborate simile between smoking and hell. First, "so are the vanities of the world a smoake and vapour," and smoking gives pleasure, just as "the pleasures of the world delight the men of the world. Thirdly, It maketh men drunken and light in the head, so doe the vanities of the world, men are drunken therewith. Fourthly, He that taketh Tobacco, saith he cannot leave it, it doth bewitch him; even so the pleasures of the world makes men loath to leave them, they are for the most part so inchanted with them."[144] Tobacco, just like sin, trapped men with its pleasure. A century later the Puritan minister Henry Burton likened heresy to tobacco, describing Pelagianism as "that great and bewitching Heresy," just as "I have heard many say of Tobacco, complaining how they are bewitched with it, when they would same leave it, but have not the power."[145] Jessica Warner has shown that English ministers crusading against drunkenness used very similar language, describing it as "an enticing, bewitching sin" and drunkards as "addicted to this bewitching vice."[146]

Sugar's role as a sweetener for medicines also provided a metaphor for pleasure masking the foulness of sin. In a work published posthumously in 1656, Thomas Hooker, the Puritan minister who helped found Connecticut, tried to explain how a well-intentioned Christian could fall into sinfulness. Despite intelligence, good judgment, and a sound conscience, "yet he doth not perceive the plague and venome" in a sin, judging it instead for the immediate reward and pleasure it will bring. "As it is with the bitterest pills when they are sugred," he continued, "so it is with many base and wretched lusts, which are the very gal of bitterness, and cary deadly poyson with them, they are so Sugared, and covered over with applause and credit in the world." Hooker likened Satan to a cunning apothecary who sugared his poisoned pills of sin.[147] The moralist Thomas Goddard described the road to damnation as "first drinking a sugared draught of sinful delights," but one that leaves the drinker unsatisfied, so he drinks again and again until he finds himself in chains and in despair.[148] The sugaring could also be literal, as when the Huguenot physician Duncan pointed out that it was sugar that made the hot drinks pleasing to the taste. "Pleasure is the fatal Bait which deludes us to swallow the Hook by which the Enemy of our Life and Salvation does catch us," he elaborated, so the quality "which makes Coffee, Chocolate and Tea to be so much admired, ought to be the Cause why it should be hated."[149] Without sugar, they would simply be benign—and bitter—medicines.

Later in his essay, Goddard seized upon opium as a metaphor for sin, describing pleasure as a "pleasing but dangerous Opium to the soul."[150] The drowsiness of opium lent itself more than any other drug to the description of Christians falling half-knowingly into temptation, sin, and damnation. In a passage discussing whether the soul possessed the free will to do good, the chemical physician Joan Baptista van Helmont explained that it should, unless it was "charmed into a lethargick inactivity by the opium of originall sin."[151] The popular London Puritan minister Thomas Adams explained that it was possible for sinners not to realize their sinfulness: "Such a one spends his dayes in a dreame . . . when the Divill, an ill Surgion . . . first casts his Patient into a mortferous sleep." In order to prevent religion from shaking the Christian awake, "Satan gives him some Opium."[152] Another English minister, Stephen Jerome, responding to an outbreak of the plague in 1625 by calling for repentance before God's judgment, decried those who "sleep in their sinne so deadly," unaware of their damnation, "as having drunke Poppy or Oppium." Not even the trumpets and thunder of the Last Judgment could wake them, "so strong are their sleepy drugs, so powerfull sinnes charmes, so pleasing and bewitching the worlds Musicke."[153] Samuel Rolle likened wine to opium, explaining that the reason men get together and drink wine so much is to divert themselves from paying attention to their sinfulness: "Many do use it but as opium to the conscience."[154]

This language evoking the satanic, bewitching enslavement to drugs—language used by Sylvester and Hurtado as well—emerged as a powerful set of metaphors as soon as tobacco entered western Europe. As the priest Matteo Pinelli put it (writing under the pseudonym "Alessandro Sanlorini da Prunalbeta"), "Tobacco is the iron and the nose a magnet."[155] James I also referred to its "bewitching qualitie," which made those who begin smoking want it more as they become used to it, just as drunkards increasingly want more and stronger drink.[156] The Spanish friar Tomás Ramón suspected that there was some sort of implicit pact between tobacco and its users in Andalusia when it appeared there. "They go around so blind and passionate," he wrote, "that once they have tried it they do not know how to let it out of their hands." One priest claimed that even if the pope forbade tobacco, it would survive: "And its use goes so strongly among those who use it, that they would kill themselves for it, and they make it their business to persuade others of its worth, offering it to everyone they encounter." Ramón, who went on to call smokers "bewitched, or enchanted by the devil," was able to persuade some learned men in Seville to give it up, but they took it up again after a couple of days, unable to abstain any longer.[157] The Huguenot refugee David Papillon also called tobacco "bewitching," as did Ben Agar in his collection of James I's sayings.[158] The anonymous author of *Tobaco-mastix* in 1677 likened the smoke-and-snuff-inhaling nose to a god: "It has become an abusive [god] like the Devil, getting adoration of much of the world as from Subjects; wheedling Christendom it self out of its wits, and . . .. tam'd its Inhabitants into a loyalty to folly." "Reek-mongers," as *Tobaco-mastix* called them, were also slaves to smoke, and smoking was a monstrous, unnatural thing, like heresy or homosexuality, its users dedicated to "that Belzebub and Dunghil-god." The author continued: "But when he is extricate and free from that slavery, sure he will look back with disgust on his former Distraction; for 'tis the waking only that can tell his dream."[159] The use of the supernatural metaphor lingered into the eighteenth century. In 1750 Dr. Short wrote that smoking tobacco "is so enchanting, that they who are once accustomed to it, can hardly leave it off . . . without the great Mortification, and a kind of Violence or Force done to their Inclination." Indeed rather than go without tobacco, they would take surprising risks and commit "shocking Crimes."[160] Note here that in this conception of addiction the power lay not with individual choice, as in gluttony, or with society as a whole, as with custom and luxury, but within the drug itself. Nevertheless the idea of entrapment remained a premodern one, different from the physiological or psychological kind of entrapment found in the modern rhetoric of drug addiction. Lawrence Spooner had blamed tobacco itself for his own entrapment and credited his freedom from it not to his own actions, but to God, who alone is powerful enough to break tobacco's bonds.

Observers applied this spiritual language of sinfulness, bondage, and bewitchment to the other psychotropic drugs. The Carmelite friar and later bishop of Durango in New Spain José Vicente Díaz Bravo published a treatise in 1753 considering whether chocolate would break an ecclesiastical fast. One reason he thought it might be food was that people wanted to consume it several times a day: "Because I have noticed that it is a dominant aliment, and in habituating oneself to it, it rules, and has power over actions, so it is not taken when the person wants, but always when the Chocolate desires it."[161] Observers of coffee and tea called them "bewitching," as so did eighteenth-century moralists who castigated gin.[162] The "Tea Doctor" Bontekoe warned that those who chose beer, wine, and distilled spirits instead of tea would become "slaves of sin."[163] The eighteenth-century writer and moralist Eliza Fowler Haywood, in her anti-gin work *A present for women addicted to drinking*, urged the friends of women who had fallen into a constant "tipling" to do everything they could to stop them and "deliver the Minds of our Fellow-Christians from the Slavery of Vice."[164] Stephen Hales, one of the early proponents of the medical theory of alcoholism during the Gin Craze, liberally applied spiritual metaphors even while advancing the idea that there was an element of disease to habitual drunkenness. "There is such a predominant bewitching of Naughtiness in these fiery Liquors, as strongly and impetuously carries Men on to their certain Destruction," he noted, despite the natural human inclination toward health and longevity. People given over to distilled spirits were so deeply sunken "that they seldom have so much as a Heart to be set free. Now when a Man's Will and Affections are thus depraved, and he is delighted with the worst of Slavery, there are little Hopes of him." A man such as this, Hales thought, had to be, "as it were, forced into his Liberty."[165] Hales described drunkards as people who "even Glory in their Shame"—a particular aspect of desperate sinfulness that would be picked up by Charles Lamb, who, in addition to giving up tobacco, was himself an inveterate drinker.[166] Lamb likened alcohol to a Correggio painting in which three women attend to a man sitting at the foot of a tree. The three women were allegorical: "Sensuality is soothing him, Evil Habit is nailing him to a branch," and the third, Repugnance, is letting a snake bite him. "In his face is a feeble delight, the recollection of past rather than perception of present pleasures, languid enjoyment of evil with utter imbecility to good, a Sybaritic effeminacy, a submission to bondage, the springs of the will gone down like a broken clock, the sin and the suffering co-instantaneous . . . remorse preceding action." Lamb offered up a description of the entrapment of sin and drinking together, both of them a form of slavery simultaneously willed and unwilled.[167]

This third category of explanation for the compulsive use of tobacco and other drugs differed than the first two categories in its emphasis on the power of the drug. Voluptuousness, luxury, custom, fashion, and vice were timeless problems of society. They existed in the settings of the Old and New Testaments and in the moral thought of Classical Greece and Rome. Anyone anywhere could be lured into the excessive use of drugs and alcohol by these avenues. The enslavement of young women drinking gin, the enchantment of smoking, and the fatal pleasure of opium ascribed power not to general conditions of humanity but to the drugs themselves. Like the emphasis of Rush and his predecessors on the unique dangers of distilled spirits, these observers moved the focus of their concern away from individual choice or the corrupting nature of society and onto the unique bond between consumer and drug. Agency here rested in the drugs themselves and their sugared, drowsy pleasures.

Western Europeans feared that exotic drugs like tobacco would alter their bodies to match the gendered, racial, and religious aspects of the people from whose lands these drugs came. Discovering the medical qualities of the new drugs, usually learned from exotic peoples themselves, made the new stimulants safe for consumption; as part of the pharmacopeia, the drugs helped to discipline their bodies and countered the threats that disease posed to bodily integrity. But while European physicians, pharmacists, and natural scientists shared a common language with which to assess the medical properties of tobacco and its fellow drugs, they had to leave medical language behind in order to understand the unusual grip that alcohol and drugs had on their users. They arrived at three strains of rhetoric, distinct but overlapping, to explain what today is known as addiction. One strain focused on the consumer, building on the notion that drugs were pleasurable and slotting the new drugs into ancient categories of gluttony, vice, and debauchery. A second emphasized problems with society as a whole and put them into the categories—also very old—of fashion, custom, and luxury. A third focused on the power of the drugs themselves, placed into categories derived from religion and magic, mastery and slavery. All three strains gestured toward the compulsive qualities of drug and alcohol use without employing the language used today to describe addiction. All three strains emphasized the ambivalent nature of the drugs, at once controlling and taming the body's humors (or, for iatrochemical physicians, salts and alkaloids) while untethering the consumer's behavior from conscious will.

These ways of understanding compulsive drug use challenges both the idea that the early modern period was one of increasing discipline, and the way that we think of addiction. One important pillar of Michel Foucault's conception of early modern discipline is the idea that medical experts helped shape the reality of medicine and bodily experience by shaping the discourse of illness and health. With psychotropic drugs, however, control over the language that tried to explain abuse and dependency evaded physicians' control. David Clemis, looking at the origins of the medical model of alcoholism, argues that, far from controlling the discourse, the medical profession simply began to contribute its expertise to understanding addictive behavior, and the traditional moralists who had traditionally dominated the conversation accommodated them without ceding the field, at least through the eighteenth century.[168] However it was discussed, the rising consumption of pleasurable, seductive new drugs posed a powerful countervailing force to the mastery over one's own behavior that theorists like Michel Foucault, Gerhard Oestreich, and Norbert Elias all posited as a key theme of early modern European history.

CHAPTER 4

Do We Take Physick Every Day?

Early Modern Wellness and Self-Medication

Born in 1714, one year before the Peace of Utrecht transferred his hometown of Mons and the rest of the province of Hainaut from Spanish control to Austrian, Nicolas François Joseph Éloy earned his medical degree at the University of Louvain in 1736. After further study and practice in Paris and his hometown, in 1752 Mons appointed Éloy as municipal physician. In 1754 Princess Anne-Charlotte of Lorraine, the abbess of a Mons convent, hired him as her medical advisor, a position he later filled for her brother Prince Charles-Alexandre of Lorraine, the governor of the Austrian Netherlands. The history of medicine remembers Éloy primarily for publishing a two-volume *Historical dictionary of ancient and modern medicine* in 1755, but he authored several other books before his death in 1788.[1] Among them was a curious 1781 monograph titled *An examination of the public health question: Whether the habitual use of coffee is beneficial or should it be ranked among those things which are indifferent for the conservation of health.*[2] Why did this distinguished physician bother to write a book questioning a drink that by then had been established in European diet and customs for a century?

Coffee has attracted a great deal of attention, thanks to its role in fostering a new site of information exchange, the coffeehouse, which has become a symbol of the emergence of the Habermasian public sphere. For historians, the coffeehouse is a landmark on the path to new, larger, more democratic, and more manipulable forms of information flow, beginning with moveable type and moving on to cheap newspapers, mass electronic communication like radio and television, and, finally, the Internet. Coffee thus points the way toward a condition of modern—or perhaps postmodern—times: the current age of social media and disinformation.[3] Brian Cowan and others have demonstrated that this is not a case of historians projecting their own anxieties onto the past; for many early modern Europeans, the new forms of discourse and sociability in the coffeehouse were in fact quite worrisome.[4] This, however, was not Éloy's concern: instead he warned against coffee's effects on the body. As demonstrated in previous chapters, coffee held an ambivalent place in consumer culture, since its exotic origins were part of its initial appeal. As coffee became engrained in European habits during the eighteenth century, different issues arose. Nervous disorders emerged as an important paradigm for understanding the body and disease, and coffee was now thought to act on the nerves and, through them, the moods of its users. This new concern is what drove Éloy to write his treatise. The rise of nervous disorders in medical thought was in part a consequence of the new cult of sensibility. Sensibility, and the broader cultural anxieties of which it was a part, were in turn closely tied to the prosperity, long-distance trade, and urbanization that characterized the increasingly consumer-driven, global European economy and society of the eighteenth century. Was Éloy right that coffee drinking contributed to the luxurious, overrefined consumption habits out of urban Europeans? Or, or as others have suggested, did it offer a cure for this enervating new lifestyle? Did the availability of luxury goods, including coffee and the other soft drugs, threaten the moral discipline and emotional regulation of European consumers? Or did psychotropic drugs offer a new way to master the body and the mind?

Coffee provides an excellent starting point for exploring the intersection between the new luxuries of cheap goods that emerged during the consumer revolution, especially stimulants like coffee on the one hand, and the eighteenth-century emergence of preventative health medicines that focused on daily diet and regimen on the other.[5] Historians have acknowledged that coffee's foreign origin caused controversy when it was first introduced into western Europe, but they have also told a story where coffee quickly overcomes that obstacle, and the only remaining difficulty lies in the coffeehouse, the site singled out by Habermas. Éloy's publication serves as a reminder that even in the late eighteenth century a lingering scrutiny remained of the bodily effects of drinking coffee; moreover, it indicates a way of linking the social history of medicine to the history of consumption. Western Europeans had taken control of coffee and its fellow psychotropic drugs from physicians and pharmacists. Many of them now took it daily, without the oversight of medical professionals, as part of a regime of dietetics and hygiene designed not so much to cure disease as to maintain health, especially mental health. Here, coffee and the other stimulants took their place along with other practices like diets, baths, mineral waters, and exercise that aimed to maintain the health of the body and, through the body, the mind. Dissenting physicians and moralists countered that these drugs were actually the cause of the physical ailments and mental anxiety that they pretended to cure—that exotic drugs simply added to the overconsumption of luxury goods that caused the nervous disorders in the first place. To borrow two concepts from our day to analyze what was going on in theirs: Should this daily self-dosing with soft drugs be labeled part of an incipient culture of wellness, or self-care, or should they be viewed as a form of self-medication and substance abuse?

Coffee: We Destroy Our Health by the Same Means We Pretend to Preserve It

Coffee arrived in western Europe originally as a curiosity and within two generations became a commodity. Travelers to the Ottoman Empire were the first to notice it, where, by the mid-sixteenth century, it had become part of daily life in Egypt and Istanbul. The so-called virtuosi, well-educated English gentlemen who delighted in collecting exotic goods and rarities, were among the first to bring coffee to Europe. Jews and Armenians, as middlemen between the Muslim and Christian halves of the Mediterranean, opened some of the first coffeehouses in Europe. The first English coffeehouse opened in Oxford in 1650, and by 1663 there were at least eighty coffeehouses in London. They became a visible part of urban life, attracting attention in the form of printed broadsheet satire as well as scrutiny by government agents. The first French coffeehouse appeared in Paris by 1672 after a visit from a Turkish ambassador that kindled interest in Eastern exotica in 1669, and the coffeehouse reached Venice in 1683. As coffee consumption rose, Europeans began to control its importation and took steps to organize its cultivation as well. By the 1660s English, Dutch, and French merchants had begun to bypass Arab and Indian traders by sailing directly to Mocha, in Yemen, the fountainhead of the coffee bean trade. In the first decades of the 1700s, the Dutch were planting coffee in Java and Suriname while the French established coffee plantations in the Indian Ocean islands of Réunion and Bourbon and in the Caribbean islands Martinique, Guadeloupe, and Saint Domingue, followed later by British Caribbean growers. In Europe the coffeehouse evolved into an institution that offered coffee and its sister hot drinks, chocolate and tea, as well as tobacco—all stimulants that began as exotic imports and became commonplace by the early eighteenth century, at least in large urban centers. Coffeehouses had also become sites of information exchange, including the controversial political and religious ideas that so worried English authorities and attracted the attention of Habermas, and they served as clearinghouses of ideas in the worlds of business, science, and the arts. Thus, by the 1700s, coffee had become firmly woven into the social fabric of cities, in foreign trade, and in the expanding overseas empires of the western European powers.[6]

The previous chapter showed how defenders of new exotic ingestibles justified their use as medicines, helping western European users fight against accusations that coffee and its fellow stimulants would alter their bodies racially, religiously, and sexually. Physicians, natural scientists, and pharmacists eagerly incorporated the new drugs into their repertoire, making them safe to use. Nevertheless, a new problem arose just as western European medicine were embracing coffee and the other new drugs: overuse. Addiction, and its early modern analogues such as gluttony, vice, custom, and enchantment, were one way of thinking about overuse. But there was something else that bothered observers—not so much the compulsive use of the drugs but the phenomenon of consumers freely choosing to abuse medicines. In 1706, when the Scots-French Huguenot refugee physician Daniel Duncan warned against the sterilizing effects of coffee on men, he meant that it would have these effects only when they consumed it daily. Coffee was healthy, he maintained, if used temperately and in the right circumstances, as a medicine to target specific physical problems.[7] But medicines were meant for the sick, and coffee could only benefit those who were ill due to humoral imbalances by adding its heat and dryness to the body. "I allow Coffee, Chocolate, and Tea are excellent Medicines every one of them," he wrote, "but does it therefore follow, that we ought to take them so often? Do we take Physick [medicine] every Day? People that are in love with those Liquors do not satisfie themselves to take it only once a Day." Duncan admitted that often enough they provided relief for real ailments, but, after they were cured, patients, now fond of the hot drinks, kept drinking them. "Must we therefore take them when we are neither troubled with that Disease, to which it formerly gave Relief, or with any other?" he asked. Overuse and abuse were not a problem for most medicines, he explained, because they tasted bad, but coffee and its sister hot drinks were pleasurable. He asserted: "We ruine our Life by seeking its Preservation; we destroy our Health by the same Means we pretend to preserve and strengthen it; we kill our selves, or at least create a Sickness by this pretended Panacea, which we call Coffee, Chocolate or Tea."[8] Duncan identified the problem in his title, *Wholesome advice against the abuse of hot liquors, particularly of coffee, chocolate, tea, brandy, and strong-waters.* Using the new hot drinks was fine; abusing them was not. What is more, when abused, they caused the very health problems that they promised to cure.

Francesco Merli, the royal physician for the army and hospitals of the Kingdom of Naples during the mid-eighteenth century, agreed with Duncan. He wondered how much the supposed benefits of drinking coffee actually came from the coffee itself and how much was imagined by those who liked drinking it. Coffee, he felt, should affect different people in different ways, and certainly some people with specific ailments might benefit from it, while others might suffer from tremors or apoplexy. But "the great use of coffee, which is thriving and expanding, seems to prove that for healthy people it has no other certain property than that of pleasure, and of making one a little more alert, and more cheerful, and more conversant by those who use it moderately. . . . I am therefore convinced that coffee has expanded so much because it is a drink that meets with public pleasure, because it offends very few, and it is useful to the lazy, who are many."[9]

Two early eighteenth-century Dutch commentators writing about coffee concurred. The anonymous author of *Clear and plain evidence of the great abuse of the foreign and exotic tea and coffee* asked rhetorically: Was it thirst that drove people to drink coffee? No, they drank it at set times, just as tobacco users had set times for smoking. This went against a golden rule of our forefathers not to eat or drink unless hungry or thirsty, he admonished, and doing otherwise throws the body out of balance. Indeed coffeehouses existed for no other reason than simply drinking coffee and tea, which would not make sense if they were only medicines, and, anyway, people gathered there not for their health but for idle chatter.[10] He warned coffee and tea drinkers to "open your eyes to the deceit of Satan," who was the enemy of their health just as he was of their souls, and to stop drinking anything unless thirsty.[11]

Similarly, the anonymous author of *The debauched and enchanted coffee- and tea-world* observed that the champions of coffee and tea called them healthy, but this is not really why they drank these drinks; it was as an excuse for women to gather together outside of the view and take control of their menfolk.[12] Unless they were related, respectable women struggled to come up with creditable reasons for leaving the house except for attending church. Medicine became a cover, a false justification for people indulging their inclination for drinking coffee for social and other nonmedical reasons. As David Courtwright has pointed out, this is a common trajectory for all recreational drug use, although Marcy Norton and others have shown that the "abuse" or recreational use of the new exotic drugs emerged simultaneously with, or even before, their justification as medicines.[13]

Every Extreme Virtue Is a Vice: Distilled Spirits, Tobacco, Chocolate, and Tea

The idea that distilled spirits could serve as medicine lingered on at least in part through the eighteenth century. In 1641, just as hard liquor was becoming more commercially available, the English clergyman Edward Kellett warned against gluttony in all of its guises, including overindulgence in distilled spirits, which he called by its traditional medical name: "*Aquavita*, or strong water, in the abuse is, *Aqua mortis*, the bayiffe of death, the executioner, leading men to destruction."[14] In 1682, in his household health handbook, Thomas Tryon acknowledged the changing view of distilled liquor when he announced that brandy and other distilled spirits were harmful to bodily health except when used sparingly, as medicine. They were invented as a medicine, he stated, "and not to be used as a Common drink, as of late years indiscreetly they are, to the destruction of many Thousands."[15] One early warning cry about gin, written by "A British Freeholder" in 1670, prefaced his concerns by admitting that "Used in Reason and with Moderation, it may be a comfortable Cordial to some Constitutions, a necessary Remedy in some Disorders," and for that reason he wished that what Parliament would legislate against "is the Abuse, not the Use of Spirits."[16] Even at the height of the Gin Craze, when distilled spirits were firmly associated with wanton use, and critics were demonizing gin, there were still some who recalled its health benefits.

For tobacco, the first complaint of abuse came no later than 1595, when smoking was just beginning in England. In a collection of the opinions of physicians weighing in on tobacco's medicinal properties, the poet Anthony Chute claimed that anyone who thought tobacco was bad for one's health must be using it too much: "Drincking it extreamly, he hath changed the good into a bad effect, since everie extreme virtue is a vice."[17] The Italian physician Giovanni Piccino wrote that if tobacco caused harm it was only through abuse, just like drinking wine.[18] In a 1658 commentary of the Epistle of St. Paul to Timothy, the English Presbyterian minister Thomas Hall lamented that "when Physicians shall prescribe one or two Pipes a day, and men shall take 20 . . . it's a kind of self-murder, and shortens mens dayes."[19] As with the other appetites, moderation in smoking was the aim. The Dutch physician Johann Ignatz Worb Beintema van Peima accused those who smoked in excess as ungodly, because everything God created is good, and God provided tobacco as a medicine; therefore, misusing it to while away the time idly was an affront to God and a sin.[20] One motivation for denouncing the abuse of tobacco was to safeguard its reputation as a medicine. With this in mind, the English physician and medical popularizer Tobias Venner subtitled his 1621 book *In which, the immoderate, irregular, and unseasonable use thereof is reprehended, and the true nature and best manner of using it, perspicuously demonstrated.*[21] As with coffee, the daily use of tobacco was worrisome to Venner, since it suggested that consumers did not really use it as medicine. More commonly, critics simply argued that if something was consumed every day it could not be a medicine. The Castilian physician Francisco de Leiva y Aguilar praised tobacco for its various health benefits, but the thrust of his 1634 book, *Disenchantment against the ill use of tobacco*, was to condemn what he described as the "confused disorder" in the way people took tobacco.[22] He complained that "it is applied without accounting for the humors because it is used at all hours, because it is continued over and over again, because it is prescribed to healthy people . . . [and] because they use it without making any distinction between regions, complexions, ages, properties, corpulence, bodily habits, or of strength."[23] Tomás Ramón, an Aragonese friar, agreed that while the "holy weed" was a powerful medicine, smoking and snuff-taking were far too frequent. "In these two ways it is used so much in Spain," he wrote, "and with such frequency, that there is almost no moment in which it is not being applied to the nostrils, the mouth, at all hours and times, while fasting and while eating, studying, and preaching." Ramón was particularly repulsed by priests who, while singing in the choir, continued to apply snuff, making faces and digging into their noses with their fingers.[24] The healthy should not take tobacco or it would make them ill, Ramón thought, and he could not understand those who would take such a disgusting thing for pleasure.[25]

Physicians and other observers were more receptive to the idea that a healthy daily regime might include drinking chocolate. In 1624 Santiago de Valverde Turices, a physician in Seville, acknowledged his colleagues who warned that the healthy should not take medicine, but he made an exception for chocolate, which, when prepared correctly, could help sustain the different humors in the body.[26] For the English at home in their more temperate realm, however, chocolate should be used only "in distress and sickness" and not "as constant food."[27] Merli described chocolate as "innocent" for those who did not abuse it, especially if they added sugar, whose salt corrected the fat of the chocolate. Nevertheless, he recognized that most people drank chocolate not for medicinal reasons but for pleasure.[28] Despite his recommendation of a daily draught, Valverde Turices realized that many users drank chocolate all the time.[29] Antonio de León Pinelo observed in 1636 that at the Spanish court "there is no order, because people are drinking it at all hours from morning to night as many times as they can, and only its cost, not their inclination, prevents it from being much more."[30] One year later, in describing chocolate's use in Spain, Fernando Cardoso wrote that it had "passed from immoderation to vice" as it spread from those who drank it for stomach weakness to ladies who could not make it through the afternoon without the drink, who had come to despise all other refreshments, and who drank it three or four times per day, starting when they woke up.[31] Chocolate had slipped so far into recreational use by the late eighteenth century that Spanish naval physician Vicente Lardizabal opened his 1788 work on its usefulness by apologizing for writing about such a commonly used commodity, and he felt compelled to remind the reader that, like wine and tobacco, it was also a medicant.[32] Similarly, Pierre-Hippoyte Boutigny, a French chocolate maker who wrote a pamphlet in 1825 to advertise his wares in part by touting its healthiness, asked how chocolate could be unhealthy if the Spanish drank it two or three times a day with no ill effect.[33] The Spanish, it seems, were renowned throughout Europe for the amount of chocolate they drank daily, both for pleasure and for health.

The Spaniards León Pinelo, Cardoso, and Lardizabal identified the main problems with the abuse of new stimulants like chocolate. Truly effective medical remedies were only for the sick and not to be taken every day. It was pleasure and fashion that made chocolate and its fellow exotic comestibles so popular, and while users might have felt that their health is improved, they really felt better because they were enjoying themselves. But the insistence of Valverde Turices, Hughes, and Merli that chocolate could be a healthy daily drink suggest another way of reading these criticisms. Users were finding a novel use for coffee: not as an approved remedy to address medical problems, but as a way to maintain one's good health, including their mental well-being, with or without a physician's advice. Recreational drinking that made the drinker feel good could go hand in hand with the health benefits of a daily intake of chocolate.

Other new stimulants found favor as part of a daily health regimen as well. The Dutch physician Cornelis Bontekoe offered a full-throated defense of daily tea drinking, batting away objections to the overuse of tea and recommending it up to "fifty or a hundred or two hundred cups at a time."[34] Tea was even good for the healthy, because while "our tea is a remedy, likewise as it is a preservative."[35] Bontekoe defended tea against those who called it harmful, pointing out that of all the common drinks, only tea was blamed for poor health, while in truth it was beer, wine, distilled spirits, and tobacco that were truly unhealthy. He wrote: "Every one chooses a beverage which imagination and custom render palatable to him; this he wants and no other, even though the drink he has chosen should be noxious to his health and shorten his life."[36] But only tea "always does one good and never hurts." In 1721 the English physician and natural philosopher James Handley advocated for frequent, perhaps even daily, use of tea, specifying bohea tea for the lungs and green tea for the kidneys, joints, and eyes. Both kinds were especially good when taken in the morning, green tea in particular.[37] Like Bontekoe he recommended it not so much to restore health but to preserve one's already good health.

It was more common, however, to advise against daily use. The Dutch author who signed his work "R. V. N." touted tea's ability to cure headaches and counteract drunkenness, but he did not favor its daily use, instead recommending moderation in eating and drinking all things, like our ancestors, who did not suffer gout as the Dutch did at the turn of the eighteenth century.[38] Contrary to belief, tea, on the whole, was bad for people's health, especially women. When people claimed to drink tea for their health, this was either a mistake or a pretense. "Lysje," "Kaatje," and "Tryntje," R. V. N. sneered, using common names for Dutch women, only passed around their warm water for fashion, sociability, and for the brandy that came afterward. Antonio

Lavedán, a military surgeon from Valladolid, blamed tea's popularity on Bontekoe and also wanted to defend its proper medicinal use against daily abuse.[39] "The long and constant use of tea as part of our regime, as it is done (in China, England, Holland, etc.), makes us forget to question whether it has any medical properties," he wrote.[40] It did, he concluded, but only for certain types of people who had specific conditions to be alleviated. Overuse was a problem: "It has been observed in populous cities like Hamburg, Amsterdam, London, and," he noticed, "that almost all the women of distinction who use tea immoderately are attacked by white fluxes."[41] Even if tea was a good medicine, it should not be used daily.[42] Moderation, as always, was the key to health. An anonymous poem, *In praise of tea*, by "J. B.," asked, "If some have vapours, by drinking to excess, / 'Tis their own faults; why don't they drink the less?"[43]

To a lesser extent, the consumption of sugar and opium displayed the same patterns. Tobias Venner advised the readers of his dietetic handbook to use sugar not to sweeten foods, but to counteract the ill effects of other medicants, with the idea that its humoral properties could provide balance to a medicinal draught. As he did for tobacco, Venner was concerned to safeguard sugar as a medicine instead of a source of idle pleasure.[44] Western European writers had a long tradition of criticizing the peoples of the Middle East for taking opium recreationally, and there was some concern about users at home doing the same. The Scots physician Alexander Philip Wilson noted that people in "eastern countries" consumed enormous amounts of opium, "and even in our own, we are every day meeting with people, who have habituated themselves to a very free use of it."[45] Certainly, by the early nineteenth century, a few celebrated individuals like William Taylor Coleridge and Thomas De Quincey were taking opium and laudanum merely for pleasure. In one sense, coffee and the rest of the new stimulants simply fell under the old medical adage that the dose makes the poison, but they also fit into a category of their own, as observers noted the great and quick increase in their use. The anonymous author of a 1736 tract defending gin tried to deflect moralizing concern away from it by asking, "Is there any thing more pernicious, than the immoderate use of Coffee and Tea, which has increased to a surprising height within a few years" and among all ranks of society? "I could mention Several other things of the like nature equally held to be pernicious," he continued, "as the immoderate use of Tobacco . . . which we use to great excess by all the different ways that can be invented." He added spice in wines, hops in beer, and "those Drugs so called and usually vended as such," whose quality is so poor that they become a poison.[46]

Thus, some physicians were allowing for the daily use of some of the soft drugs while others warned against it as an abuse of medicine. Meanwhile, it is clear that consumers were deciding for themselves how frequently to take these drugs, whether daily or not, with or without physicians' permission. The recreational use of these drugs—consuming them for pleasure—shaded into a new understanding of how they might be used to cultivate and preserve the health one already enjoyed. The daily use of soft drugs thus reinforces the arguments of historians who have recently tried to pull the history of medicine away from physicians and pharmaceutical interventions and toward the household. Indeed, most medical care took place at home—not just the practice of healing, but vernacular forms of empirical experimentation with what remedies work best, spread through networks of people sharing ideas, recipes, and books.[47] At home, Europeans privileged enough to have choices ordered their lives to emphasize fresh air, personal hygiene, and food intake as part of a daily regimen of hygiene aimed at preserving health. Recently Phil Withington has found that coffee was mostly consumed at home, not the coffeehouse, so coffee drinking folds nicely into this growing practice of home-based health maintenance.[48] The eighteenth century especially saw hygiene and dietetics attract more attention from western European elites, and coffee as a promoter of health fit right in.[49] By incorporating the new stimulants into home-based, consumer-driven daily use, western Europeans shed the discipline that physicians, natural scientists, and pharmacists tried to impose on the use of drugs, and on the oversight of their clients' health and bodies.

Coffee became an everyday item of consumption for people during the eighteenth century just as the revival of Hippocratic medicine encouraged close attention to regimen, including nutrition, sleep, and exercise.[50] Physicians and their affluent patients gave close scrutiny to their diet, and they eagerly incorporated coffee, as well as tea and the other early modern stimulants, as a subject of their dietetic concerns.[51] Geoffrey McCalman noted that there were climatic and physical reasons for Europeans, even more so than residents of the torrid zones along the equator, to develop such a "luxurious taste" for exotic drugs. "In northern sites," he argued, "a coarse and heavy animal-machine, naturally in a vapid, and approaching a torpid state, finds pleasure in whatever is apt to rouse and agitate its spirits; namely, in travelling, dancing, fencing, hunting, war, the use of spirituous liquors, tobacco, tea, coffee, foreign spiceries, and pungent homegrown substances."[52] Put another way, western Europeans incorporated the new stimulants into their daily routines as a way to regulate their moods.

Coffee and its fellow stimulants began to occupy an indeterminant position between drugs and food. Nicolas Blégny, the surgeon to Louis XIV and founder of perhaps the first European medical journal in the vernacular, published his *The correct use of tea, coffee, and chocolate for preservation and the healing of maladies* in 1687.[53] In it he referred to coffee and chocolate as both a medicine (*remede*) and a food (*aliment*), and to chocolate as a "medicinal food."[54] Two Italian participants in the debate about whether chocolate broke ecclesiastical fasts Giovanni Batista Gudenfridi and Giacomo Sanvitale, writing decades apart, entertained the idea that chocolate was neither a food nor a drink but a medicant. Gudenfridi called it "a medical nourishment, and a nourishing medicine."[55] The new soft drugs straddled the divide between foods and pharmaceuticals, and the English physician Hugh Smythson devoted a section of his 1781 home medical guide, *The compleat family physician*, to "certain Articles in common Use, which can neither be considered as Food or Medicine," where he addressed tea, coffee, tobacco, and opium. Smythson puzzled over their popularity, taking tea, chewing tobacco, and snuff as examples: tea and tobacco tasted bad, and tobacco and snuff smelled bad, and "nor shall it be contended that the general and constant use of either of those exotics, is attended with the smallest advantage." Any medicinal benefits that tea might have had "are destroyed by the constant and immoderate use of it."[56] Yet "among the higher classes, who from late suppers, late hours, and other nocturnal debauches, are without any morning appetite, the tea constitutes the breakfast, unaccompanied with bread, or any other eatable."[57] Opium earned its place in this section of his book because, despite its excellent qualities as a medicine, "an abuse of it has of late years crept into this country." Europeans living abroad in Muslim countries had imitated their hosts by adopting the daily use of opium to support their spirits and then brought that custom back home with them, requiring "large doses and frequent repetitions" to maintain the same effects.[58]

Like academic physicians, the authors of home health manuals and recipe books such as Smythson, Blégny, Charles Estienen and Jean Liebault, and George Cheyne offered advice on the place of food-medicines in one's diet. Their suggestions repeated the same advice for eating and drinking as moralists had since classical times: moderation in all things.[59] Yet their understanding of moderation might include daily use for the prevention of disease and maintenance of health. In his medical handbook of 1684, the English physician Thomas Willis recommended drinking coffee every day to purge the brain and sharpen one's mental acuity, unless one had a choleric or melancholic disposition.[60] Likewise, a century later the coffee proselytizer Benjamin Moseley observed that "the Turks, Arabians, Persians, and Egyptians drink Coffee all day long. . . . In the Dutch, French, and English colonies, it is the daily breakfast, and evening repast." Moseley approved of this daily usage, advising "the general use of Coffee in England, as an article of diet, and . . . as a safe and powerful medicine."[61] In a separate medical tract published in 1800, Moseley noted how, since the growth of sugar consumption in Europe over the past two hundred years, "there is now scarcely any person who does not mix, more or less of it, in his daily food," and that this has benefited the health of users.[62] Where others decried sugar and the drugs as enervating luxuries, they found favor with Moseley. "Since European countries have had intercourse with the East and West Indies, and a free and enlarged traffic with each other . . . Europe has greatly improved in its regimen. The popular diet before," he observed, "was crude, coarse, and unwholesome."[63] Bontekoe, of course, recommended large amounts of tea as part of one's daily diet, and chocolate, too, had its promoters. The early English commentator on chocolate Henry Stubbe himself drank chocolate several times a day for years while in Jamaica and then back in London during the mid-seventeenth century, and as long as one mixed the correct spices with the chocolate to match one's humoral disposition and did not indulge "without measure," it was a healthy daily regimen both as nourishment and medicine.[64] Writing in the mid-eighteenth century, Manuel Navas de Carrera agreed, calling it an "alimentary medicine."[65] He recommended its daily use for all and acknowledged that "chocolate is already a daily bread."[66] Tobacco, too, could be part of a daily health regimen, as evidenced by the dismay of the Lombard Pier Luigi Origoni, who argued against the belief that tobacco "is an opportune remedy for preserving human bodies from infirmity."[67] As iatrochemical and mechanical medical theories gained traction in the eighteenth century, some physicians were less concerned with diagnosing each individual patient's humoral complexion before prescribing a medicine, and these theories also encouraged their willingness to disregard the old insistence that drugs should be taken only in certain seasons and at certain times of day.[68]

As an article of daily consumption, offered not by apothecaries but by coffeehouse proprietors and grocers, coffee shifted the decision-making over therapeutic choices from physicians to consumers. Most physicians continued to favor the model by which they would assess each patient's individual complexion, or the makeup of humors (or salts and alkalines or nerves) before deciding on the right course of action. As E. C. Spary has argued, coffee enabled merchants and other nonprofessionals who promoted and advertised their products to claim authority over the health of the body.[69] Patients could choose between physicians who acted from different theoretical bases and applied different therapeutics, whether mechanical, iatrochemical, or traditionally Galenic.[70] Further, they always had access to other providers of health care, ranging from charlatans (here not meaning "frauds," but simply those who hawked medicines via advertisements and theatrical public performances), patent medicines, and a variety of "empirics," or medicants that were aimed at curing maladies without the help of a physician.[71] Coffee and its sister stimulants gave consumers one more choice in this marketplace, unsupervised by physicians and apothecaries and ambivalently positioned in medical theories, approved by some physicians but disapproved by many. Governments declined to regulate the use of coffee, instead focusing their attention on coffeehouses—still under suspicion as sites of disorder into the nineteenth century—and even encouraging the consumption of coffee to help the economic growth of their coffee-growing colonies.[72] Kevin Siena has contended that "health was just linked to righteousness," with rational individuals responsible for their own health and the unhealthy consequences of bad behavior. Temperance, self-discipline, and health went hand in hand.[73]

As Smith and Thomas Trotter have pointed out, there was a global reach to the suffering of western European consumers of drugs and alcohol. Stimulants like coffee lay at the intersection between increasing global trade, the increasing medical choices available to the elites and middling classes, and the consumer revolution—or, more precisely, between the medical marketplace and what historians call the industrious revolution," which saw more and more western Europeans allocating the time and resources of the family to enable the purchase a new type of luxury goods, often from abroad. A shift was taking place in thinking about luxuries, which were increasingly marketed not for the aristocracy but the middling classes, and designed not for durability but for rapid consumption—goods like cotton garments and chinaware as well as stimulants like sugar, chocolate, tea, and coffee.[74] For some, these new products shed luxury's traditional association with corrupting decadence and instead conjured ideas of politeness and moderation. Beginning with the Dutch-English physician Bernard Mandeville, eighteenth-century economists defended luxury purchases against the ancient claim that they drained the importing country's wealth and began to argue instead that they would quicken commerce and enrich both buyers and sellers.[75] Christine Fertig and Ulrich Pfister have noted that consumers in the German port of Hamburg were increasingly purchasing, among the proliferation of luxury products, exotic medicines like cinchona bark, jalapa, and asafetida, and they point to a heightened concern for individual care of the body driving the consumer revolution.[76] The global trade and exploration decried by Trotter brought coffee and other exotic soft drugs into an already existing medical marketplace. European botanists and apothecaries carried out a worldwide search for new stimulants to bring to the market, introducing chinchona bark, ipecac, sarsaparilla, and the like into the European pharmacopeia.[77]

The new soft drugs fit into the growing array of therapeutic goods and practices in the eighteenth century that combined the two seemingly disparate categories of health care and luxury. In 1698 the physician and natural scientist Martin Lister made a list of several bodily practices that were meant to help maintain health but were actually damaging and only taken up because they were pleasing and fashionable. This included coffee as well as "Tobacco, Strong Waters, Steel Remedies, the Drinking [of] Mineral Waters, Bathing, Tea, Coffee, Chocolate, &c."[78] But however much physicians might disapprove, laypeople kept returning to coffee and the other soft drugs—for pleasure, for health maintenance, or both—which took their place among fashionable cures alongside visiting spas, drinking mineral water, consulting celebrity physicians like the London- and Bath-based English doctor George Cheyne, taking the sea air, and an enthusiasm for breastfeeding, exercising, dieting, and medical electricity. J. B. Sassenus, an Antwerp physician, recommended tea as an invigorating drink and explicitly pointed out that it was more healthy than cold baths. In 1725 Antonio Valisneri, a professor of medicine in Padua, wrote an entire treatise comparing hot and cold drinks to hot and cold baths.[79] To Sassenus, Valisneri, and their readers, these choices simply represented equally viable options for maintaining health out of an array of possible fashionable therapies.[80] These practices helped create a sophisticated, metropolitan, Enlightenment culture of personal care and hygiene, aimed at more general feelings of well-being, mostly working through the body to target mood.[81] This array of health-care goods put medical consumers in control of their physical and mental well-being. Regular, even daily, use of coffee and other drugs was sometimes encouraged by physicians, but more often Europeans simply decided on their own to make them a part of their routine. They were fashionable goods and services available in the market economy supplied in part by overseas trade and empire and designed above all to fight mental discomfort and make the consumer feel good. Western Europeans could purchase physical and mental well-being on a scale ranging from traveling to Mediterranean climes to take the air, for the truly elite, to a regular cup of coffee, for almost anyone.

Coffee: Extreme Nervous Sensibility

As the annual amount of coffee consumed in western Europe continued to rise, and even as some of the anxieties about incorporating it into one's body lingered, the initial sharp wariness of its Turkish, Arabic, and Muslim origins dissolved into a mostly comfortable familiarity with the brew, especially in large cities such as London and Paris. It was in this context, where coffee had become normalized as a routine part of western European daily practice, that Éloy wrote his 1781 treatise on coffee and the nerves. Éloy was worried that so many people, including women, beyond the elite—even in the countryside—were drinking coffee, and "the tyrannical habit has even imposed on them a law of taking it daily."[82] Like previous commentators, he acknowledged the arguments for coffee's effectiveness as a medicine, including the power of its "volatile salt" to open the obstructions of the brain, to "restore the elasticity of its membranes and weakened vessels," and to chase away melancholy.[83] But, Éloy inquired, could such a medicine be taken daily? Were all coffee drinkers ill in a way that coffee might help? Éloy allowed that coffee could revive the bodies and minds of people who overindulged in food and drink, but he warned that for them coffee was "a seductive trap, which deceives them by preserving them in their daily intemperance," soothing the symptoms and thus encouraging further overeating and drinking.[84] Like previous writers, Éloy raised the issue of disordered sexuality and fertility: it was not true that coffee caused sterility, he allowed, but it did lead to depopulation, because it weakened mothers and their children. Young women became enervated by coffee drinking, suffering from vapors and irregular menstruation and then losing their appetites, disgusted by food. They would turn to marriage to revitalize their health, but coffee so ruined their constitutions that childbirth became more difficult, and their babies were either stillborn or born so weak that they could not survive. Those babies who lived found that their troubles were not over, since coffee-drinking women could not nurse their newborns and therefore sent them out to wet-nurses. Even that option would disappear in time, Éloy warned, if the habit of daily coffee drinking continued to extend into the countryside, for then there would be no one left to nurse the babies.[85]

Éloy worried about similar things as writers before him when he aired his anxieties about women, gender, and sex and his concern that coffee as a medicine would be used daily, and by people who were not ill. But much of his treatise took a different tone, reflecting developments in medicine in the late eighteenth century, as the nerves came to dominate the understanding of sickness and the body.[86] Concern for the nerves did not displace older paradigms of medicine such as the humoral model that held sway over medieval medicine, or the iatrochemistry that gained traction in the seventeenth century. Instead it was layered on top of previously existing models, as were other new paradigms such as the neo-Hippocratic revival that appeared in the early eighteenth century, with physicians tending to combine various elements of each doctrine in their own medical theories and therapeutic practice.[87] Éloy mixed the language of nerves with that of vapors, as when he complained that "the abuse of [coffee] has altered the vigor of the common people so much that nervous maladies are now as well known among them as to those reared in indolence and opulence."[88] Women, especially, suffered under the regime of coffee, with damaged reproductive organs, vapors, and general enfeeblement, and the most surprising thing of all was to see peasant and artisan women stricken by vapors, just like their social betters.[89] Daily coffee drinking, he stressed, caused "extreme nervous sensibility."[90] Coffee caused men, too, to suffer from nervous attacks: "Most of them would be wanting only to be put into bed, their head in a bonnet, to fool spectators into thinking they were women, so much do they resemble them with their simpering grimaces."[91] Worst of all, coffee started a vicious cycle, as people afflicted by "vertigo, dizziness, hand trembling, panic terrors, and bouts of melancholy" turned to coffee to alleviate their symptoms, scarcely realizing that "it is to the abuse of coffee that they should attribute all these evils."[92] Thus coffee was both the cause and the purported cure of the nervous maladies of the day.

The rise of nervous diseases was especially captivating to some physicians—and moralists—because it was deeply intertwined with the problems of civilization in the growing affluence and urbanity of the eighteenth century as well as with the new cult of sensibility. Faced with a seeming epidemic of nervous ailments among the elite in places like London and Paris, commenters affixed blame to the growth of luxury, artificial social manners, and decadent overconsumption, including excessive intake of both food and alcohol and fashion and leisure activities such as gambling, theatergoing, and novel-reading. The way forward was to return to a more natural lifestyle, like that of one's forebears or the Rousseauian "natural man" of Enlightenment thought. The new cult of sensibility was, among other things, a program of moral reform that rested on a Lockean ability to change one's own behavior by changing one's environment. It depended on the reformation of manners toward a more natural disposition and style of emotional communication, and a reorientation of consumption away from the vicious baubles of luxury toward a virtuous austerity. Sensibility had medical aspects, too, promoted by celebrity physicians like George Cheyne in England and Pierre Pomme in France, that aimed to soothe the nerves by restoring simpler habits of eating, exercise, and daily habits in general.[93] For example, the Edinburgh physician Andrew Wilson took issue with Rousseau's position that it was the manners of the ancients that made them more robust; Wilson believed that the mind follows the body, and that Rousseau was wasting his time trying to imagine educational systems that would mold his fictional Emile or Heloise into models of clear-minded vigor. Instead it was the luxurious exotic foodstuffs from Asia and America that had led to the flood of "Hysteric and Nervous Diseases" in western Europe, and the most important thing that parents could do would be to stop giving sugar to their infants.[94] It is easy to see how sensibility's moral and bodily reforms would target drugs like coffee and its fellow soft drugs tea, distilled spirits, and opium.

People who successfully navigated the demands of sensibility, especially women (a particular focus of the new manners), were able to fashion themselves as morally refined, elite members of society, distinct from the ordinary. There is no wonder that patients might interpret nervous disorders, connected as they were to the perils of highly cultivated civilization and its reform, as a badge of superiority, and, indeed, the positive reaction of laypeople to the theories put forward by physicians helped nervous disorders come into focus in eighteenth-century medical thinking.[95] And if the disorders that patients complained about, and that physicians treated and described in writing, lay on a spectrum between purely physical disease and mental illness, the emergent attention to the nerves and sensibility marked a shift on the spectrum away from the physical toward mental health.[96] Increasingly, consumers used the new exotic drugs not just to rectify or preserve their bodily health, but, by their workings on the nerves, to regulate one's emotions or mood as well.

Éloy was not the first to worry about coffee's effects on the nerves and mood, and its association with the perils of city life. As early as 1663, when coffee was first becoming popular in England, *The maidens complaint against coffee* associated it with fast-paced, cosmopolitan life in London. In it the character Snapshort found his brains addled by all the foreign languages he heard at the Royal Exchange, drank some coffee to try to ameliorate it and found that it made his disorientation worse. Only good English ale could resettle his brain.[97] In 1705 the English physician Thomas Curteis remarked that too much coffee weakened the nervous system.[98] Half a century later the Paduan physician Giovanni dalla Bona complained about the illnesses with "unusual and extravagant symptoms" like "hysterical convulsions" that especially affected women. Their sudden emergence, he believed, was due to the abuse of coffee, with a fashionable drink leading to fashionable illnesses.[99] Antonio Lavedán recognized coffee's virtue when drunk occasionally as a medicine, especially for the nerves and the "animal spirits," but warned of the evils of its daily use.[100] Writing in 1796, he acknowledged that in Spain it was really only common in the largest cities, like Madrid, Cádiz, and Barcelona.[101] But for those urban dwellers who drank coffee every day, Lavedán emphasized its damage on the nerves. He listed a number of classes of people, including scholars who took coffee to stay awake, who would suffer "trembling, enfeeblement, and premature aging."[102] Guillaume Massieu cautioned that if poorly prepared, coffee was "especially dangerous for the melancholy and the hypochondriacs."[103] Hypochondria had not yet taken on its contemporary meaning as a psychological condition where one fears nonexistent diseases; it was originally thought of as a disease of the spleen that caused emotional turmoil, among other things, but by 1798, when Massieu was writing, hypochondria had become categorized as a nervous disorder.[104] On the other hand, some observers believed that coffee helped the nerves. For example, in a treatise published in 1752, the Spanish professor of mathematics Arias Gómez touted coffee's ability to stimulate the nerves.[105] In 1785 Benjamin Moseley, a coffee booster connected to British Caribbean plantations, pushed for coffee to become a part of daily regime that preserved healthy nerves against "those inconveniencies, habits, and diseases . . . so injurious to health and beauty, filling the large towns and cities with chronical infirmities."[106] It was tea that consumers should beware of, Moseley believed, since that other hot drink truly did ruin the nerves. In 1792 Alexandro de Moya published a dialogue set in a coffeehouse that featured one friend defending coffee to another against the charge that it "attacks the nerves."[107] These men seem to have been articulating the motivations of daily coffee drinkers, in the belief that coffee helped manage the effects of civilization and luxury. Even Éloy thought that daily coffee could blunt the effects of excessive eating and drinking.

In the early nineteenth century, the Napoleonic military physician M. de Reynal provided a good example of the ambiguous role of coffee in the refined lifestyles of the late eighteenth-century elite. On the one hand, it eased digestion, helped the blood circulate, fended off drowsiness, brought gaiety to the mind, and "restore[d] some of their elasticity to loose, stretched out nerves."[108] In general, he wrote, it "produces artificially that which nature does much better and more constantly by itself in those who enjoy perfect health."[109] On the other hand, "nothing is more characteristic to it than that it opens the door to nervous diseases."[110] Ever since the introduction of coffee to western Europe, Reynal declared, it was clear that each generation had declined in health and vigor, and their nerves continued to deteriorate. Those who avoided coffee "are scarcely exposed to this crowd of symptoms that the nervous maladies bring along with it," while "the passionate lovers of this liquor are sensitive, infirm, subject to trembling, to nervous maladies, to the embarrassment of the abdomen, so if coffee does not destroy in us the principles of life, it consumes little by little their vigor; and by attacking animal spirits, the very substances of the nerves, it renders them useless to society."[111] Worst of all,

> let us add that the soothing qualities of this drink gives us the illusion in many circumstances and conceals from us the precipice, they are deceptive appearances that plunge us further into the sensation of our miseries; it is thought to dissipate dullness of the head, but it throws us into trembling and the vapors; it alleviates our feelings for a while, but little by little it destroys the source [of health]; we imagine we have found the secret to healing our

maladies, but it perpetuates their cause to the point of rendering them incurable.[112]

If coffee formerly had an ambivalent place for consumers who were both attracted to and repelled by its exotic origins, now that ambivalence was about its role in the maturing consumer culture and the emerging focus on dietetics in the eighteenth century. Did coffee contribute to or alleviate the physical effects on the body of overconsumption and overrefinement?

Tea and Chocolate: This Deceptive Comfort

This palette of concerns, about nervous disorders and a medicine that both soothed and caused the problems it was meant to palliate, was not unique to coffee. Daniel Duncan assailed tea and chocolate along with it, and in 1728 the Florentine physician Giovanni Batista Felici warned that although many claimed that chocolate invigorated those who drank it, "this deceptive comfort" caused its users to plunge back into "extraordinary languor" five or six hours later.[113] Decades before his attack on coffee, Éloy published a similar work, on tea, *Reflections on the usage of tea in which, after having presented the history of this foreign drink, gives essential warnings for taking it profitably*. He cautioned that although tea was a useful medicine, people of all conditions were drinking it, more frequently and at all times, which is of course not at all how one should use a medicine.[114] If people insisted on drinking tea every day, the quality of the tea and the time of day was important; if the tea was too astringent, the tone and strength of the nerves would suffer, finally becoming irritated to the point of loosening.[115] Éloy was mostly concerned with women in the towns and cities of Flanders and Holland, whose devotion to tea could be read on their faces by the pallor of their skin, and who were no longer able to nurse their babies the way they should. "Having shown that the abuse of tea renders women pallid, exhausted, and listless, what should be expected of such a mother, than a child feeble and unenergetic?" he asked. [116] As he would observe later about coffee, however useful tea could be as a medicine, it was overused, damaging to the nerves, and dangerous for mothers and their babies.

Another warning on tea and the nerves came from the Methodist leader John Wesley, whose "Letter to a friend, concerning tea," first printed in 1749, derived from personal experience. He had noticed he was suffering "some Symptoms of a Paralytick Disorder," including a trembling hand, that disappeared when he temporarily stopped drinking tea.[117] Finding that many of the tea drinkers around him had "their Nerves quite unstrung," he started advising against the drink while permanently giving it up himself.[118] Wesley recorded the objections from those he advised—for example, "But I cannot leave it off; for it helps my Health. Nothing else will agree with me." To this he argued that the people of England were able to keep themselves in good health before tea's arrival a hundred years earlier, and in truth tea was a trap. "When I first left off Tea," Wesley explained," I was half asleep all Day long; My Head aked from Morning to Night: I could not remember a Question asked, even till I could return an Answer. But in a Week's Time all these inconveniences were gone."[119] Like Éloy, Wesley argued that while his contemporaries believed that tea was essential to maintain their daily health, it was causing the very symptoms it was meant to relieve.

The celebrated Quaker moral reformer and physician John Coakley Lettsom found that most healthy people were unaffected by tea, but others of a weaker constitution "find themselves rather fluttered" for a while after tea at breakfast, or affected by "involuntary trembling" after tea in the afternoon.[120] These symptoms affected the higher classes more than the lower, since tea's effects were stronger the higher the grade of tea and the more expensive it was.[121] The higher grades, however, "affect the nerves" and cause drinkers to be "agitated by the most trifling cause, shutting a door too hastily, the sudden entrance even of a servant, and other the like causes." Some even "are constantly seized with great uneasiness, anxiety, and oppression" as soon as they take just one cup of tea, and Lettsom recalled one "young man of a delicate constitution" who suffered from "depression of spirits" and "melancholy" such that suicide was feared. The subject drank great quantities of tea, and as soon as he stopped, the mental symptoms also ceased. A few weeks later he resumed drinking tea and returned to "his former dejection and melancholy, with loss of memory, tremblings, a proneness to great agitation from the most trifling circumstances, and a numerous train of nervous ailments," after which he immediately stopped drinking tea again.[122] We might look at the cults of sensibility and nervous disorders in the eighteenth century as a kind of fashionable trend, but this anecdote conveys an element of real human suffering.

It was not just Éloy who believed that nervous disorders hit women who drank tea especially hard. J. N. Surgeon's 1745 publication on tea singled out "tender and delicate females" who found themselves suffering one to three hours after drinking tea from "anxiety, and a sense of weight on the praecordia." These were symptoms of "an oppression upon the nerves," as well as trembling, spasms, hysterics, and melancholy. Worse, some women then reached for a dram for relief.[123] An anonymous English moralist found that as tea made its way down the social ladder in the late eighteenth century to "the poor country cottager" so, too, did hysterics, a malady once unknown but now found by physicians everywhere in society. This observer linked the malicious gossip spread by women drinking tea to the way that it "unstrings the nerves" and caused ill temper, especially when joined with sugar. The effects of tea on the nerves could be read on the face: "Where now are the pleasing smiles, the dimpled damask cheek, which were accustomed to dance on and adorn the jocund face of the artless, cheerful, innocent Country Girl? Instead of these, succeed the haggard, yellow, meager visage."[124] In Spain, too, it was the same, as Lavedán remarked that if people with the wrong temperaments drank tea they would experience "the agitations or irritations experienced by hysterical women."[125]

The English physician and botanist William Woodville made a direct connection between tea drinking, the growth of luxury in England, and the rise in nervous disorders. "Since our wealth has increased and our navigation been extended, we have ransacked every part of the globe . . . to indulge in luxury and provoke excess."[126] The habits of the wealthy made things worse, as they surfeited themselves on food and drink and then abandoned exercise, gambling or listening to music instead, moving through the city with coaches and chairmen instead of walking. "It is any wonder that the diseases which proceed from idleness and luxury, should increase in proportion, and keep pace with those improvements of the matter and cause of diseases?" Woodville inquired. Indeed wherever and whenever history provided examples of wealth and excess, the attendant medical disorders could also be found. Greek, Roman, and medieval Arab physicians saw the same problems, although not as frequently as in Woodville's time, and they did not use the term "hysteria." The ancient peoples of the Mediterranean were protected somewhat by their stronger constitutions, but for Britons in the eighteenth century, "there is no disorder incident to the inhabitants of this island and climate more common, of late especially, than paralytic afflictions, nor of a more difficult cure when they happen to people of original or acquired weak nerves. . . . The causes I must totally attribute to the increased luxury of the age, and particularly to the use of tea."[127]

Gin, Opium, and Tobacco

The nerves became a theme that those writing against hard liquor emphasized during the English Gin Craze, as the English physician Hugh Smith wrote in his 1789 *Essay on the nerves*, warning that, after tea, distilled spirits like gin were the second leading cause of nervous disorders.[128] Among the letters to his patients that he published as a health guide in 1714, the physician Richard Carr warned one of his correspondents that her son's habit of drinking distilled spirits every morning concerned him. Morning draughts might lead to any of a number of maladies, but especially to "threaten the Nerves themselves; for Spasms, Tremors, Palsies, Convulsion and Epilepsies, frequently ceize up on those who are guilty of this Folly."[129] Like tea, gin was thought to be especially bad for women and their nervous systems, as John Coakley Lettsom explained in his *History of some of the effects of hard drinking*.[130] Charles Lamb added another connection between distilled spirits and the nerves: "it is to the weak, the nervous; to those who feel the want of some artificial aid to raise their spirits in society" that he writes, those who feel compelled to drink brandy and are more susceptible than those with "stout nerves" to suffer from its excesses and to be unable to stop.[131]

The Scots physician and surgeon George Young noticed something similar about opium in 1753, in part from his own surprisingly free experimentation with the drug. For patients who suffered from "lowness of spirits," he found that opium would first give "a flow of spirits . . . but they find them proportionally depressed, after its influence is over."[132] Under the influence of opium, one patient swung between exhilaration to despair when it wore off, when "he would behave more like a true penitent: he fancied he was dying, and wanted the assistance of a clergyman" until he received another dose of opium.[133] Young hesitated to prescribe opium for nervous disorders simply because they were so poorly understood. Mostly he believed that women who displayed symptoms like "hysteric pain" or "hysteric vomiting" were really suffering from strong negative emotions, and the best opium could do was to relieve the pain until the underlying emotional cause of distress had passed.[134] The Irish physician and reformer Samuel Crumpe concluded his own 1792 study of opium with a summary of the debate by modern physicians as to whether opium was a stimulant or narcotic, and whether it worked by affecting the nerves or the blood. Crumpe took an unusual position by concluding that opium was a stimulant, but he fit well within the mainstream by characterizing the idea that opium worked through the blood as an antiquated, slightly ridiculous theory.[135]

Tobacco, too, was a foreign stimulant that had become deeply entrenched in western European habits by the eighteenth century, only to be caught up in new worries about its effects on the nerves. In 1726, when Francis Daniel Mutain published a book about the use and abuse of coffee, tea, chocolate, and tobacco, he claimed that the latter was harmful to "the elderly, children, and those with weak nerves."[136] By the 1790s the English surgeon Edward Teare could write an entire treatise that focused on tobacco's dangerous effects on the nerves.[137] Snuff in particular was thought to be bad for the nervous system, as John Hill argued in his 1761 *Cautions against the immoderate use of snuff.* Not only did snuff immediately affect and destroy the nerves of the nose, ultimately eliminating the sense of smell, but by mixing with the saliva it also "corrodes and destroy the nerves" throughout the entire body.[138] In 1700 the anonymous French author of *The good use of tobacco in powder* explained that all pungent ingestibles damaged the nerves when used in excess. Furthermore, because the nerves of the nose were connected so strongly to the rest of the body, snuff could cause vapors, and users were attacked by "hysterical and melancholy passions," among other nervous disorders.[139]

All these new soft drugs—tobacco, opium, distilled spirits, and tea—were linked to the nerves just like coffee, mostly for their ability to damage them and either cause or exacerbate nervous disorders, but sometimes as a cure. Also, as Éloy and Reynal noted for coffee, they were touted as both the remedy and the cure for nervous disorders. For example, in 1780, the physician Hugh Smith (who blamed Bontekoe for tea's popularity) identified tea as the cause of "melancholy, palsies, epilepsies, night-mares, swoonings, flatulencies, low spirits, hysteric, and hypochrondiacal affections"—indeed, an "innumerable train of nervous afflictions."[140] Furthermore, Smith asserted darkly, "the hysterics, which used to be peculiar to the women, as the name itself indicates, now attacks both sexes indiscriminately."[141] Again tea provided a false cure: "This, like every other stimulus, either by constant use loses its effect, or unnerves the system it is meant to strengthen."[142] Describing the body under the influence of tea, Smith added: "Instead of being supported by nutritious ailment, its nerves are enfeebled, its spirits diminished, and all its functions enveloped with the gloom of melancholy. Even in the afternoon, when nature is exhausted by care and fatigue, we fly for refreshment to tea, which, instead of bracing, still further relaxes the unnerved system."[143]

The author of *An epistle to the fair-sex on the subject of drinking* identified spirits and drunkenness as a scourge among women of all classes, and, in addition to its corrosive effects on morality and physical health, he noted its cyclical effects. If a "young Woman of Quality" was lured into drinking gin by her friends or relatives, "she is continually troubled with Vapours, to relieve which she has constant Recourse to that which is the Cause of them, and thereby increases, while she endeavours to asswage them."[144] Around 1790 John Coakley Lettsom agreed that distilled spirits were both a cause of illness and the pretended cure. In his *History of some of the effects of hard drinking* he warned that women, in particular "those of delicate habits," were tempted into drinking to relieve the symptoms of "nervous debility." However, "the relief . . . being temporary," they found themselves forced "to keep up their effects, frequent access is had to the same delusion, till at length what was taken by compulsion, gains attachment, and a little drop of brandy, or gin and water, becomes as necessary as food."[145] Thus, nervous disorders led to alcohol as a remedy, leading in turn to dependence. Decades earlier, at the height of the Gin Craze, the anti-gin crusader Stephen Hales broadened the point to include all drinkers and to health beyond the nerves. "And as to the Health of these miserable People," he wrote, it is "greatly deprav'd and sottishly given in Exchange, for a false, unnatural Sensation of it, which each fresh Dram seems to give for the present; while it is, at the same Time, really undermining and destroying their Healths."[146] At first spirits made the stomach feel good, but then "the unhappy persons are thereby, in a little Time, reduced to a cold, languid, and dispirited State of Mind, which gives them so much Uneasiness, that they are impatient to get out of it, by fresh Supplies of the same deadly Liquor; which, instead of curing increases their Disease more and more."[147] Yet gin and brandy drinking continue to spread, "for it makes its Way into the World as a Friend to Mankind, and insinuates itself . . . under the Notion of helping Digestion, comforting the Spirits, and chearing the Heart"; meanwhile it "produces the direct contrary Effects."[148] Even tobacco was a false cure and an actual harm, as Philaretes observed in 1602. The health effects sought by purging with tobacco brought on debility because tobacco is such a strong drug, "an extreame and desperate medicine."[149] He likened it to the poison of the scorpion, thought to be cured only by itself: "This onely difference seemeth to be between those two poisons, That the venome of the Scorpion hath his perfect and absolute cure from the Scorpion itself, but that of Tabacco hath onely a certaine ease and palliation for a time by the fume of Tabacco received; but after perfect and absolute cure, this Tabacco by it selfe a thousand times resume or reiterated, admitteth none."[150] Smoking produced a vicious cycle of purge, further ill health, then purge again.

Using drugs that make one feel better at first but then worsen the conditions that caused the original distress sounds like the modern phenomenon of "self-medicating." Alcohol, cannabis, and harder drugs like heroin and cocaine are all ways that people today seek relief from anxiety and depression, but in self-defeating ways that end up worsening the underlying causes of their suffering. Early modern critics observed the users of soft drugs doing the same thing—turning to gin or tobacco to brighten their spirits or calm their nerves, only to worsen their moods. Further, these critics tended to pinpoint the true underlying causes of physical and mental malaise as the overconsumption of luxury goods, as one of the problems of overrefined modern urban life. Similar to Rousseau's condemnation of the inherent falsity of eighteenth-century commercial society, where polite behavior and consumption patterns alienated people from one another and from their own true selves, drugs pulled people away from their natural mental states into a depression that they characterized as melancholy, hypochondria, or a similar nervous disorder. Like the glittering promise of sophisticated cities like Paris or London, soft drugs were a trap that lured consumers hoping to brighten their mental states, only to betray them.

Coffee already serves as a harbinger of modernity for historians, thanks to its role in fostering an emergent public sphere. Éloy's tract shows the way for the shift of attention from the coffeehouse to the actual ingestion of coffee, and it might also point to other aspects of modernity, such as the wellness industry and self-medication. Today's health-care marketplace explodes with fashionable new cures every year—juice cleanses, mindfulness apps, keto diets, aromatherapy, crystals, and, ironically, the old humoral therapy of cupping. Most of these revolve around the consumption of luxury health items, and few of them are prescribed by physicians but instead are chosen independently by medical consumers.[151] Despite their countercultural or New Age origins, they have become a big business, as in Gwyneth Paltrow's GOOP.[152] Furthermore, the wellness culture aims not only to improve bodily health but also to fight stress and anxiety and improve mental well-being, even as anxiety and mental well-being suffer from consumerism, just like coffee and its fellow soft drugs did in the eighteenth century. The history of coffee shows that the history of "wellness" might extend even further back, as in today's emphasis on the individual's personal responsibility for his or her own wellness, usually with a moral judgment attached, and in the connection between wellness and consumerism.

But the uses of coffee and other new stimulants for daily self-care created ambivalence over whether the daily, proactive use of these drugs was a healthy way to discipline the consumer's body and mind, or if it displayed an undisciplined abuse of medicine. Was this behavior evidence of consumers taking control of their own mental well-being, or of a self-sabotaging cycle of self-medication? Many critics thought that the new stimulants offered merely a short respite from physical and mental ailments, but then in the long run worsened them. The pleasure and immediate mood-altering effects of soft drugs did nothing to address the real causes of eighteenth-century malaise: the effects of global capitalism, and the luxury consumption that it encouraged, on individuals and on western Europe as a whole. By ingesting stimulants—many of them brought from exotic locales all over the world—people seeking relief from anxieties and physical symptoms of surfeit, luxury, and consumerism were simply adding more fuel to the fire.

Gerhard Oestreich and Norbert Elias argue that the increasing emotional self-control displayed by Europeans during the early modern period emerged either because of the external pressures of the growth of the Neostoic state, which sought to discipline its subject, or the increasing interdependency of a more complex society, which necessitated emotional self-regulation for Europeans to negotiate without provoking conflict. Historians like William Reddy and Barbara Rosenwein have disproven the view held by both that premodern Europeans had an emotional regime that was loosely disciplined or even primitive, allowing for the naive, childlike venting of emotions.[153] Certainly emotions have changed over time, yet even if Oestreich and Elias are correct that self-discipline was increasing during the early modern period, the idea that individuals were choosing commodities from the medical marketplace with the aim of self-soothing is wildly different than the models of causation that they had in mind. Additionally, Max Weber believed that self-denial was at the heart of the cause of the growth of capitalism in Europe. However, Europeans were indulging in psychotropic drugs to regulate their mood, often without the permission of physicians, and the growth of this wellness marketplace was itself a product of the emergence of global capitalism. Consumers targeting nervous disorders with the exotic new drugs meant that western Europeans were taking knowledge and cultural products from foreign, sometimes subordinate, peoples to ease the anxieties of modern urban and commercial life. The adoption of the medical knowledge and cultural practices of an exoticized non-West and then packaging those cultural artefacts into commodities that are then exoticized and sold to calm the minds of an anxious elite certainly have a long history, stretching from coffee and tea in the eighteenth century to reiki, ayahuasca, yoga, and the micro-dosing of psilocybin today.

CHAPTER 5

And So the Game Goes Round

Women and Sociability

In 1701 the provocative Amsterdam printer Timotheus ten Hoorn published a book, The *debauched and enchanted coffee- and tea-world*, that featured fictional young women in Dutch towns such as Amsterdam, Rotterdam, the Hague, and Utrecht and the misadventures that followed from gathering over coffee and tea.[1] The anonymous author lamented that the misuse of tea and coffee was a spectacle of the modern age, increasing since the introduction of the hot drinks forty or sixty years previously, so much so that women were now entrapped in a "water frenzy." The Netherlands had become another China or Japan, he complained, despite tea's failure to cure any illnesses at all.[2] Tea had spread so quickly in his homeland because it had become fashionable, just like perfuming oneself with *eu de Paris*, and while its devotees claimed to drink tea for its health, they really drank it simply because it gave women an excuse to meet and socialize. It was the harm that they did to women, the author claimed, that turned him against coffee and tea, and most of the book consists of a series of cautionary, fictional tales about women falling into trouble thanks to drinking tea or coffee together.[3]

One story revolved around Lea, the wife of Timothy the wool merchant; Maria, the wife of Tobias the grain merchant; and Diwertje, the wife of Rynier Adriaanse. In trying to prevent their wives from gathering,

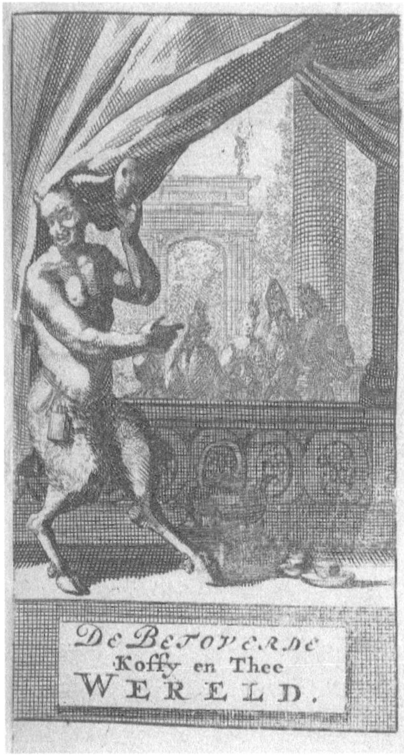

FIGURE 5.1. *De gedebaucheerde en betoverde koffy en thee wereld* (Amsterdam: Timotheus ten Hoorn, 1701), frontispiece. A devil pulls off his mask and gestures to the genteel women who are enjoying coffee and tea, demonstrating the easy slide into depravity that these new drinks encourage. Reproduced courtesy of the British Library.

the three husbands arranged to keep them busy with visits to church. Nevertheless, the women kept meeting. One day while they were drinking tea with brandy, Tobias came home unexpectedly just as the young wives had begun singing lewd drinking songs. Right before he entered, the women realized he was approaching and hid their glasses and brandy bottle under the table, trying to look sober and merely drinking tea so he would not suspect they had been singing and dancing. When Lea realized that Tobias had heard them through the door, she explained to him they had just been repeating a ribald song they had heard elsewhere, and they were now ashamed they had laughed at such things. The lie worked, and the women fooled Tobias, but the story exemplified the themes of ten Hoorn's entire volume: women's sociability becoming scandalous when outside men's supervision, with tea leading to sexual impropriety, although in this case it was just singing about risqué activities and not action. Other stories from the book described tea parties as ruses to facilitate unmarried women meeting young men, thereby ruining their reputations.[4] By drawing an explicit comparison between women drinking tea at home and Dutch men going to coffeehouses, the author concluded that coffee and tea had taken from Dutch women their best qualities: service to God, modesty, and honor. Men and boys, he complained, frequented the coffeehouse to talk, discuss news, smoke pipes, and play games, wasting their time and money. At coffeehouses, weavers and other low-status men addressed each other as "my Lord" or "Monsieur" and talked about politics, theology, and war, assuming "a ridiculous gravity" and dawdling away their time, or worse, using the coffeehouse as a place to meet prostitutes. Tea was just as bad for men, since conversation with women at the tea table corrupted them and made them lazy and effeminate. Such a useless drink, created by easterners who had been conquered by the Dutch, a drink with no purpose fit only for cowards and slaves, had replaced native Dutch beer.[5]

Ten Hoorn's publication highlighted two important points that applied not only to tea but also to the rest of the early modern stimulants. First, the new drugs changed the social behavior of their users, and, second, critics were especially concerned with how those changes impacted women. Tea provides a good entry point for investigating these changes, thanks to the palpable anxiety that women's participation in the new rituals of the tea table caused among critics. But ten Hoorn's juxtaposition of tea and coffee serves as a reminder that the coffeehouse, and the work of historians to uncover the way it affected sociability in early modern England, can help explain what was so new, so troubling, and so exciting about tea. As Jürgen Habermas has argued, the coffeehouse produced both enthusiasm and alarm because it created a new space for men to get together and discuss ideas, unpoliced by the established church or state. Tea performed a similar function in western Europe, providing a new place and time—the tea table—to gather. Unlike the coffeehouse, however, the tea table welcomed women, sometimes with men but sometimes alone, unsupervised by husbands or fathers. While politics and religion were the dangerous topics of discussion among men at the coffeehouses, critics feared that, in the absence of husbands or fathers, women would be tempted to gossip, compromising the reputations of those not present, and to discuss or even arrange for illicit sex. Thus it was the site and setting where the new drug was consumed, more than the drug itself, that generated anxiety about the disordering of traditional sociability.

Historians have found that, in England, contemporary defenders tamed the coffeehouse, making the space acceptable by encouraging polite self-discipline among patrons. Teatime experienced a similar rehabilitation as women adopted a similar project of self-policing to make the tea table a safe space for women to converse. For all the worry provoked by women gathering together, self-discipline was the answer.[6] Similar patterns of a new stimulant reshaping social relations and causing anxiety occurred with the other drugs, especially gin. One powerful current running through discussion of the new drugs was the way in which the adoption of their use spread through existing social ties, after which one's social behavior then reoriented itself around the drug use. These changes were welcomed by some and provoked profound concern in others, leaving early modern Europe with a strong sense of ambivalence over drugs and sociability.

Coffee: What News Have You, Master?

It might be best to consider the coffeehouse before the tea table, since it is the most well studied of the new sites of consumption, and because it has served as such a powerful symbol of modernity. Coffeehouses have attracted attention as a symbol of the Habermasian public sphere, partly because they were controversial for encouraging free political speech (which was Habermas's focus), and partly because earlier British historians highlighted the survival of the coffeehouse in the face of the Stuart regime's attempts to eradicate it as part of a patriotic, teleological narrative in which the Whigs rescued England from tyranny.[7] In 1675 Charles II tried to outlaw the retail vending of coffee (and chocolate and tea) because of coffeehouses' role in fostering free political speech, and although this measure failed to become law, threats to close them down persisted for several years until the regime settled on a system of licensing and browbeating coffeehouse proprietors as a way to contain the threat.[8] Brian Cowan has shown that critics reviled coffeehouses not only for nurturing sedition but also for the way they encouraged general disorder: rumor, libel, and prostitution, among other ruptures in sociability.[9] In an attempt to rescue the coffeehouse from its reputation for disorder, defenders like Joseph Addison and Richard Steele, the publishers of the *Spectator*, urged an ethos of self-policing, advocating for the creation of a polite society of sober, dignified men engaged in a knowledgeable discussion—as opposed to a rancorous debate—of public affairs. "Polite" here does not simply mean cordial, but signifies a new style of manners that emerged in western Europe during this period, manners that suited commercial and urban society and replaced the courtliness and honor codes that typified feudal society. Above all else, politeness demanded self-control in the face of the temptations of individual freedoms, money, and the luxuries that money could buy.[10] The *Spectator* modeled the kind of civil discourse that its authors believed should be the only kind of conversation taking place in coffeehouses, and their attempt was so persuasive that later scholars like Habermas took it for an objective description of how men actually behaved there.[11]

Cowan also points out a class dynamic in the coffeehouse, as its supporters tried to push nonelite and uneducated men out of the institution to help preserve it as a site for measured and learned discourse. An earlier chapter of this book featured the anonymous author of *The character of a coffee-house with the symptomes of a town-wit* complain about the mixing of social classes in the coffeehouse; critics also lamented that coffeehouses encouraged lower class men to talk freely of matters of which they had no knowledge. *The character of a coffee-house* mocked a working-class patron for buzzing all around the room, asking each customer he met: "What News have you Master? Then with a grave whisper (yet such as all the Room may hear it) he discovers some mysterious Intrigue of State told him last night by one that is Barber to the Taylor of a mighty great Courtiers man, relating this with no less formality than a young Preacher delivers his first Sermon." The author went on to damn the clientele of coffeehouses as nonelite men who, instead of deferring to their social betters, presumed to mingle and discuss grave matters with them as equals.[12] Similarly, the London satirist Thomas Brown, in his 1702 guide to London, emphasized the social disorder of coffeehouses, first explaining that they were sites to find prostitutes and going on to say they fostered conversation between men unacquainted with one another, and that the fumes of the coffee entering their noses, eyes, and ears "has the Vertue to make them Talk and Prattle together of everything but what they should do."[13]

Brown's mention of prostitutes gestures to social critics' firm disapproval of women's presence in the coffeehouses. Even the women who worked there as serving maids could raise concern, as they did for Daniel Defoe. The novelist and Whig polemicist alleged that the servers were insolent and inclined toward licentious sex, encouraged

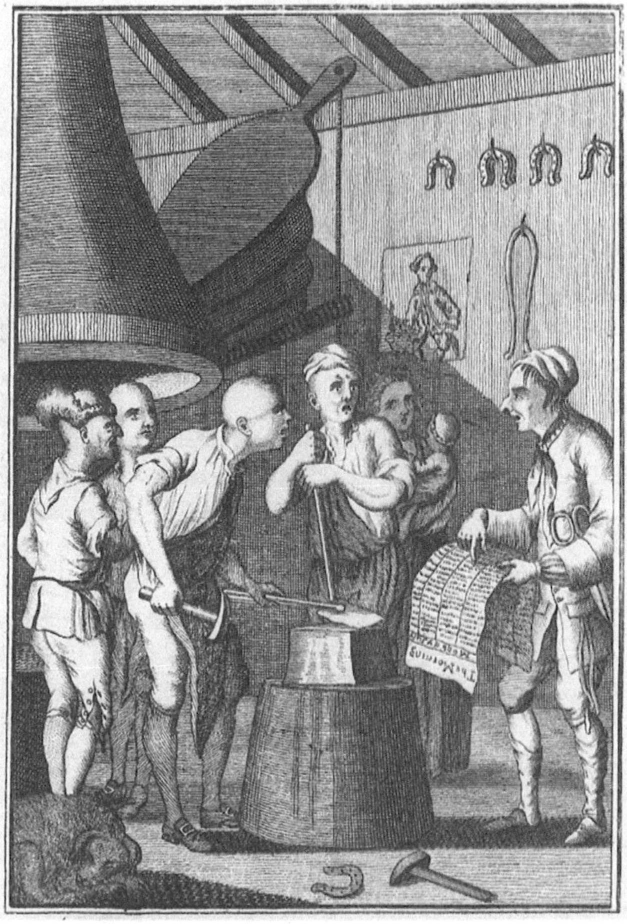

FIGURE 5.2. "The blacksmith lets his iron grow cold attending to the taylor's news," 1772. While these working-class men and women are not at a coffeehouse, their slack-jawed credulity demonstrates that these working-class men had no business discussing the news. Unpoliced discussion of current events needed to be restricted to elite men who exercised the self-discipline of the new culture of politeness. Reproduced courtesy of the British Museum.

as they were to flirt with customers. As he put it in 1725, "I was at a Coffee-House t'other Day, where one of these Ladies kept the Bar, and had bespoke a Dish of Rice-Tea; but madam was so taken up with her Sparks, that she had quite forgot it. I spoke for it again, and with some Temper, but was answer'd after a most taunting Manner, not without a toss of the Head, a Contraction of the Nostrils, and other Impertinencies, too many to enumerate."[14] When commenting on proper coffeehouse etiquette, Steele contrasted "Eubulus," the wise and discreet wealthy man of affairs who judiciously advised his friends on their own business matters—subjects about which he was knowledgeable—with characters like the haberdasher opining on the ongoing war with France, "Tom the Tyrant," who saw fit to correct the government's policies, and the law students who attended the coffeehouse to discuss opera and silently evaluate each others' clothing.[15] Steele, Addison, and other defenders of the coffeehouse promoted the self-policing of Eubulus as an alternative to the state stepping in to regulate or shut down coffeehouses, but both the defenders and critics broadly viewed the unpoliced conversation of the nonelite, not just politics, to be the problem.

An additional critique censured coffeehouses for displacing a more traditional social site with its own mood-altering drink: the tavern. The general line of attack is summed up by the title of the anonymously penned 1675 *Ale-wives complaint, against the coffee-houses, in a dialogue between a victuallers wife and a coffee-man, being at difference about spoiling each others trade.* The alewife hurled invective against "our English Turk," the coffeehouse proprietor, who sold his "Heathenish Liquor" coffee as well as chocolate and "your Tea that will make one vomit that drinks it," leaving men impotent.[16] Champions of coffee promoted its threat to the tavern as a virtue; the anonymous author of a 1675 tract noted that it provided not only a sober alternative to the alehouse but also a less expensive way to socialize, since customers were allowed to nurse a cup of coffee for hours, and, indeed, the price of beer was rising in late seventeenth century England.[17] Defenders of alehouses also accused coffeehouses of breeding disloyalty. High-church Tories in particular viewed them as sites of Whig and Dissenting sedition, in sharp contrast to taverns, where men drank alcoholic toasts to the health of the king.[18] Coffeehouse defenders countered that self-policing patrons engaged in reasoned, consensus-building discussion, and that it was wine, brandy, and ale that encouraged subversion.[19] The anonymous publisher of a broadsheet in 1674 claimed that God's providence had arranged for coffee to arrive in England just after the Civil War to soothe the contentious effects of "Drink, Rebellion, and Religion," replacing "the sweet Poison of the Treacherous Grape" with "this All-healing-Berry."[20] Another anonymous publication that same year celebrated the calming effects of "that harmless and healing Liquor, which Indulgent Providence first sent amongst us, at a time when Brimmers of Rebellion, and Fanatick Zeal had intoxicated the Nation, and we wanted a Drink at once to make us Sober and Merry."[21] In "A Dialogue between Two Horses," a satirical poem composed by the metaphysical poet and polemicist Andrew Marvell to celebrate the restoration of Charles II, Marvell urged, "Let the City drink Coffee. . . . For Wine and strong Drink make Tumults encrease, / Chocolate, Tea, and Coffee are Liquors of Peace." He then urged Charles to revoke his edicts against coffeehouses since "there's ten times more Treason in Brandy and Ale."[22] Ironically, Phil Withington has shown that in Britain, coffee was increasingly consumed at home, not in the coffeehouse, which in turn featured many products beyond coffee including alcohol, tea, chocolate, and, of course, tobacco.[23] So, it was the coffeehouse as a site for a novel form of socializing, more than coffee itself, that caused so much contention among its critics and defenders.

Many of these specific concerns were limited to the unique political and cultural context of late Stuart London, but throughout western Europe observers viewed coffeehouses as models of an emerging, modern civility, one that could be good or bad. In Milan in the mid-eighteenth century, Pierro Verri, Cesare Beccaria, and their friends created a club as a place to discuss enlightened reform, and, to broadcast their ideas, they set up a journal, *Il caffè*, which pretended to report what the authors heard in coffeehouses, just like Addison and Steele.[24] The Italian Jesuit Alfonso Muzzarelli published a poem in 1774 in which he imagined the goddess Diana entering a café and meeting prototypes of different kinds of people from all over Europe.[25] The anonymous *Le porte feuille galant*, a kind of French *Spectator* published in 1700, described Parisian coffeehouses as places where honest men and women could gather and converse, mixing people from all walks of life: "charming men, elegant women, polite abbots . . . soldiers, news-writers, officials, provincials, and foreigners." Like the London version, the Parisian coffeehouse was a site for participating in and observing new forms of social mixing among refined city residents.[26] Alexandro de Moya's *El café*, a two-volume work published in 1792, used a Madrid coffeehouse as a setting where people from all over Europe and all walks of life could come together to discuss private affairs or public business: war, economics, science, or poetry.[27] These observers imagined continental coffeehouses in the same ways as an idealized London coffeehouse, stripped from the real-world disordered socializing, class-mixing, and unpoliced conversing that occurred in actual coffeehouses.

We Chiefly Spend Our Time in Visits, and Tea-Talk of This and That

When European travelers to China and Japan, especially Catholic missionaries and Dutch traders, first noticed tea, they also noted East Asians' high regard for it. Unlike the societies that Europeans found in the Americas, China and Japan impressed Europeans with their large cities, great wealth, and long history, and westerners also grasped the role that tea played there in medicine and elite luxury consumption.[28] In 1637 the directors of the Dutch East India Company asked their employees to import tea to fuel the tiny but growing market for the exotic drink, and by mid-century small quantities could be found for sale in Paris, London, and several Dutch cities. By the 1680s tea drinking was familiar among English elites, led by the cosmopolitan, novelty-seeking intellectuals called "virtuosi," and England began to impose taxes on tea in England in 1660.[29] 1700 marked a turning point for tea importation into England, as less than fifteen thousand pounds of the dried leaves had been imported in total before 1700, but 1701–4 saw the arrival of over two hundred thousand pounds.[30] European merchants first obtained their tea from South and Southeast Asia, especially the Dutch colony in Java, but in 1713 the English East India Company was able to purchase it directly from southern China, thanks to a change in Chinese trade policies.[31] England replaced the Netherlands as the chief importer of tea, even selling some to the Netherlands, and also became the chief tea-consuming country in western Europe, purchasing some 60 percent of all tea imported from Asia, with the Netherlands right behind.[32] By the 1750s tea brought from Canton to Europe and its colonies had reached almost seven million pounds per year, and over twenty million pounds per year by 1770.[33] Tea's spreading use in western Europe played a role in the retail revolution, which saw the emergence of modern shops selling groceries and other ready-to-sell goods, including tea sets and utensils. In 1700 tea services first appeared in London household inventories, and by 1725 60 percent of all such household inventories listed them. Enabled by its affordability, by the 1780s it was common even for poor households in the English countryside to make tea a routine purchase.[34] The cheap price of tea was driven by competition between the East India Company and its Dutch, French, Danish, Swedish, and Flemish rivals, as well as by the smugglers who profited from undercutting the high English taxes on tea.[35] In 1785 the British government slashed its tax rates on tea, effectively ending smuggling and allowing twelve million pounds of it to be sold per year in England alone.[36] By the 1790s, about 40 million pounds of Chinese tea reached Europe per year.[37]

In a 1721 poem, Peter Motteux, the writer, Huguenot refugee, and one-time editor of the *Gentleman's Journal*, and thus a promoter of politeness and the emerging public sphere in England, praised tea in terms quite similar to coffee. Like alcohol, it cheered and fortified the drinker. Like coffee, it "settles the Heads of the Young" and "cools the Brain of the hard Drinker" while lacking "the Headiness of our strong Spirits."[38] The Duchess of Newcastle, Margaret Cavendish, a scientifically minded writer and trenchant critic of society, also weighed in on the similarities of coffee and tea, especially on its trajectory from a pharmaceutical item to a consumer good that promoted sociability. As early as 1666, in her magnum opus, *Observations upon experimental philosophy*, she observed that while physicians might promote tea as a medicine, "Tea and Coffee, are now become mode-drinks, and their chief effects are to make good fellowship, rather than to perform great cures."[39] In 1722 a writer calling herself "A. N." published a pamphlet purporting to be a summary of a recent conversation between her and other women over tea. She described the tea table as a place where women could speak on a "Variety of Things, concerning Men and Matters, as of our Betters and others, likewise our Selves as to our Births, Breedings, Educations, and the like common Affairs of Human life." The tea table was becoming an important site for socializing that encouraged women to exchange information, and A. N. quoted Royalist pamphleteer Roger L'Estrange as claiming that while our great-grandmothers spent their time at the spinning wheel, "in our Age, we chiefly spend our Time in Visits, and Tea-Talk of this and that."[40] Like coffee, tea quickly made its way from a medicine to a social drink, only in this case its imagined consuming public was made up of women at home, not men in coffeehouses.

By the nineteenth century, tea had became a symbol of domestic serenity, associated with middle- and upper-class women. Woodruff D. Smith describes teatime in England, centered on the family and directed by women, as a performance of respectability, and argues that its role as a marker of gentility is what drew the English to drinking tea.[41] Beth Kowaleski-Wallace points out, however, that in seventeenth-century England, just as in *The debauched and enchanted coffee- and tea-world*, tea began as a disruptive force, mistrusted for the way that it brought women together in new ways, crossing class boundaries in the new, densely crowded cities, leading them away from their domestic duties and into a new social space where they could exchange information (pejoratively called "gossip") without the oversight of men.[42] The lines of communication between women that tea created meant that gossipers could secretly attack their neighbor's reputations. Tea might also throw unsupervised young women into the company of young men, creating opportunities for sexual scandal, as in *The debauched and enchanted coffee- and tea-world*. Tea threatened to remove women from traditional habits of orderly sociability into a new, disordered social regime.

Critics of tea's corrosive effects on sociability even included Cornelis Bontekoe, the Dutch "tea doctor" who did so much to popularize tea in his *Treatise on the most excellent herb tea* in 1678. Eight years later, in a posthumous volume, he expressed some misgivings. Not only were urban gentlemen and women drinking tea, but so were common people, who did so to excess. Bontekoe admonished: "It cannot be viewed otherwise than that men want to drown tea in brandy." Tea drinkers were wasting their time and losing their livelihoods, using tea as a pretext for leaving their homes to spend money while shopping. Young women especially were susceptible to start out drinking tea and then, once they were out of men's sight, move on to wine and even tobacco.[43] In 1722 a scold under the pseudonym "Whipping Tom" (taken from a sensationalized nickname for an unidentified man who had assaulted women in nighttime London by whipping their buttocks) published an attack on fashionable clothing and manners among young women in London, especially the working class: "Every Servant-Wench before she handles her mop and Pail, must have forsooth a dish of this Indian or Chinese liquor: There is scarce a scull in any Market about London, or Mechanicks Drab, but what must have her Load of hot Water and Sugar, five or six Times a Day, to the no small Charge," he added, sexualizing tea drinking, "of the poor contented Cuckolds their Husbands." For Whipping Tom, tea was a threat to gender and class expectations, and it even disordered the way that women carried their bodies: "Then as many Postures must be us'd in drinking a Dish of Tea, as taking a Pinch of Snuff. . . . Then to hear insignificant Chit-chat, and dull impertinent Discourse," he continued, "which these Tatterdemalions, your Exchange-Girls and Shop-Keepers Froes have over their Tea, would make the lunatic Inhabitants of Bedlam laugh at 'em." He ridiculed women of leisure at their tea as well, "for to be sure a great deal is to be gather'd from them, when enquiring of their Gentlewomen, how the Doctor lik'd such a Lady's last Water, how this Monky slept last

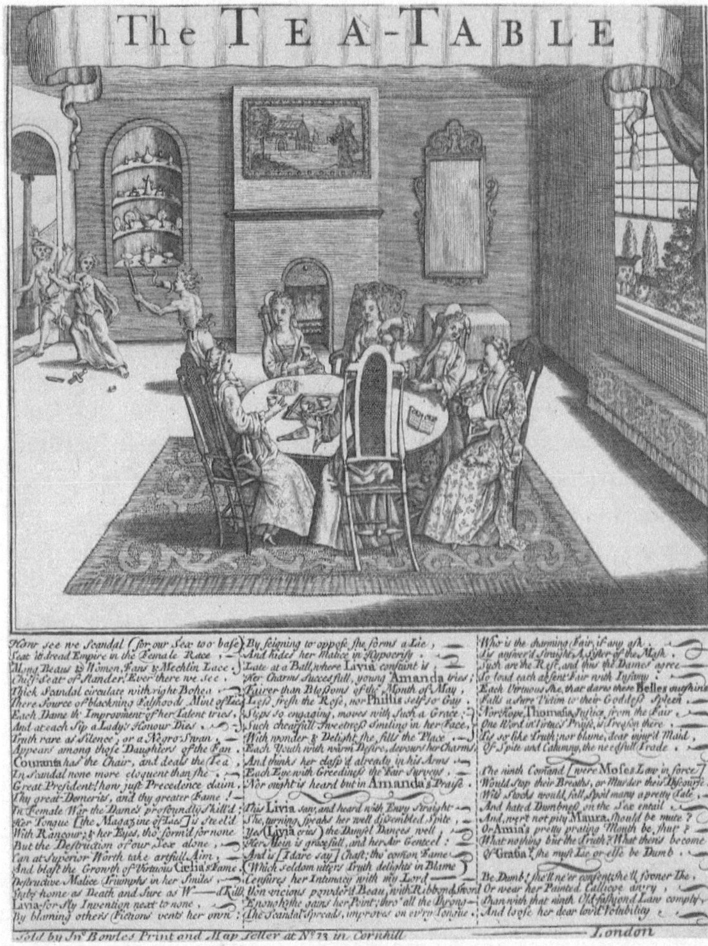

FIGURE 5.3. "The Tea-Table," early eighteenth century. The elite women here seem to be partaking in the new polite pastime of a tea party, but signs of disorder abound. To the left, allegorical figures depict "Envy" chasing "Justice" and "Truth" out of the room. To the right, two men listen in, trying to hear what women about when unsupervised by men, and a devil lurks under the table. Reproduced courtesy of the British Museum.

Night, that Dog this Morning, that Parrot talk'd to Day; oh!"[44] Tea was a symbol of the social pretentions of working-class women as well as the empty domesticity of elite women.

Malicious gossip, illegitimate sex, and the inappropriate social climbing of the working class were three constant themes in early eighteenth-century English anti-tea literature. Some of the criticism was mild, as in an anonymous writer's poem, "The Tea-Table," published in 1746, which gently chastised women who were not content to stay at home and had to go out for tea, engaging for hours in idle gossip about other women they knew.[45] More commonly critics imagined the gossip as vicious, causing scandal and ruining reputations of men and women who, absent from the table, were unable to defend themselves. The anonymous poet who styled "Tea, a poem" after Alexander Pope's *Rape of the lock* in 1743 depicted tea as growing in a grove that recalled both antiquity and East Asia, but the goddesses who attended to the tea plant were "Folly," "Envy," and "Pride," not the typical Olympic deities. These malicious tea goddesses were keen to sacrifice "Reputation" as a victim on an altar to tea, overseen by "Scandal," leading to a war between them and another goddess, "Truth," who rushed in to assist Reputation.[46] A similar classicizing poem, "The rise and progress of tea," imagined that the nectar the gods drank while conversing in the *Iliad* and the *Odyssey* was tea, fostering gossip among the goddesses at Olympus. The poem portrayed the goddesses as jealous of mortal women attracting the gods' romantic attention, and in punishment they sent it down to earth to spread dissent and jealousy among women there, too.[47]

Simon Mason, who was probably a London apothecary, took this further in his 1745 treatise, *The good and bad effects of tea consider'd.* While Mason spent most of his attention on the physical effects of tea, he spared some ink for excoriating "the Chair or Washer-woman, who, to be fashionable, must have Tea for Breakfast," and who then begged her mistress for more tea later in the day before moving on to drinking gin. Tea and gin led to "much Gossiping, Lying, Backbiting," including speculation on "some Neighbour, whose Wife has been too free with such a certain Man" and similar sexual rumors. They also shared information, much like the young women of *The debauched and enchanted coffee- and tea-world*, on how to subdue and tame their husbands, praising men who acquiesced to everything their wives demanded and slandering those who did not. They would stop at nothing, he continued, "to ruin his Reputation and his Business; this is the only Way to bring him to Poverty, and is the sure Way to bring him to humility and Subjection." Further, drinking tea led to drinking gin, which in turn led to women's vulnerability to sexual license and exploitation. [48]

Outside of England things were much the same. *The debauched and enchanted coffee- and tea-world* was not the only Dutch publication to warn that tea led women astray. Abram de Vri published a fictional account of women getting together for a tea party in Amsterdam in 1702. Klara hosted her four friends, telling them how she sweet-talked her husband to leave the house so they could gather, which led to a discussion of the best ways to get their husbands to leave them alone and how helpful a maidservant could be for this kind of deception. Meanwhile they drank tea, chocolate, and also brandy, ending up singing drunkenly, and, after her guests left, Klara's maid Neel had to help her get into bed to recover before her husband returned.[49] The next time they met at Marretje's house, where they discussed sex, both marital and extramarital, their husbands, and gossiped about their neighbors while drinking tea, coffee, and sack. There, too, they broke out into song, and when asked about food they were eating, Alegonde recited a ribald poem: "Carrots and cabbage are good for cooking / Eggs and Spanish wine are good for f[ucking]."[50] Another Dutch moralist, apparently a physician, who went by the initials R. V. N., remarked that "lovers of Venus" went fishing for women at tea and coffee parties, especially when brandy accompanied the hot drinks. One acquaintance told him he was surprised to see a healthy young man such as himself rail against coffee and tea because it was such a good way for men to gain access to these women. "Now that tea and coffee are in fashion," the author's friend continued, "more whores are made in three years than before in fifty."[51]

In the imagination of its critics, tea induced women to leave their houses and indulge in malicious slander, sexual misconduct, and the consumption of alcohol. It is hard to know how accurate the depiction was of gossiping, licentious women at tea; the anti-tea rhetoric drew heavily on age-old misogynistic tropes in European culture, and moralists had portrayed women gathering without men as gossipers centuries before tea arrived in Europe. Furthermore, tea had its defenders as well, who believed that far from disordering women's social lives, it helped discipline them, or could do so if employed the right way. The writer and reforming critic of women's manners Eliza Fowler Haywood published *The tea-table* in 1725, in which she conceded that when women gathered at tea, "Scandal, and Ridicule seem here to reign with uncontested Sway." *The tea-table* provided an alternate model in the form of a tea party presided over by the refined "Amiana."[52] Just as Addison and Steele modeled a polite form of self-policing sociability at the coffeehouse to save it from discredit, Haywood did the same for tea. Indeed Haywood modeled her own magazine, the *Female Spectator* (1744–46), on Addison and Steele's *Spectator* from decades earlier, using it to promote their goal of shaping a polite, self-disciplined society in England.

Haywood laid it on thick when she described Amiana's virtues, but she made it clear that the most important quality for anyone hosting a tea party was to ensure that none of her guests spoke ill of a person absent from the table.[53] *The tea table* was devoted to an imagined conversation at Amiana's table, with genteel men and women discussing love, personal character, and the good and ill romantic fortunes both of young people they had known and of fictional characters. This conversation, plus a description of the virtues of the participants and the poor manners of some guests who left early (which enabled the remainder of the party to carry on with truly polite discourse), provided a clear model for how people should behave at tea—what to discuss, and how to do so properly. It was the opposite of the character, behavior, and speech of the characters featured two decades earlier in *The debauched and enchanted coffee- and tea-world.*

Another defense of women at the tea table came from the physician James Bland in 1733. According to Bland's *An essay in praise of women: or, a looking-glass for ladies to see their perfections in*, tea created a space where a virtuous, improving sociability could thrive among women. Unlike men, drinking wine and talking all at once "like geese," women at tea were given to sweet expressions of wit and edification.[54] If gossip occurred, Bland argued, tea had nothing to do with it: "Tatlers would be Tatlers still; and they would no less inveigh against their Neighbours over any other Liquor," and indeed would behave worse if drinking alcohol.[55] Against the argument that tradesmen's wives were squandering the money earned by their busy husbands and wasting time that could be put more profitably to use in business or some industrious behavior like spinning, Bland upheld the necessity of tea for the social life of families engaged in trade. Women of modest means could not hope to serve luxury wines when hosting gentlemen who visited their shops, but tea offered a respectable yet affordable way to display hospitality. Tea also strengthened the bonds of female friendship, which then would lead to their friends becoming lifelong customers. "And so by the frugal Management of the Tea-Table," he wrote, "a Man may gain no small Credit, Interest, and Reputation. . . . Friendship has all along been got and retain'd by Eating and Drinking."[56] All tradesmen had long been in the habit of sealing agreements and finalizing payments by drinking together, and tea was the most innocent drink that could be shared.[57]

In 1734 Duncan Campbell published *A poem upon tea*, where he played on many of the same themes about tea, including its ability to brighten wits, its potential for providing sober entertainment, and its strong association with women. He depicted a female character defending tea against the criticism that tea led to gossip: while drinking wine, she alleged, men urged each other on to greater vice, but tea disposed women differently, keeping them reasonable and careful lest they give offence to one another. She added another virtue of tea: it allowed the young to practice in engaging in virtuous conversation. "The little Miss that scarce can wattle, / At Tea will learn to smile and prattle," she wrote.[58] The power of the tea table to socialize young girls, teaching them correct behavior and conversation, became another important defense of tea. A subgenre of imagined tea parties developed that involved young women and girls, similar to Haywood's fictional gatherings at Amiana's but even more pointedly didactic. The anonymous author of 1750's *A new tea-table miscellany* offered a series of poems that were imagined to be read and discussed at teatime. "Some have represented the Tea-Table as the theater of obloquy, the nurse of detraction, and . . . the inexhaustible fund of slander and defamation," the author acknowledged, but it did not need to be so, thanks to English women "gladly listening to the dictates of an Addison and a Steele."[59] The miscellany contained dozens of witty poems and tales featuring young women and innocuous romance, without any serious barbs that could give offense. In 1796 Richard Johnson published *Tea-table dialogues*, in which a governess presided over the teatime conversation of adolescent girls, whose names—"Mary Sensible," "Eliza Thoughtful," "Jane Bloom," "Ann Hopeful," and "Dinah Sterling"—betray the tenor of the book. The governess, "Mrs. Goodwill," gently steered the conversation, checking the girls' immature emotions and guiding them in correct speech and manners.[60]

Eventually Johnson, Haywood, Bland, and the others who promoted the tea table as a space for genteel young women to practice self-discipline won out. The ritual of teatime became part of polite society, especially in England, and, like the coffeehouse, more important to western European culture than the beverage itself. Tea was prestigious enough that elite women took charge of its ceremonies, either directing the servants conducting the service or actually pouring the tea themselves. Tea became feminine, and as much a part of constructing the emerging private or domestic sphere in the eighteenth century as the coffeehouse was for the public sphere. Knowledge about tea—the gradations in quality and price, the method of serving, and especially all the silver and porcelain serving items, which were constantly changing in fashion—constituted part of its politeness. Not only did a family need to have the money to purchase the mahogany table, the silver and the china but they also had to possess the taste and manners to ensure that they purchased the correct things and used them the correct way. Markman Ellis and his coauthors suggest that instead of thinking of porcelain as becoming popular as a way to drink tea properly, perhaps tea owed its increasing popularity to the way it created an excuse to bring out the porcelain and show it off.[61]

David Hancock has described the idea of "conversation" in the early modern period as a collaboration between people, an exchange of information, and a reciprocal relationship where each participant revealed their knowledge about an issue, articulated their own position, and then sifted through the competing claims to discern the truth.[62] The coffeehouse was a site that promoted such conversations about public affairs, either seditious or polite, depending on one's point of view toward coffeehouses. Throughout the medieval and early modern periods, prescriptive literature portrayed women discussing their neighbors' reputation as gossip—as a vice. But it should be easy to look beyond the misogyny of premodern Europe to see gossip instead as a conversation, staged by women (and men), and aimed at establishing the truth about their neighbors' character.[63] In an age before modern banking, when everyday commerce relied on networks of credit, when there was not yet any distinction between "credit" as financial creditworthiness and "credit" as whether one was true to one's word, this kind of character assessment was no idle pastime but, rather, a relay of important business information, which helped to impose work and spending discipline on one's neighbors.[64] If, unlike the scolding voices in works such as *The debauched and enchanted coffee- and tea-world*, respect is granted to women's conversation and their ability to form moral judgments, a picture emerges of women at the tea table policing the ethics of their neighborhood and enforcing the bounds of their moral communities, just like men did at the coffeehouse in matters of in business, arts, and letters. If coffee fostered the discussion of the public affairs of state, arts, and letters, tea fostered the women's discussion of the public affairs of people closer to home, including their moral standing and creditworthiness. Whatever men thought of it, the tea table gave women a place to gather, exchange information, and strengthen the ties of friendship and neighborliness on which every household relied.[65]

Gin Shops the Nurseries of All Manner of Vice

The juxtaposition of the civility of the tea table, once it had been reformed by politeness, with the barbarity of gin drinking became a commonplace in eighteenth-century England.[66] Historians have focused on two aspects of the Gin Craze: the anxiety that arose over alcohol, social class, and women, and the attempts of the government to rein in consumption through licenses and taxes. It was the most famous early moral panic created by drugs or alcohol, provoked by the fear and loathing of English elites for the perceived drunkenness and disorderliness of the urban poor, and especially of women who drank so much that they neglected sexual modesty and good motherhood.[67] One aspect of the Gin Craze that remains understudied is the threat gin posed because of the way, like tea, it brought women together. Dram drinking was imagined to spread through women's networks, and in turn women who had taken up gin began to reorient their social lives around its consumption.[68] Most of the information about gin drinking and women comes from London, but *The debauched and enchanted coffee- and tea-world* show that anxieties about women drinking distilled spirits were not limited to that center of the Gin Craze.

An epistle to the fair-sex on the subject of drinking, anonymously published in 1744 at the height of the Gin Craze, prominently featured the topic of female sociability. The author opened by decrying the "Corruption of the Present Age" and the "Degeneracy of Manners," which he attributed mostly to women drinking brandy and gin.[69] The rest of the book explored the various social positions of women to describe the special ways that drinking would ruin each type, starting with unmarried women, including "a Young Woman of Quality," the "Daughter of a rich Tradesman," and "a common servant," and then working its way through married women, from "a Married Lady of Quality" through the "Wife of a Clergyman," and then to wet-nurses, widows, and every type of woman in between. In the first example, a young woman of quality might be "misled by the Example of some foolish Relation, or drawn in to share the secret Pleasures of some Companion or Governess." Notice how the author assumed that the influence of one woman would lead to vice in another. The consequences were also social, as people of high status "draw the Eyes of all Observers; and when once her private Folly is found out . . . it is quickly whispered through the malicious World, and her Reputation is totally lost" before she has even begun to suspect that others know.[70] The scenario for a gentleman's daughter was similar: once she started drinking, the family's chief servants would discover it and encourage her. From there the other servants would find out, "and then a thousand Traps are set to catch her. If she visits her Nurse, the Compliment is the favourite Liquor; if her Milliner, it succeeds the Tea; and if her Mantua-maker, it is great odds that it comes instead of it."[71] All of her social activities conspired to encourage gin drinking.

The daughter of a merchant, which described so many young women in London at this time, was much at risk of "this Contagion. She may be very early solicited by some of her acquaintance to amuse herself this way . . . to laugh and be merry. And tho' she has . . . strict Principles," she would probably be "laughed out of these right Notions" and told they are only for those who had to work for a living. "Then Examples are cited; She is told, that Miss Such-a-one and the Deputy's Lady drink together, and are never the worse thought of. . . . When she is once initiated, the Itch grows upon her; she . . . talks of nothing but Country Jaunts, and Parties for taking the Air," and she would begin to visit the pleasure gardens of Vauxhall and Ranelagh three nights a week to drink and socialize.[72] The thread that connected the examples of the *Epistle* was the influence of those in a woman's social network, including servants, family, friends, and acquaintances made through that new leisure pursuit for English women: shopping. Ellen Hartigan-O'Connor points out that in the days before the department store, shopping for household items was an important task that called on all of a woman's social resources to find out where the best-quality goods could be found, what the current prices were, and how to manage her credit and debts with various shopkeepers. Women needed their social networks to help manage their households.[73] In the eyes of misogynistic scolds, however, shopping was an idle pastime that led to vice, including gin tippling.

Once started, drinking began to bend social behavior around itself, as the woman looked for excuses to leave the house to drink and seek out others to join her. The social aspect of gin and brandy was thought to be so strong that the author's first point of advice for ending a woman's drinking habit was to withdraw her from all company.[74] Similarly, William Henry's *Earnest address to the people of Ireland, against the drinking of spirituous liquors*, printed in Dublin in 1753, decried whiskey's effects on social life for men as well as women. By making a drinker seem "a King in his own Eyes," he "forgets Respect to his Superiors . . . and acquires . . . a Dog-like Impudence," and, by inflaming the brain, liquor led men into anger and quarrels and women into promiscuity and prostitution. Henry painted a scene of unmarried women who, when going to market, "led by the elder Women! . . . are hurried to the Whiskey-House," where they would sit and drink in mixed company of men and women, "until their Passions are all on Fire."[75] Again, social ties led to drinking, which then disordered sociability.

Henry's emphasis on the site of drinking, the "Whiskey-House," points to a deep vein of commentary: alarm over the disordered nature of the places where people drank distilled spirits. There was a long history of disapproval, stretching from the medieval period, of alehouses and taverns as sites that fostered disorder, but at the same time they were recognized as necessary institutions that could also foster healthy social life.[76] This tension remained through the eighteenth century. In *Le tableau de Paris*, Louis-Sébastien Mercier offered his broad overview of Parisian life during the 1780s in which he scorned taverns as dissolute places where the dregs of society met, although, as Thomas Brennan points out, the clientele of Parisian taverns were mostly quite respectable.[77] In the eyes of English observers during the Gin Craze, gin made the sites of drinking even worse, intensifying the evil effects of alcohol on the places that sold it while shedding all the respectable and useful aspects of the alehouse. The anonymous writer of *A dissertation upon drunkenness* in 1727 opened his book with this condemnation: "Of all the publick Mischiefs, Miseries, and Inconveniences, attending the People . . . there cannot, in my Opinion, be a greater than the present scandalous Number of Taverns, Coffee-Houses, Alehouses, Brandy-Shops, and other kinds of Brothels, for vending and retailing Liquors." All of the arts, sciences, and trades have been lost, "and the whole Kingdom become nothing but a Brewer or Distillery, and the Inhabitants all Drunkards."[78] London was filled with people hawking drink, to the point of almost becoming one giant dram shop itself, such that living "a regular sober Life" had become impossible.[79] The *Dissertation* alleged that gin, brandy, and ale even corrupted coffeehouses, which used to be for genteel coffee drinkers, and had now become places for craftsmen to drink alcohol. Taverns had become sites of gross disorder as well: "The vile obscene Talk, Noise, Nonsense, and Ribaldry Discourses, together with the fumes of Tobacco, Belchings, and other foul Breakings of Wind, that are generally found in an Ale-Room, where the Companies sit promiscuously together, are enough to make any rational Creature amongst them almost asham'd of his Being: But all this the rude Rabble esteem the highest Degree of Happiness."[80] Drunkards never felt shame in their sinfulness, thanks to the companions in drinking whom they could always find, and together they "habituate themselves to this Sin, that they at length run into it with Greediness."[81] In short, drinking led to anger, quarrels, profanities, blasphemy, and violence, or a reversal of all good sociability, and, again, social ties led to drinking, which then bent social ties around that activity.[82]

For all that, taverns, inns, and alehouses possessed established rules and norms for conviviality, including buying rounds, drinking toasts, and cultivating what Mark Hailwood calls "good fellowship." They also followed guidelines to help decide who could and could not legitimately enter and drink.[83] In other words, they had a long-standing tradition of etiquette and rituals that disciplined the manner in which patrons consumed alcohol and that enforced the boundaries of a moral community. In the absence of such traditions in western Europe, how would the consumption of gin and tea be disciplined? Who could legitimately access the new drugs, and when and how? Physicians and natural philosophers had created rules for using the new drugs as medicines but not for their recreational use. Not only did they need new rules, but their emergence also threatened to replace the old psychotropic substances, beer and wine, their sites of consumption, and the moral communities that formed around their use. The number of satires on coffee published in England and pitched as arguments between proponents of ale and coffee, like *The ale-wives complaint, against the coffee-houses* (1675), is just one indication of the threat the new exotic drugs posed to the traditions of alehouses, taverns, and inns.[84]

The trial of the spirits, an attack on gin and the gin trade published in 1736 by an author calling himself "Philanthropos," singled out gin shops as "seminaries of Mischief" and "the Alma Mater of Rogues and Strumpets." Respectable families who otherwise shied away from gin sellers were nevertheless vulnerable to their influence due to their servants, who were drawn in by gin shops when out of their masters' houses.[85] An English magistrate calling himself "T. S." published a rebuttal to *The trial of the spirits* that same year in which he countered that gin was not really the problem; everyone, rich and poor, who wanted to drink would find a way, and that they certainly did so before gin became common, and that the real issue was the ubiquity of "scandalous Tippling-houses."[86] Focusing on the disordered site of consumption, T. S. proposed that the government solve the problem through tightening the licensing system for establishments that sold alcohol. Also in the same year, in response to the Gin Act of 1736, which required gin retailers to pay £50 per year for a license, "Jack Juniper" published *The deposing and death of Queen Gin*.[87] This satirical ballad featured Queen Gin sitting on a barrel in a brandy shop, lamenting the loss of "liberty" among gin's drinkers. The shop, now in danger of shutting down, had been a place for disreputable members of society to congregate; now where would

> The Cast-off Mistress, the despairing Maid,
> The Officer disbanded, Gamester broke,
> Or Bankrupt Tradesman
> find a place to mingle?[88]

The deposing and death of Queen Gin called attention not so much to gin but to the gin shop in particular, which offered a mirror version of what the coffeehouse was meant to be, a place where "Ragged Men and Women" instead of the polite and respectable came to socialize.[89] A "Country Justice of the Peace," who also weighed in on the dangers of gin to England in the mid-eighteenth century, pointed out that gin shops "entertain all Sorts of Persons without enquiring from whence they came," thus licensing a "Torrent of Gaming, Extravagance, Lewdness, and Irreligion . . . among all Ranks of People."[90] Like the coffeehouse, the gin shop created a new public space where people could come indiscriminately and exchange information. Unlike the coffeehouse, the dram shop had no Addison and Steele to encourage self-discipline. Instead it had Queen Gin.

William Henry went further, hinting that gin led to the reversion of society to a precivilized state. Spirituous liquors threatened people's lives, families, and "their Hopes of Posterity," as well as property, business production, and public order, "the Preservation of which is the great and ultimate End for which Men first entered into civil Societies."[91] Gin and the shops where it was sold had become so dangerous that, in some critics' eyes, beer and taverns now seemed beneficial in comparison. Nathaniel Blackerby, a magistrate in Westminster, held that disorder in London had increased so much because gin was a drink "quite different from that of other Liquors." This was a commonly held belief, and Blackerby took it one step further at a 1738 speech to other justices of the peace for Westminster by praising beer.[92] Famously, William Hogarth illustrated the distinction between gin and beer in two 1751 prints. *Beer Street* featured happy, well-fed, and prosperous

Londoners, in contrast to the emaciated and depraved denizens of the St. Giles slum in *Gin Lane*. In *A dissertation on Mr. Hogarth's six prints lately published'd, viz. Gin-Lane, Beer-Street, and the Four Stages of Cruelty*, which appeared in the same year that the prints were published, the Scots surgeon and writer Tobias Smollett emphasized the way that gin disordered women's relations with others. Serving women and wives from the middling classes who lived near slums frequented dram shops, or rooms attached to chandler's shops and herb stalls where gin was sold, up to "ten Times in a Day," under the pretense of running errands.[93] Women of means were able to send out for gin and drink it privately, but doing so brought the disorder of gin shops inside the house. From the start of the day, gin caused the lady of the house to turn on her servants, "at whom she scolds, raves and rages like a Bedlamite." "The poor Children are kick'd and tumbled about like so many Footballs," but their mother soon sent them to school to give herself more time to drink, either at home or while visiting "some drunken Gossip in the Neighbourhood." She then returned home, having failed to prepare dinner for her husband, whom she scolded in turn, causing him either to beat her, leave to go drink himself, or indulge her, letting the disorder of his household grow worse. "Look on her Children," Smollett urged, "and you will see such a Parcel of poor little diminutive Creatures, that you will fancy yourself in the Country of the Pigmies." What is more, "one is bandy-legg'd, another hump-back'd, another goggle-ey'd, another with a Monkey's Face . . . and all of them wearing some visible Mark of their Mother's Folly."[94] While the family of the gin-drinking woman displayed the visible marks of poor motherhood, the children of a beer-drinking woman were plump, lively, and healthy.[95] Like coffeehouses, gin shops displaced the beer-and-ale-serving tavern with new, dangerous sites of sociability or, worse, perverted the normal relations inside the house. Unlike coffeehouses, there was no effort to discipline the behavior and clientele of dram shops until the nineteenth century. The British government attempted to limit the production and sale of gin, but not the manner and context in which it was consumed.[96] Also unlike coffeehouses, the sharpest criticism of the effects of gin on social order focused on women.

The perception that gin corroded women's morality and destroyed family life featured prominently in popular literature like ballads, broadsheets, and satires during the eighteenth century. However, some writers defended women drinking distilled liquor. Elite women drinking punch or madeira wine inside their houses drew little criticism, but even nonelite women were welcome in taverns and alehouses. Certainly any woman who left the house could draw suspicion for sexual misconduct, gambling, and other offenses, but Tim Reinke-Williams finds that, throughout the period, it was normal for women to frequent London taverns, even with unrelated men, without disapproval. Moreover, nonelite women sold beer and wine in inns, taverns, and alehouses, again without drawing the disapproval that occurred when women were hawking gin in the street.[97] In 1734 Stephen Buck published a poem called "Geneva" that praised gin for its generally beneficial effects on sociability, claiming that sharing a glass of gin brought husbands and wives back to loving affection for another, and that gin could take more credit for witty conversation than "insipid Tea."[98] While Buck was undoubtedly at least half joking, he was probably also half serious.

After the Gin Craze died out, critics still drew attention to the ability of normal social ties to draw new people into drinking, and then for drinking to disorder that sociability. James Yates, a Unitarian minister in Glasgow, published four sermons in 1818 that denounced distilled liquor. Drunkenness was particularly insidious, he stated, because it has its origin in "innocent, amiable, and becoming" social ties. Friendly sociability induced some to urge their companions to drink more, and that same conviviality led them to go along, "until all have taken a greater quantity of intoxicating liquor than they would have done." Then, once people have made a habit of drinking to excess, they "will employ their influence and authority in favour of the continuance and general prevalence of that vice, to which they are themselves addicted" as they seek company for their excesses.[99] Companionship with drinkers further eroded resistance to drunkenness: "Every time a man yields to the importunity of gay and jovial companions, he renders himself an easier prey to their future attempts upon him; his disgust at the effects of drunkenness is gradually destroyed; his resolution grows weaker, and his taste for spirituous liquors continually increases."[100] In an anonymous 1813 essay titled "Confessions of a Drunkard," the English Romantic poet and man of letters Charles Lamb testified to similar forces working on him. He described how in his mid-twenties he began to drink after falling in with a group of friends who drank, in part to match the witty conversational style that was required in the group. He dropped this circle of friends and with them the excessive drinking, but later found another cadre of friends who smoked. Smoking led to drinking, and then Lamb found himself reordering his social life around alcohol: "My favourite occupations in times past, now cease to entertain."[101]

Lamb began with beer and wine, but ended with brandy. Some viewed distilled spirits as the worst of all possible alcoholic drinks while others saw them as a wholly different type of drug, in a different category altogether as wholesome beer and ale. Either way, gin drew people out of an ordered sociability into a disordered one. The deepest fear was that women would be drawn out of the home and into dram shops, or would bring gin into their homes and disorder relations within the household. Like tea, distilled spirits brought women together; in this case social ties between women helped foster gin drinking as friends, family, servants, and shopkeepers encouraged women to drink, to the point that they rearranged their social networks around drinking gin. Men like Charles Lamb experienced the same pattern of social ties, first encouraging and then coalescing around drinking, but the moral panic centered primarily on women. Gin drew women away from the proper management of their children and servants and led them into scolding their husbands and gossiping. As with tea, many of these sites of drinking gin took women away from the oversight of men into unpoliced all-female spaces that stimulated improper talk about sex. Worst of all, gin, like tea, threw women together with men eager for sex and encouraged sexual license, premodern Europe's most unmistakable mark of female immorality. Not only was gin a stronger and more fast-acting type of alcohol than beer or wine, but it also existed in a world without any kind of disciplinary manners or rituals to constrain its use. Unlike coffee and tea, no new code of manners emerged to regulate the use of gin, and for some it made beer seem respectable in comparison. Historians have noted the intensely gendered aspect of the moral panic surrounding gin in eighteenth-century England, but have not commented on the way that gin's creation of spaces for women to socialize unsupervised by husbands, fathers, or older women who could act as moral arbiters made it similar to coffee and tea.

Tobacco: An Inexpiable Breach against All the Royal Laws of Civility

Even before the arrival of tea, coffee, and gin in western Europe, tobacco had become closely associated with sociability and male companionship. Tobacco quickly became connected to drinking—as Lamb's regretful experience suggests—and with taverns, and later with coffeehouses as well, although by itself smoking could still foster togetherness.[102] Throughout western Europe, smoking pipes and taking snuff became normal behavior among men, both alone and in groups, and many observers believed that tobacco helped social relations. As early as 1614 the Scots physician William Barclay recognized that tobacco, which was still presenting mostly as a medicine at that point, "is the only medicament in the world ordained by nature to entertaine good companie: insomuch that it workesth never so well, as when a [*sic*] it is given from man to man, as a pledge of friendshippe and amitie."[103] A comic play written by Thomas Tomkis for Cambridge students and printed in 1607 featured the character "Olfactus," who, while praising tobacco, noted along with its pharmaceutical benefits that it was a "firme knot of good fellowship, Adamant of Company."[104] In 1606 the poet and soldier Barnabe Rich agreed; even while satirizing tobacco and mocking those who claimed it was a panacea for all maladies, he conceded, "It cannot be denied, but it makes men sociable."[105] In 1617 Richard Braithwaite observed that among "our young English Gallants," the first thing they said upon meeting an acquaintance was: "Will you take a pipe of Tobacco?" Right when it first appeared in western Europe, tobacco became engrained in male sociability. Lauren Working argues that the Inns of Courts were places where elite young men in Jacobean London learned how to converse with civility and wit, made friends and allies for their future political careers, and learned to smoke tobacco. All of these behaviors were part of an integrated project that shaped these young men into a colonizing political elite in a city that had recently become a capital, not just of England but of an Atlantic empire as well.[106]

The connection between tobacco and friendship persisted and was not confined to England. In 1700, the anonymous French author of *The good use of powdered tobacco* quoted another writer who observed that both coffee and snuff were "admirable inventions for filling the gaps in conversation." When one tired of talking or of listening, they allowed for the taking of a breath before starting again.[107] At the end of the eighteenth century, the Spanish physician Antonio Lavedán remarked that tobacco fostered courtesy, causing people to say, "God bless you," to snuff takers who sneezed, as well as creating a need for people constantly to be asking each other for tobacco.[108] The Italian physician Giovanni Piccino had even more glowing words for tobacco's effects on human relationships in 1635: "You perfect friendship, effect peace, forbid enmity," and make all of human experience better.[109]

More commonly, critics disapproved of tobacco's effects on male sociability. John Deacon accused tobacco of encouraging "carowsing and quaffing" and "excessive and riotous banqueting" in England, among other "foule and shamefule disorders."[110] In his 1616 dialogue, *Tobacco tortured; or, the filthie fume of tobacco refined*, a character wonders about smokers, "our carousing companions, who so viciously, so vainely, and so wildly do use the inward taking of filthie Tobacco fumes, as an intoxicating poyson to make themselves, and other their swaggering associations more dangerously wilde and mad with the venimous and deadly contagion thereof?"[111] Around the same time, Joshua Sylvester contrasted churches, colleges, and courts—places that were inappropriate for smoking—to the theaters, brothels, and gambling houses where tobacco made itself home amid "Blasphemers, Ruffians, Atheists" and "Damn'd Libertines."[112] Like gin much later, as soon as tobacco arrived in England it disordered orderly sites of sociability and, further, found itself in disorderly ones, making them even more disorderly.

A vein of thought appeared in Spain that smoking and snuff were so physically disgusting that its use menaced civil order. The physician Leiva Aguilar focused on its disgusting qualities, complaining that "it is against ethics or the doctrine of moral virtues, and against civic and urbane life, which teaches, and obligates one to keep one's modesty, and clothe oneself in cleanliness and interact without troubling others." Leiva Aguilar stated that to live among people, unlike a monk, one has to behave with others in mind, "because God created man as a social animal, and a companion, or partner, and what partner would one be who . . . causes disgust or discomfort?"[113] Writing one year later, the Spanish friar Tomás Ramón agreed: "This frequent use of tobacco is against all urbanity and humane practice." Going around all day grimacing while stuffing filth into the face with one's fingers and then expelling it through sneezing and drooling was extremely rude.[114] This criticism found adherents in both Britain and the Netherlands. The anonymously authored *Tobaco-mastix or thee common use of that weed in all the wayes of preparing it* complained that the stench of tobacco and the faces made by those who used it "is a Treason and inexpiable breach against all the Royal Laws of Civility."[115] *Tobaco-mastix* attacked tobacco in a way more commonly associated with coffeehouses: "That Drinking, Swearing, Lying, Whooring, Mischievous Plotting, Nastiness, botches and Bubo's, idleness, Backbiting and coyning of News, as interest carries, are the attending evils, and devils-guardian to Nicotian (for a great part) all will acknowledge, but he that is drunk with its venim."[116] Like coffee, tobacco brought people together and encouraged them both in vice and the unpoliced exchange of (mis)information. In 1692 the Dutch physician J. I. W. Beintema van Peima categorized tobacco use as a kind of drunkenness, which was a common criticism in the Netherlands, and likewise argued that the dirty nature of tobacco ruined normal human social life. "Tobacco gatherings," he wrote," are usually but practice-schools of idleness, back-slapping, slander, and thievery."[117] The Jacobite journalist Nathaniel Mist was one of many others who connected coffeehouses with smoking, gossiping, and news-mongering. He included a satirical letter in his journal feigning outrage that a French observer called the English people idle, "because they spend half their time in taking Tobacco," in coffeehouses, "seeing how the World stands, and settling the Affairs of the Nation."[118]

Sugar: Sad Partners in the Sinful Act

Whether they welcomed it or reviled it, observers noticed how tobacco bent sociability around itself. Whether they believed that tobacco encouraged friendship or broke the bonds of civility, observers could all agree that it affected social life in profound ways. This was true of the other drugs as well, although there was not as much commentary surrounding chocolate, sugar, or opium. Most notably, the boycott against slave sugar in late eighteenth-century England, when sugar had found its way into the pantries of all but the poorest families in England, encouraged a reordering of social ties, and, again, as with tea and gin, it was women who were the focus of the changes. In *An address to the people of Great Britain, on the propriety of refraining from the use of West India sugar and rum*, William Fox pointed to the corrosive effects of slavery on normal human social life, contending that "in every pound of sugar used, the produce of slaves imported from Africa, we may be considered as . . . tearing parents from their families, and children from their parents; breaking every bond of society, and destroying every source of human happiness."[119] Forgoing sugar from the Caribbean allowed women to sidestep Parliament, act as moral agents, and safeguard the ties of family in Africa.

The boycott also reoriented the moral community that formed around the tea table. Activists encouraged women to reflect on the tensions between the way that tea, and, with it, sugar, fostered the domestic life of their families in England while destroying social life in Africa and the African diaspora. Reformers had been trying to tame the tea table by expelling gossip, alcohol, and conversations about (or actual occasions for) illicit sex. By the end of the eighteenth century, they had succeeded in making the tea table into a setting for domestic conversation, a space for the family and for friends close enough to be treated as family members where dissention was discouraged.[120] Introducing imperial affairs and debating the moral value of teatime was a disruptive and intentional breach of those conventions, and all the more powerful for being so. Antislavery activists writing to encourage abstention from Caribbean sugar denounced women who purchased it as "sad partners, in the sinful act" of chattel slavery and the slave trade.[121] The boycotters were trying to upend what had become accepted as a normal and acceptable ceremony in order create a new moral community centered around the ethical consumption of sugar, just as the defenders of tea had done decades before.

False Politeness, Misdirected Kindness, Good Humor, and Sociality

The new stimulants changed social life: they attacked the old sites, ceremonies, and articles of consumption that fostered sociability while creating ones. The coffeehouse, the tea table, and the dram shop replaced the tavern with its beer and wine, and, later, the new tea table that abstained from West Indian sugar replaced the old one now reframed as immoral. Tobacco, meanwhile, changed and intensified the social behavior of the tavern and coffeehouse and introduced its own new methods of socializing that revolved around smoking and snuff. In short, the new drugs bent sociability around their use, attacking older manners either implicitly or explicitly. After self-reflection, Charles Lamb was able to see how this affected his own life, but he was not the only one who commented on the way that intoxicants reshaped social life. As early as 1615, the Puritan poet, pamphleteer, and satirist George Wither complained in a poem that tobacco had insinuated itself into everyday polite chitchat:

> Now it is as common at each meeting,
> As how d' yee, or God save yee for a greeting;
> Hee's no good fellow that's without the Pox,
> Burnd pipes, Tobacco, and his Tinder-boxe.

Even those who did not smoke still carried tobacco, Wither remarked, to share with others.[122] Lawrence Spooner, in chronicling how he fell back into smoking after abstaining for twenty years, explained that after a grave illness his wife persuaded him to smoke a little as a medicine to help him get his strength back. He did so, but a desire to be pleasing to his companions and smoke with them caused him to slide from medicinal use of tobacco to regular heavy smoking. Once he had begun smoking sociably, he found more and more occasions to do so:

> And if I did but chance to meet my Friend,
> The Pipes were call'd for, then to work we went,
> Till one or two apiece were idly spent.
> Then part with that Friend, and strait meet another,
> A Neighbour, Kinsman, or an only Brother;
> And then the same again, the Pipe and Pot.[123]

Tobacco even changed one's social relationship with one's own self. As Antonio Lavedán observed, snuff, taken from time to time while going around alone, alleviated loneliness.[124] As Marcy Norton has pointed out, tobacco fostered a kind of companionship with oneself.[125]

Most famously, coffeehouses wound sociability around itself by creating new spaces for new associations of like-minded men to form. The *Memoirs of the Bedford Coffee-house, by a genius* recalled how like other coffeehouses it served as a information-gathering site for political, financial, and foreign news, but, due to its location at the piazza in Covent Garden, it served especially as a meeting place for actors and their followers.[126] This type of specialization was not unique to London. Étienne-François Bazot composed a satire on the cafes of Paris in the years after Napoleon's downfall in which he was able to map out the social geography of the city by naming the cafés in each neighborhood, their clientele, and the things they discussed and read. Aristocrats gathered at the Café Valois at the Palais Royal, talking of their adventures in war and exile during the revolution and reading the *Outidienne*, the *Gazette de France*, and the *Journal des Débats*, among other periodicals. Unemployed military officers congregated at the Café Lemblin, also at the Palais Royal, pitiably waiting for something to occupy their time—and so on.[127]

In the eighteenth century, gin was the ingestible that drew the most notice for bending sociability. *The tavern scuffle: or The club in an uproar*, whose author called himself "Slyboots Saynought," appeared in 1726 and featured a debate between a distiller and a brewer as to whether gin or beer was the better drink for England. The brewer complained that women encouraged each other in drinking gin: "The Mother teaches the Daughter, the Maid follows the Mistress, the Prentice learns of the Maid, and so the Game goes round." Tea was also a venue for drawing women into gin drinking: "Wherever the Tea-Kettle is, there the Dram-Bottle be."[128] Once the women were drinking gin, all normal social intercourse was ruined, and sexual license followed:

> Go along the Streets, and you shall see every Brandy Shop swarming with scandalous Wretches, swearing and drinking as if they had no Notion of a future State; there they get Drunk by Day-Light, and after that run up and down the Streets swearing, cursing, and talking Beastliness like so many Devils; setting ill Examples, and debauching our Youth in general: Nay, to such a heighth are they arrived in their Wickedness, that in a manner, they commit Lewdness in the open Streets; young Creatures, Girls of 12 and 13 Years of Age, drink Geneva like Fishes, and make themselves unfit to live in sober Families; this damn'd bewitched Liquor makes them Shameless, and they talk enough to make a Man shudder again. . . . This fills our common Fellows with lewd Notions, and filthy Diseases; and to maintain these Trulls, some Rascals starve their Families, others go a Thieving, and stick at no Wickedness to go on in their riotous way of Life.[129]

Gin entered poor women's social networks and then made them into prostitutes, bending women's behavior around its pursuit.

Even the British government's attempts to curb gin led to disordered social relations. For its enforcement, the 1736 Gin Act relied on paying people to report neighbors whom they suspected of selling gin without the proper license.[130] Not only did the Gin Act fail in its aims, merely forcing the sale of gin underground and steering the profits away from honest taxpayers to criminals, but, by encouraging informants, it disordered neighborliness. This at least was the claim of one social critic, the anonymous author of *A short history of the Gin Act*: "Former Friendships have been forfeited; old Acquaintance sacrificed; all Obligations forgot; and the very Ties of Nature have been without avail, when they stood in the way of a Wretch's Design to gain one sordid Guinea."[131] *A short history* told story after sad story of honest people betrayed by those they trusted, such as a father and son, both victualers, who had treated one particular customer with great kindness, giving him free meals and letting him stay at their houses, only to have him encourage them to serve him gin and then turn around and report them to the magistrate.[132] Government-encouraged informing created an anti-community, dissolving the normal bonds of neighbor and family for gain, rewarding criminals for persecuting honest men, and allowing the dishonest to ruin the reputations of the neighborly and helpful. People who claimed to be ill and begged shopkeepers to sell them illegal gin as medicine played an especially conspicuous role in the *Short history*.[133]

Another sign of the power of stimulants in the early modern period to reorient social life around them was the plea by those who, in trying to break people away from one or another of them, to stop consorting with other users. The Anglican priest, scientist, and temperance advocate Stephen Hales warned in 1734 that people trying to avoid gin "must carefully avoid the Company of Dram-Drinkers . . . avoid such Company . . . shun such Conversation; for if once we give Ground and comply, we are lost; the Sin will, by little and little, prevail upon us, as it did on them."[134] In "A letter to a friend, concerning tea," in which John Wesley tried to encourage tea drinkers to stop, he parried some their potential objections. One excuse was "I can't bare to give Trouble," indicating the way that tea had become engrained in the social landscape of England.[135] It was so unimaginable to live a normal social life without tea that refusing it was thought to be offensive. Wesley advised his reader as a last resort to just pour milk and water in one's cup while serving others tea. The English Presbyterian minister Thomas Hall admonished his readers to shun drunkards and especially to avoid alehouses, where the devil tempted men to become intoxicated on both alcohol and tobacco.[136] Social ties led to distilled spirits, which in turn bent social life toward itself in a vicious cycle. Hales, Wesley, and Hall all feared how difficult it would be to extract oneself from the social ties that promoted the consumption of stimulants. Charles Lamb certainly would have agreed, having fallen into habitual drunkenness twice, thanks to two different sets of friends.

Tea, distilled spirits, and the rest of the early modern drugs were too deeply entwined in western European social manners to avoid easily. Consider the journal that the Scots writer James Boswell kept when he visited London as a young man in 1762, hoping to make his future. In it he recorded his social engagements and tended to note what people drank. Tea was the normal refreshment whenever he met a social equal or superior, as with his genteel friend from Scotland, Lady Betty Macfarlane, although punch was sometimes served, or wine. He sometimes went to coffeehouses to meet his peers, either for tea or coffee. When he went slumming, beer was on the menu, as when he visited a "low inn" before attending a cockfight as part of a day he spent pretending to be English. He also treated some sentries with whom he chatted at Buckingham Palace to pints of beer, and he once met an impoverished man while taking a meal at an alehouse and paid for his meal. Each social setting had its own corresponding drink. Perhaps most revealing of all, while pursuing the actress whom he called Louisa, they drank tea together, and sometimes with her brother as well. But when he tried to arrange a meeting in which he planned to have sex with her, she asked, "What? to drink a dish of tea, Sir?" He replied, "'No, no, not to drink a dish of tea.' (Here I looked sheepish.)"[137] Just as *The debauched and enchanted coffee- and tea-world* warned, women and tea drinking slipped easily from harmlessness to sexual license.

For Boswell each different social situation called for a different stimulant, and he was unusual only because he included such great detail in his diaries as he cataloged the social geography of his drug use. Tea and all of the other new soft drugs were inseparable from sociability. New users learned to consume them through existing social ties. Use of the new exotic drugs then threatened the old rituals and ceremonies of alehouse and tavern, which was exciting to some and intimidating and strangely novel to others. Defenders of the tea table attempted to rescue its reputation by disciplining the behavior and speech that occurred there. The new soft drugs needed this kind of discipline, as western Europeans needed to decide which times, places, and people were permitted for the consumption of the new drugs. Just as inns, taverns, and alehouses provided the setting and rituals for the proper use of beer and wine, tea and its fellow newly arrived stimulants needed new rituals and ceremonies in order to conquer critics' ambivalence about the disruption of previously settled norms around drinking. While the defenders of coffee and tea successfully established new settings, gin and sugar were more problematic. The consumption of distilled spirits by the poor in the streets remained contentious until the emergence of gin palaces in the nineteenth century, and sugar faced attacks during the antislavery campaigns in Britain beginning in the late eighteenth century. As new norms emerged, users stumbled their way toward inventing the necessary rituals and ceremonies of consumption: what to discuss and what not to at the tea table, who was permitted in the coffeehouse, how to share snuff and smoking tobacco, and whether to serve one's guests slave or free sugar.

Even while the new drugs became increasingly popular, the ambivalence about the ways that they reoriented social life around their use continued. One great source of that ambivalence was the use of the new drugs by women. No matter how conduct-books urged women to behave at the tea table, critics saw it simply as a forum for malicious gossip and sexual license. Perhaps at the root of the unease was simply women engaging in conversation unpoliced by their superiors—similar to the coffeehouse, but with the fears concentrated on domestic disorder and sexual license rather than political and religious unrest. On the other hand, perhaps the tea table (and, for the nonelite, the dram shop) was as exciting for some women as the coffeehouse was for men, not only for the effects of the new stimulant but also for the possibilities for the exchange and creation of knowledge.

If men did not see women as rational actors, or their conversations as productive generators of social knowledge, neither did Habermas (except in supporting roles, as the hostesses of Parisian salons). Somewhat justifiably, his treatment of the public sphere ignored women, but it also overlooked their ability to produce knowledge in their own emerging domestic sphere, as well as their ability to police themselves through politeness. Nor was the coffeehouse the only site of drug consumption needing new rules to guide social interaction. The tea table, taverns, the dram shop, private parties where rum punch or chocolate were served—all of these places created new communities with their own rituals and ceremonies to govern behavior. More research would undoubtedly show that dram shops, and cartmen and women hawking gin in the streets, created their own sphere of self-regulated interaction and conversation, as a few satirists suggested. Unlike Habermas, historians today should take seriously women, their social networks, their knowledge production, and their drugs.

Chapter 6

Who Should Poison the People?

The Ethics of Commerce

In 1753 William Henry, an Anglican priest in Ireland, published *An earnest address to the people of Ireland, against the drinking of spirituous liquors,* in which he criticized gin distillers as a threat to the nation even more dangerous than the Jacobite Rebellion eight years earlier. Henry condemned distillers for using grain and potatoes as the basis for their liquor, thereby taking food away from the people. Bad harvests threatened Ireland with famine every four or five years, he explained, and if it were not for the importation of foodstuffs from Britain and America, the Irish would die. Yet distillers, "these Grave-diggers, these Cannibals, these Man-eaters, who prey upon the very vital Blood of their Country, will not lay it to Heart!"[1] Distillers thrived by consuming Ireland's grain to make gin, at the expense of their fellow countrymen.

Decades earlier, when the Gin Craze was first beginning, another Anglican clergyman, Edward Chandler, the bishop of Coventry and Lichfield, gave a sermon to the Society of the Reformation of Manners at St. Mary-le-Bow, London. In it he attacked the "Strong-Water-Shops" that sold gin, lamenting their ubiquity in the city, and the consequences for Londoners of the inundation of gin. "They are multiplied into such Numbers," he wrote, "and distributed into such convenient distances for the destruction of lives and corruption of the manners of the lower people, in all parts of the town. . . . More of the common people dye of consumptions, fevers, dropsies, cholicks, palsies, apoplexies contracted by the immoderate use of brandies, and distilled waters, than of all other distempers beside."[2] While the Gin Craze has attracted historians' attention mostly for the way that moralists heaped scorn upon the poor, especially women, for indulging in disorder and vice through consuming gin, Henry objected to the producers, and Chandler objected to the vendors, men who profited from spreading hunger, disease, vice, and misery among the working classes. "It is thus the Patrons of Debauchery," Chandler continued, "do cater for the pleasures of the unenterprising sinners."[3] Further, most critics focused on England, especially London, the epicenter of the Gin Craze, but Henry was concerned with Ireland, and both he and Chandler expressed their anxiety in patriotic rhetoric, concerned that by wreaking havoc among the working classes gin threatened the entire nation's safety and wellbeing, rendering profit-seeking distillers and retailers treasonous. Men like Henry and Chandler pioneered a new strategy against vice, attacking the manufacturers and vendors of liquor for profiting off their own people's immiseration, an approach that, as Mark Lawrence Schrad demonstrates, would become standard practice for moral reformers in later centuries.[4]

Henry and Chandler's jeremiads went against the grain of some of the most influential thinkers of the eighteenth century, who lauded the growth of commerce as a civilizing and benevolent force. At a time when western Europe experienced economic growth, a rise in global trade, and the early beginnings of industrial capitalism, writers from Bernard Mandeville to Adam Smith tended to pull these trends together into a celebration of what can be called "commercial society," or, as the Baron de Montesquieu labeled it, *doux commerce* ("sweet, gentle commerce").[5] There were even some who praised gin and its sister drugs, reasoning that they helped spur a Smithian virtuous cycle of increasing wealth and industriousness, benefiting the national economy, despite the ill effects they might have on some individual consumers. But there were two major objections to this optimistic view. First, some asked, like Henry and Chandler, whether their production and sale created commodity chains connecting consumers and producers alike to evils like slavery, debauchery, and national ruin. The boycott of slave sugar relied on this reasoning, tying those who enjoyed sugar, tea, coffee, and chocolate to plantation slavery and the transatlantic slave trade. Second, many critics suspected that the temptation of the new soft drugs, and the addictive sociability that they created around them, pulled men and women away from their work, creating sites of anti-industriousness like the tea table, coffeehouse, tavern, and dram shop, that eroded a disciplined use of time and labor dragging down the national economy. Was it ethical to produce such drinks at all? These issues surrounded the new soft drugs in western Europe, but gin provides an excellent entry point, because, while the slave sugar boycott is the most well studied, Henry and Chandler point to a similar attempt to blame gin distillers and vendors for profiting at the expense of the nation decades before antislavery became a popular cause.

The new psychotropic drugs forced Europeans to examine whether commercial society was good, whether those who consumed a product were responsible for the conditions of its production, and whether increasing consumption made people work more or less. These issues cut to the heart of the economic changes taking place in seventeenth- and eighteenth-century western Europe and the supposed increase in self-discipline that accompanied the growth of a capitalist economy. There was no general agreement on these matters, and gin and its sister drugs highlighted observers' profound ambivalence about commercial society. The drugs were not only symbols of global capitalism, but also drivers of its growth, since commodity chains featuring the manufacture, transportation, and sale of drugs sprawled from Europe across the globe. Early modern psychotropic drugs forced Europeans to confront the ethics of commerce during the earliest stages of global capitalism.

Daniel Lord Smail has pointed out that Max Weber's insistence that the birth of capitalism rested on self-denial was wrong, and that in fact a consumer revolution driven by self-serving hedonism fueled the growth of the early modern economy.[6] Drugs and alcohol played an increasingly important role in this growth as well as in the tax revenues of the growing early modern state. If one accepts that consumers used the drugs to regulate their own mental and physical state of wellness and to orient their sociability, then both capitalism and the modern state were built in part on the emotional and social needs of western Europeans.

Of all the chapters in this book, this one will be the most focused on the English experience because the Gin Craze made gin more of a moral issue there than elsewhere. But distilled spirits, and the moral issues they raised, were everywhere. In 1698 the English physician Martin Lister noted that that, in Paris, "there is no Feasting without the Drinking at the desert all sorts of Strong Waters." They had become fashionable among elite men out on campaign during the wars of Louis XIV and then brought back to Paris, where they helped both men and women "become fat and corpulent."[7] Throughout western Europe the new exotic drugs became integrated into trade, production, retail sale, and taxation, while outside Europe explorers and botanists scoured the globe in a race to find useful commercial and pharmaceutical products, tying the production of knowledge about the natural world to medicine, commerce, and state power.[8]

Whether Our Own Manufacture Shall Supply Us and Our Own People Employ'd?

In Western Europe, distilled spirits were widely produced and sold in western Europe by the early eighteenth century. Europeans had learned to distill alcohol from their Muslim neighbors during the Middle Ages, although at first it was rare and expensive, more the stuff of alchemy than commerce. By at least the thirteenth century, however, distilled spirits had entered the European pharmacopoeia as aqua vitae. By the sixteenth century brandy, from the Dutch *brandewijn* or "burnt wine," was becoming cheap enough for recreational use, and it was common enough in German-speaking lands to be regulated, mostly to protect beer and wine vendors from competition.[9] In the seventeenth century, distillers in non-wine-growing regions began to use grain to make gin and whiskey and to turn molasses and other byproducts of sugar production into rum. Commercial production began to grow considerably, and the sales of fortified wines like madeira, sherry, and port increased throughout the Atlantic world.[10] Gin came into prominence in the London market after 1689, when the new king, William III of Orange, brought England into conflict with France, shutting down imports of French brandy. The English began importing gin from the Netherlands instead that took its name from the Dutch *genever*, after the juniper berries that were added for taste. Soon England had developed its own commercial distilling industry, and English gin production rose from half a million gallons in 1688 to more than two and a half million by 1720.[11]

The Gin Craze soon followed, from roughly 1720 to 1751, and, as Jessica Warner explains, the moral panic over poor Londoners drinking gin formed only a rough match with the actual rise in gin consumption. Gin production was rising well before 1720, doubling from almost half a gallon of gin consumed per person per year in 1700, and began falling before 1751, peaking in the 1740s at 1.3 gallons per person per year. Parliament passed several laws trying to regulate the production

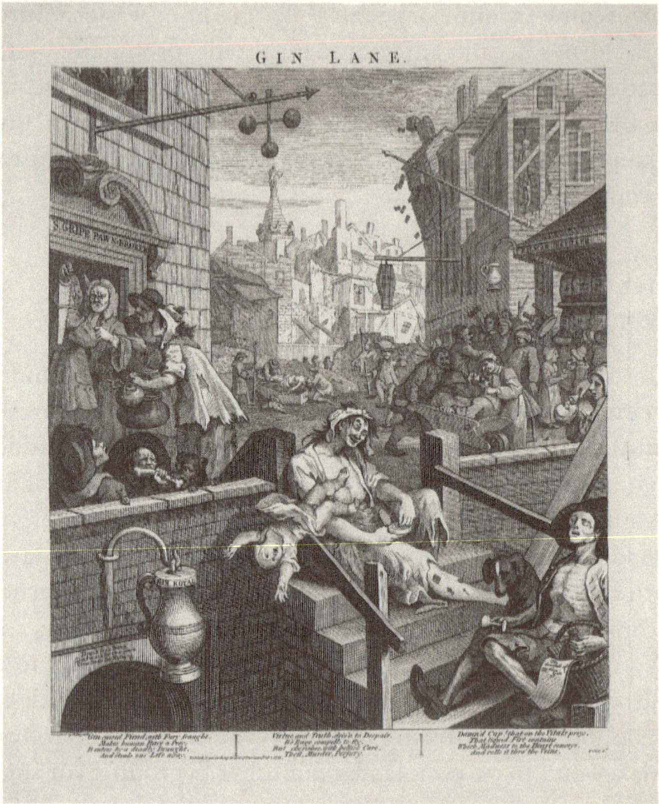

Figure 6.1. William Hogarth, *Gin Lane*, 1751. Hogarth's print depicts the way in which gin created gross disorder among the London working classes, especially among women. In addition to economic ruin, all healthy sociability is destroyed, with riot, poverty, and neglect taking its place. Reproduced courtesy of the British Museum.

and sale of gin, taxing it and demanding a license to distill, but by the 1740s the British government had abandoned the goal of social control in favor of encouraging the sale of gin to pay for the War of the Austrian Succession. The willingness of the government to drop its attempts to curb gin drinking suggests that it was not so much gin, but the unprecedented growth of London, with thousands of poor men and women pouring in from the countryside every year into slums, with no ties to family or neighbors to discipline their behavior, that most alarmed the authorities.[12] Indeed the consumption of beer, ale, and wine had also risen in seventeenth-century England, and taverns and alehouses drew increasing concern as sites of disorder.[13] Because there was no professional police force in London (or anywhere) in the eighteenth century, the laws relied on neighbors informing on each other, which led to riots and increased disorder. As both its consumption and government scrutiny waned in the late eighteenth century, gin gained respectability, along with rum, whisky, and other distilled liquors, and in the nineteenth century cocktail culture helped rehabilitate its social standing, including the malaria-fighting gin and tonic.[14]

During the late seventeenth and eighteenth centuries, just as distilled liquor became commercially viable, market forces were infiltrating into more and more aspects of the lives of Europeans, shifting from physical sites of exchange located in towns and cities into a metaphor governing a society in which everyone bought and sold things, including labor, from and to everyone else. The increasing salience of market-oriented thinking and behavior attracted enormous attention from commentators like Smith, who claimed that by the eighteenth century people were so dependent on the market to provide for their own material needs that every man had become a merchant, exchanging goods or his labor with others.[15] Smith and many other Enlightenment figures celebrated commercial society for its civilizing tendencies, believing that the market fostered politeness and liberalism. Markets, after all, brought people together peacefully to make mutually beneficial deals and contracts, in contrast to the coercive tyranny of absolutist governments and the established churches that Enlightenment philosophes deplored. As the Dutch-English physician Bernard Mandeville put it in 1714 in *The fable of the bees: or, private vices, publick benefits*, the vice of selfishness indirectly helped the public welfare and expanded the economy. Tradesmen and merchants did not provide goods and services out of an altruistic desire to help their fellow men, but from a selfish desire for gain. Mandeville's praise of self-interest cut against a centuries-old tradition of moral condemnation of luxury consumption as a vice that corrupts society. Commercial society still had its critics, like Jean-Jacques Rousseau, who argued that Mandeville and his followers simply glorified the old vice of luxury. Commercial society also degraded men by making them dependent on others for their own subsistence, Rousseau contended, eroding a manly form of autonomy and freedom. Having everyone act as merchants led to insincerity, exploitation, individualism, and selfishness. Luxury engendered greed and envy, corrupting the manners, social relations, and ethics of all those involved in the market. Historians who have chronicled this debate have ignored the gin industry, unable to hear the voices of those like Henry and Chandler who pointed out how commerce could also profit from spreading vice, misery, and death.[16]

Supporters of commercial society could argue that the manufacture, importation, sale, and taxation of stimulants promoted the broader goals of furthering commerce and civilization. In his preface to *The use of coffee, tea, and chocolate*, Philippe Sylvestre Dufour explained that divine providence had distributed "certain plants and drugs to some countries, which she has denied to others; so that she might better promote mutual commerce between all nations, and better cement civil society together."[17] Coffee, tea, and chocolate fit into the emerging Enlightenment idea that doux commerce civilized both consumers and sellers while also increasing the wealth of every country. In 1700 William King noted that the use of psychotropic drugs spurred virtuous cycles of consumption that helped the economy grow: "I have been told, Coffee hath greatly encreased the Trade of Tobacco and Pipes, Earthen Dishes, Tin Wares, News Papers, Coals, Candles, Sugar, Tea, Chocolate, and what not?"[18] James Bland observed much the same thing later in the century while defending tea drinking as an innocent or even beneficial pastime for women: "The Tea-Table is a Promoter of several Trades, nay, I may venture to say, almost all Trades in General." Not only did all men benefit by the friendships, cemented with tea, that their wives made with tradesmen, merchants, and their own wives, but grocers also benefited through the sale of tea itself and sugar, while "the Silver-Smith and Copper-Smith must be employed, and so must the China-Man, and Joyner. The Coal Trade is augmented thereby; and those that sell Snuff are never the worse, the Milliners get by it, and no one can make it appear that any Employment is worse for it."[19] To these men, sugar, tea, chocolate, and coffee were part of the alchemy that turned the private vice of luxury into the public benefit of increased common wealth, creating opportunities for those catering to the tastes of the consuming public.

Even Mandeville himself, one of the most important prophets of commercial society, used similar logic to defend gin. In a commentary he wrote after his initial publication of *The fable of the bees* in 1714, he acknowledged that "nothing is more destructive, either in regard to the health or the vigilance and industry of the poor, than the infamous liquor." Gin spread misery, squalor, poverty, and death, both among its drinkers and the small-time retailers who sold it to their neighbors in London's slums. But, Mandeville assured his readers, gin increased the wealth of England as a whole, providing a large portion of the royal revenue in taxes, propping up land rents, and raising the demand for tools, cattle for tilling, "and above all, the multitude of poor that are maintained, by the variety of labour, requited in husbandry, in malting, in carriage and distillation." Taking this broader view enabled the observer to "see good spring up . . . from evil."[20] Similarly, Dufour, King, and Bland demonstrated the two lines of argument used to defend the consumption of the new drugs: first, that they helped create wealth instead of wasting it, and, second, as wealth-creators they fell into the category of the "new luxuries," which promoted virtue instead of vice.

Traditionally, luxury goods were associated with aristocrats adorning themselves and their surroundings, at court or in their rural residences, with imported goods like spices, silks, and fur that served to distinguish themselves physically and visually from the nonelite. Of course the rhetoric of luxury was one way that early modern commentators could explain what today is called "addiction." In the late seventeenth and eighteenth centuries, however, a new idea of luxury emerged, associated with cities, the domestic sphere, women, and comfort. The new luxuries engaged the senses—the feeling of silk and cotton, the smell and taste of tea, coffee, chocolate, and tobacco. Instead of demarking social rank, luxuries brought the elite and middling classes together, both groups now sharing the same taste. The impulse to tame coffee and tea through the new social codes of politeness acted to domesticate the new luxuries. Moreover, consumers used luxury goods to create new identities for themselves as polite, educated, urbane consumers of taste, perhaps suffering together from nervous disorders from the elegant anxieties of sophisticated society.[21] In fact, the new exotic drugs were so different from the traditional understanding of luxury and were becoming so widely used that one could argue that they were not luxuries at all. One anonymous author defending sugar, for example, argued that

> Necessaries, what he cannot well exist without; what is absolutely necessary, not only to his Being, but to his Well-being: I reply, in this Sense, Sugar is, by Custom, now become a Necessary. . . . And such a kind of Necessary, in England, among the Females, are Tea and Sugar, by Custom, become, as Snow [for cooling drinks] is in Naples. You cannot hire a common Maid Servant, to do all Work, but expects her Tea. . . . In short, Tea, and consequently Sugar, are now become so much Necessaries of Life, that I believe there are very few poor Men in the Kingdom, but sensibly feel the extravagant advance of Sugar.[22]

It was not just British political economists who championed the new luxuries. In Milan Pietro Verri published "Considerations on luxury" in his periodical, *Il caffé*, supporting the idea that luxury consumption was not a vice but a virtue because it promoted economic growth.[23] The physician Michele Nicolò Chiazzari justified writing about tobacco in 1819 by observing that, while it was unknown to Europeans just a few centuries earlier, it had now spread all the way to Russia, and for everyone, rich and poor, "it is a pleasure, or rather a need."[24]

This logic could even be used to blunt the assault on slave sugar. In the 1790s the anonymous author of *A vindication of the use of sugar, the produce of the West-India islands* argued that although slavery was immoral, its abolition would not be possible for many years "without incurring greater evils than those of slavery itself" because of Britain's great need for sugar. "Sugar has been called a superfluity," he wrote. "Undoubtedly at its first introduction it was so. But the constitution, from long habits of luxury, becomes so much changed as to render that at last necessary, which originally owed its introduction to caprice and effeminacy. . . . The artificial wants of polished society are scarcely less necessary to be provided for than the claims of rude, uncultivated nature."[25] Britain was so entrenched in its sophisticated, commercial ways that the effect of removing sugar from the diet of its people would be worse, according to this writer, than plantation slavery. Not everyone concurred: one anonymous writer countered that "if the Universality of any customary Luxury was to make us consider such Luxury as a Necessary of Life, why not admit Dram-drinking, Gaming, and other debaucheries by the same rule? . . . Tea and Sugar are Luxuries, not Necessaries, and it is, perhaps, a misfortune to Society that they are so cheap as to make them universal."[26]

The production and sale of stimulants also received crucial support from an important source that sometimes aligned with, and at other times contradicted, those who championed commercial society: mercantilist economic ideas. Mercantilism, more commonly called "cameralism" outside of Britain, was not a unified theory and still less a unified set of practices.[27] It was a collection of impulses and projects designed to increase exports, decrease imports, secure a favorable flow of specie, and dominate international shipping, all in the service of amplifying a country's common wealth and individual prosperity. Mercantilist writers can be said to have invented the concept of "the economy" as an interlocking exchange of goods and services inside a political boundary. Epitomized by the projects of Jean-Baptiste Colbert, who oversaw the financial and economic policies of Louis XIV's France in the late seventeenth century, mercantilist theorists and actors were not opponents of free markets, as laissez-faire opponents stereotyped them. But they did believe that markets needed more state intervention than writers like Mandeville and his successors believed, especially to protect domestic manufacturing against foreign imports. Mercantilist instincts survived through the eighteenth century, intermingling with ideas that promoted the free markets of the ideal commercial society, both of them trying to maximize a country's wealth. As much as mercantilism aimed to increase the wealth of the country, it also aimed to increase the revenue and power of the state.[28] James I of England provided an early example of the power of mercantilist thinking on drugs and alcohol when, shortly after publishing his *Counterblaste to tobacco*, the Crown's regulatory regime shifted toward encouraging the growth of tobacco production in the Chesapeake and sale in England to encourage Virginia's economic survival. Early modern governments maintained a limited ability to monitor and intercede in economic activity, but they possessed an insatiable appetite for income. Imports like tobacco, chocolate, coffee, tea, and sugar arrived at ports that provided convenient choke points and therefore became easy targets for tax collectors. By the time of the reign of James's son Charles I, tobacco had become such a noteworthy contributor to royal revenue that there could be no thought of banning its use, as James had wanted, and indeed the English Crown tamped down on farming tobacco in England itself in order to funnel the demand for the weed through ports and royal customs, where it was more easily taxed.[29]

Mercantilist logic provided a powerful weapon for those who supported the sale of the new stimulants. During the Gin Craze, Daniel Defoe defended distillers by reframing the issue around the promotion of domestic manufacturers. Faced with the accusation that gin debauched the poor while depriving them of bread, he replied that "the Question does not seem to lie here, Whether the spirits shall be distill'd and consum'd among us, and whether the Poor shall drink them? But, Whether the Dutch shall furnish us with them, and cheat and impose upon us . . . or whether our own Manufacture shall supply us, our own Growth be consum'd and our own People employ'd?"[30] Defoe's concern for supporting domestic producers was entirely in keeping with post-1688 Whiggish political economy.[31] The objection that he was countering, that the diversion of grain to distilleries starved the poor, derives from what E. P. Thompson labeled the moral economy of precapitalist

Europe. Traditionally, the poor had a right to fair market prices to grain even in times of dearth, and the ruling class acknowledged their responsibility for maintaining low prices and punishing those who attempted to profit from the scarcity of grain. Opposed to this was a new idea, favored by the champions of commercial society, that the price of grain and bread should move up and down as supply and demand dictated, since a free market in grain would—eventually—produce more grain and eliminate famine and scarcity altogether.[32] "As for the Excesses and Intemperances of the People," Defoe wrote, "and their drinking immoderate Quantitys of Malt Spirits, the Distillers are not concern'd in it at all."[33] Making a quality product and selling it honestly was all that could be asked of distillers, like any other businessmen.[34] As another observer put it, even allowing that drunkenness was the worst vice, and that the most vicious drunkenness came from drinking spirits, "if Spirits are drank . . . why should not the Nation, which suffers so much in other Respects by this pernicious Practice, avail itself of it by a tax."[35] The pseudonymous Saynought Slyboots believed that criticizing gin was really just pleading on behalf of alehouses, who were losing customers to the new drink.[36] Meanwhile, the English government passed legislation imposing taxes and licenses on gin distillers eleven times between 1700 and 1771, hoping to reduce its consumption.[37]

In 1736 *An impartial enquiry into the present state of the British distillery* set its defense of distillers in the context of the entire array of stimulants for sale in England. The *Enquiry* conceded that gin encouraged immorality and disorder but thought that the economic gains from its production and sale outweighed the losses. Coffee, tea, and tobacco were all "pernicious" like gin, but unlike gin they sent specie out of Britain to pay for them. Moreover, gin was not unique in its destructive powers; beer and ale could also become bad for the working poor: "There is nothing but what the Vicious Inclinations of Man may abuse." Yet banning these drugs would cause more harm to the nation than good, destroying the livelihoods of thousands involved with "importing, Exporting, ending and Retailing" of the hot drinks and of sugar. Government intervention to safeguard public morality would be a mistake—or, as the author put it, "it may be an Experiment of Evil Consequence to a Trading People to attempt an Absolute prohibition of things of that nature." Especially bad for the economy would be banning gin, since distilleries were "more Useful to this Kingdom than the Mines of Peru, which only employs Slaves; and the possession thereof has drawn a people once the most considerable and formidable in the

World to a Wretched state of Indolance and Poverty: whereas the British Distillery, like a real Treasure" supported landowners, who paid most of the countries' taxes, as he put it, and sent wealth flowing through all the other tradesmen involved with its production and sale.[38] Likening the manufacture of a commodity to a gold mine was a common mercantilist trope, put to use here to defend the wealth created by distilling.[39]

Mercantilist ideas also encouraged the production of exotic drugs and other raw materials in one's own colonies to consume at home. Not having to import tobacco, for example, from a rival's colonies would limit the amount of specie flowing to one's rivals. This became more urgent as the wars between European powers increasingly incorporated blockades and economic warfare during the eighteenth century, culminating in the Napoleonic Wars. But these concerns began much earlier, as soon as chocolate and tobacco arrived from the Americas. In 1615 an English commentator complained about the poor quality and high price of tobacco from the Spanish Caribbean sold by Portuguese merchants in London. His plan was to cultivate the leaf in England, where there was indeed a tobacco-growing boom in southern England during the early seventeenth century.[40] Five years later Edward Bennett expressed his alarm that although English merchants should be bringing in hard currency from Spain for all the goods that they shipped there, instead they returned with nothing but Spanish tobacco. The French and Dutch managed to get silver for their exports, but the "Spaniard & al other Nations say tauntingly to us, when they see al our goods landed . . . that al wil be paid in smoak." Bennett called for a ban on importing tobacco into England, there being no other way to avoid the loss of silver, since "our people will buy it what soever it cost."[41] The Spanish Crown, too, benefited from tobacco, operating a monopoly on its sale in Castile from 1636, and it eventually became the single most important source of revenue for the royal government, exceeding even the silver that came from America's mines.[42] France also had a royal tobacco monopoly, and it depended on the tax revenues it extracted from tobacco imported from British America so much that the French Crown more or less killed off domestic production in France and even in the French colonies of Louisiana and Saint Domingue.[43] Italy, without colonies of its own, was left to try to cultivate tobacco in its own lands, as Niccolò Gavellli urged in 1748.[44]

Tea also had a rich history of taxes, smuggling, and mercantilist debate about how best to profit from its import, especially in Britain. The English and the Swedes tried to grow tea well enough to harvest it in

England, Sweden, and the Americas. All of these attempts failed, and not until the British began growing it in India would Europeans break the East Asian monopoly on tea.[45] As tea gained in popularity in Britain and its colonies, the economic fortunes of the English East India Company, and of the contributions that the EIC could make to the British state, became increasingly tied to tea's price and taxes. But as the taxes grew higher, the temptation for the Dutch and others to smuggle tea into Britain also grew, and contraband product accounted for more than half of all the tea consumed in the British empire in the eighteenth century.[46] A writer calling himself a "Man of Kent" published his idea for a solution to tea smuggling in 1756. He estimated that more than 1200 tons of tea were smuggled into the southeastern counties of England yearly, costing the government £195,000 per year, all to the benefit of the Dutch and French, "our Enemies in Trade and Navigation." (He also noted his satisfaction that the domestic production of gin had almost eliminated the smuggling of brandy from France.)[47] Nevertheless, despite initial success in leveraging the profits from tea into tax revenue for the British Crown at home and economic and political power for the East India Company in India, British governing authorities miscalculated the right balance of taxation and monopoly while trying to tighten its control of the North American colonies in the mid-eighteenth century, inadvertently blundering into the Boston Tea Party and the American Revolution.[48] Concerns like this were not unique to Britain; the anonymous Dutch author of *Speculative historical notes on today's new taxes on coffee, tea, chocolate, and other medicinal drinks* considered how the Netherlands should weigh the potential medical harms and benefits of tea and its fellow drugs on Dutch citizens with the revenues they could provide.[49]

Coffee and sugar elicited the same mix of concerns. At the end of the eighteenth century, Pierre Joseph Laborie, a refugee from the Haitian Revolution grateful to Britain for giving him a refuge, offered to teach his hosts how to develop coffee plantations in their Caribbean colonies, relieving Britain of the need to import coffee from other countries.[50] Meanwhile, back in the metropolis, French dependence on British colonial exports moved a writer who called himself "Monsieur C. de T" to recall in 1824 a German project to fight against the British, "the tyrants of the sea. Sugar and coffee have become needs, so to speak, everywhere, and they exhaust the specie of the nations which, having few or no colonies, are forced to purchase these commodities second hand." Discussing homegrown substitutes for sugar, tobacco, and, above all, coffee, he considered chicory, holly berries, almonds, horse chestnuts, and even a slurry made from potatoes.[51]

In 1700, after a hesitant recommendation of sugar as a healthy ingredient in foodstuffs, the English physician Thomas Tryon added an observation about its role in society. "How mightily Sugar advances the Kings Customs," he wrote, "not only in respect to the Imposts laid upon it self, but by occasioning many Foreign Commodities to be imported; which before our Sugar Settlements were not thought of," like chocolate, coffee, and tea.[52] As Tryon observed, sugar played a unique role boosting trade, manufacture, and government revenue connected to several interlocking stimulants. Even an antislavery article from 1775 in the Dutch newspaper The *Patriot* leaned on this kind of mercantilist thinking. The author castigated the imagined reader of the piece, "Alintera," a young lady drinking coffee with her lover. Not merely did her purchase of coffee and sugar condemn others to slavery in plantations across the Atlantic from their homes—the author wanted Alintera to imagine that she and her beau could be ripped away screaming from her house to be sold overseas—but everything about coffee consumption enriched foreigners and starved the Dutch poor, even the Saxon porcelain in her hand that she chose over homemade delftware or china imported by the Dutch East India Company.[53] Other commentators simply wanted more sugar produced in their own country's colonies without regard to the morality of plantation slavery, like Joseph-François Charpentier-Cossigny, who wrote a tract suggesting that the sugar, rum, and other colonial products that had been produced in Saint-Domingue before the Haitian Revolution could profitably be transferred to the French Indian Ocean colonies of Réunion and Ile de France.[54]

Opium was subject to the same mercantilist calculus of gain versus loss. In 1788 an anonymous southern Italian physician or apothecary wrote a tract suggesting that opium processed from poppies grown in Puglia could work just as well as opium from the Levant. He documented his attempts at gathering opium from the heads of local poppies and experimenting on local patients, finding Pugliese opium to be of higher quality than imports.[55] The quest for domestic sources of imported goods reached an even greater urgency just after this publication, as the French Revolution began, spurring global warfare that cut much of Europe off from foreign products intermittently for the next twenty-five years. Italians elsewhere promoted poppy cultivation for opium production in their own principalities, Tuscany and the Papal

States.[56] The same logic would later propel the English East India Company to foster the cultivation of poppies in English-held India for export to China, thus launching a century of friction between China and Europe, with the growing social problem of opium addiction in China leading to the two Opium Wars.[57]

Mercantilist writers believed that economic exchange was a zero-sum game, in which one party's gain was the other's loss. Champions of commercial society like Mandeville and Smith thought that both sides gained whenever there was a free exchange of good and services. But both wanted economic growth for their own countries, and both eagerly welcomed the production, sale, taxation, and consumption of soft drugs in early modern Europe and its colonies. Some recognized that there was a cost, both to individuals and to society, for the promotion of the new drugs. But many political economists believed that the benefits outweighed the cost, especially since the costs were scarcely avoidable—consumers would consume drugs and alcohol regardless, so the state and economy might as well profit from them. As Edward Chamberlayne proposed in 1667, England should raise heavy taxes "upon all such Commodities as occasion either Excess or Luxury, Wantonness, Idleness, Pride, or Corruption of Manners." Among these goods he included "all Wines, all strong Drinks, Tobacco, Coffee, Chocolatte, Sugars, Spices, Plums, all sorts of Sweet-meats, Orange, &c." in addition to other dry goods like silk, lace, ribbons, feathers, cards, dice, coaches, sedans, perfume, and cosmetics.[58] Either luxury would decrease, or government revenue would increase. There were still others who did not care at all for the damage early modern drugs and alcohol did so long as it furthered the economy.

The Most Wicked Saying in the World

By highlighting the connections between the consumption of drugs and their production and sale, backers of commercial society and of mercantilism were presaging a recent trend of modern historians: the commodity chain history. Historians have begun exploring the network of producers and middlemen who came together in complex webs to create finished consumer goods. They have traced the commodity chains of refined products such as madeira wine and mahogany furniture to the workers who made them, like enslaved woodcutters or entrepreneurial vintners.[59] These interconnecting links fascinated early modern observers of commercial society such as Smith, who introduced *The wealth of nations* with the example of a woolen coat, explaining how the labor of hundreds of men from all over the world combined to create it: shepherds, ship builders, coal miners, dye makers, tailors, and so on.[60] Contemporaries like Smith tended to view the links forged by commerce as a purely positive phenomenon, with doux commerce bringing people together to their mutual satisfaction. But historians have countered this optimistic eighteenth-century view with the knowledge that plantation slavery and the transatlantic slave trade constituted key links in many of these commodity chains. They point to the sugar boycotts of the late eighteenth century as the first turn against the sanguine view of trade, when anti-slave trade activists insistently drew the attention of sugar consumers—and of the drinkers of chocolate, coffee, and tea that sugar made palatable—to the human suffering that went into their creation.

The slave sugar boycott began when the English abolitionist William Fox published *An address to the people of Great Britain, on the propriety of refraining from the use of West India sugar and rum* in 1791. He did so at a time when the Haitian Revolution had all but stopped sugar imports from that French colony, sending demand for sugar, and enslaved workers, skyrocketing in the English colonies of Jamaica and Barbados. Fox's intervention came after decades of growing unease about consuming the products of slavery, beginning among North American Quakers like John Woolman, who linked slavery to the production of all the luxuries that became available during the expansion of commerce in the Atlantic World, and the broader corrupting influence that these luxuries caused.[61] Fox used the *Address* to highlight the processes that brought sugar to the tables of England in exactly the same way that Smith had for the wool coat, but, instead of celebrating it he emphasized that sugar consumers were responsible for setting in motion the enslavement of millions of Africans.[62] To historians, two things stand out about the anti-slave trade movement: first, that focus of the antislavery activists toward fell on women. Because they were increasingly responsible for the domestic sphere, and therefore in charge of food purchases, women were important participants in the slave sugar boycott—a fact celebrated by modern historians.[63] Second, the boycott has garnered attention as the first important new attack on the benignity of consumer society, different from the traditional attack on luxury or the critique by Rousseau, who believed that commercial society emasculated consumers and encouraged insincerity. Instead, the anti-slave trade campaign directly linked sugar users to the depravity of Atlantic slavery and the slave trade. Here they turned the tropes of Smith and the other defenders of commercial society on their head; rather than celebrate how the purchase of a woolen coat brought people from distant lands together in a community of prosperity and voluntary association, they underscored how sugar purchases created links of oppression, misery, and slavery.[64] Slave sugar gave the lie to Mandeville's famous quip that the private vice of greed led to public benefits; the gluttonous individual desire for sugar led instead to the immiseration of millions.

For example, in 1792, William Allen described the commodity chain of sugar, from the impressing of sailors to protect the slave ships to the Middle Passage to the plantations, using sensory language to portray it as "a chain of Wretchedness every link of which is stained with blood!"[65] One cannot claim, he asserted, that the individual consumer of sugar has a small portion of guilt compared to the whole system. "No plea whatever can diminish the Aggregate of Guilt by which the Slave Trade is distinguished—and it becomes us to say of every part of this system, and of every thing connected with it—Here's the smell of blood on the hand still" (paraphrasing the guilt-ridden Lady Macbeth), "and all the perfumes of Arabia cannot sweeten it."[66] Any true Christian must listen to duty, and, when presented with West Indian products, "turn indignant from the sight, and exclaim with David, upon an occasion not altogether dissimilar—My God forbid it me, that I should do this thing: shall I drink the blood of these men!"[67]

If sugar boycotters tried to make consumers feel responsible for the sins of producers, critics of the gin industry like Henry and Chandler used the commodity chain to show how producers and sellers were responsible for the ruin of the consumers. Like sugar, gin was an immensely profitable driver of capitalism as it emerged in the Atlantic world, celebrated by mercantilist writers for its ability to prop up grain prices for landowners, to create wealth in London, and to increase tax revenues. Also, like sugar, gin led some to doubt the morality of commercial society and question especially those who sought private profit while causing the degradation and suffering of others. In 1736 an English writer calling himself "Philanthropos" wrote a tract addressed to Robert Walpole, the leader of Parliament, which was considering another round of anti-gin legislation. Philanthropos announced that his goals were to show how gin hurt the people of Britain and to refute the idea that distilling helped the landed interest and increased tax revenue. The rapid and extreme drunkenness that gin created first caused drinkers to "forget all Obligations of paying their just Debts, and by that Means to expose their Children to . . . Want and Poverty." Once gin drinkers had spent all their money, they turned to crime to fuel their next gin binge: "Desperate attacks, High-way and Street-Robberies, attended sometimes with the most cruel, unheard of Murthers." After each drinking bout came weakness, so that anyone who continued down that path, "instead of being a useful Member of the Community, he is actually become a scandalous Burthen upon it," and eventually England would lose its soldiers and laborers.[68] Moreover, landowners would actually lose money as distilling grew, because the impoverished working class would purchase less beer and bread. Trade in meat, wool, and even tobacco would suffer because gin drinkers had no money for clothing, nor any energy for eating or smoking.[69] Philanthropos urged Parliament to weigh the losses of gin against the gains. "Mankind, in a Trading Nation especially, live upon the Vices and Extravagancies of one another," he conceded in a nod to Mandeville. Philanthropos argued that the government should only tolerate vices that provide more good than bad. Even if the tax revenues from distilling did increase, it could never compensate for gin ruining the workers, driving them into workhouses and hospitals, sending women into prostitution or "houses of correction," whipping up violence and crime in the streets, and disabling soldiers. "Will this Revenue attone for the making us a poor ruin'd Nation?" he asked. "When we shall have no Hands to carry on our Manufactures and Merchandize, no Hands to Cultivate our Lands?[70] Note that Philanthropos aimed his invective not so much at gin itself, nor at its consumers, but at those who manufactured and sold it, as the title spelled out: "Upon the Pernicious Consequences of the Gin-Trade to Great Britain."[71]

Likewise, Thomas Wilson published a treatise in 1736 titled *Distilled spirituous liquors the bane of the nation* in which he sounded the alarm about the entire working class, impoverished and diseased from gin, "so that in a Generation or two We shall not have People able to do the Servile Offices, or to cultivate our Lands."[72] Gin was worse than war or plague, he argued, because these "rage for a while, and then they cease; but This merciless Destroyer threatens Misery, Sickness, and Want, to all the Generations that are to come."[73] Servants and workers had been corrupted, both in bodily strength and in morals, as they now demanded higher pay for doing less work than before. "'Tis a certain and known maxim," Wilson continued, "that the Strength and Riches of any Nation, arises principally from the Number, bodily Strength, and

Labour of its Inhabitants." But employers in London complained that now they needed to hire more laborers to perform the same amount of work, "besides the hourly Fear they are under some Mischief, from a drunken ungovernable set of People."[74] Concern for the poor as a social problem was part of a trend in the eighteenth century as the increasing prominence of political economy in Enlightenment thought turned thinking about the poor as a moral problem—the moral failing of the poor themselves and the failure of the rich to provide charity for them—to a practical one. The focus was shifting from individuals to the abstract issue of poverty.[75]

Wilson went on to directly attack those who defended the gin industry for increasing the public wealth, or, as he put it, "under the subtle Pretence of promoting the Trade and Consumption of our home Product, whilst in reality it is destructive of that and every thing that is Good." Furthermore, would not a healthy and hardworking laboring class spend more money in the long run? "Surely the saving of Lives and increasing and mending the Breed of the Nation, would in a few Years abundantly compensate for such pretended Disadvantages, when the Consumption of all kinds would be much greater from a numerous healthy Race, then from a ragged Company of walking Ghosts."[76] English workers needed to renounce luxury and sin and go back to drinking beer and eating bread and cheese. Here Wilson squarely attacked economic arguments for promoting gin. Instead of consumption, "Thrift, good Husbandry, and Sobriety are Virtues which render a Country Rich and Powerful. What is true in private Persons will hold as to the Community . . . That Private Vices are publick Benefits, will be found to be the most . . . wicked Saying in the World."[77] Like Philanthropos, Wilson believed that private vices led to public ruin.

Population growth was another concern, and Wilson pointed to the government-published Bills of Mortality, arguing that they showed that gin was depopulating London and all of Britain.[78] Thanks to its hot and dry qualities, Wilson explained, distilled spirits blunted fertility, in addition to its moral effects on motherhood. Not only did gin lead to mothers neglecting children, but also "the immoderate Love of such Poisons seems to be communicated to their Children from the very Womb that bare them."[79] Fifteen years later, at the height of the Gin Craze and during another flurry of discourse about it, Isaac Maddox, the bishop of Worcester, expressed these natalist concerns. Gin, he argued in a sermon, was "dis-peopling our Country of Thousands that might have proved useful Members."[80] Like Philanthropos and Wilson,

Maddox decried the increasing numbers of people made idle and useless, damaging the nation. His main worry was the degeneration of children from one generation to the next. "Still more dreadful is it to see Children," he preached, "even Babes hanging at the breast, with those pining, meagre, hagged Looks, that do at once declare their Misery, and the horrid Guilt of their unnatural and cruel Parents."[81] The concerns about population, natalism, and the health of the lower orders were firmly supported by mercantilist thought. A country's strength was in its population, and mercantilists concerned themselves with issues that would foster a large, healthy working class, like preventing tilled fields that produced food from turning into pasture for sheep or trying to prevent the poor from emigrating to the colonies. Warnings about gin's effects on the health of workers voiced the same anxieties about the health of the nation.[82]

Other critics kept a steady focus on the choices made by those who sold gin. In 1760, William Henry published another open letter, perhaps afraid that the licensing of gin sales, which had become strict in the middle of the century, would relax in order to provide more tax revenue for the Seven Years' War. Henry gestured toward Lockean principles to help guide the government. "The Safety of the People take Place of all other Considerations," he argued. "According to this Rule, if Spirituous Liquors are ruinous to the People; if they destroy their Lives, their families, their Hopes of Posterity, their manufactures, their Properties, and public Order; the Preservation of which is the great and ultimate End for which Men first entered into civil Societies," the government should put an end to them.[83] If disallowing gin meant that the government would lose tax revenue, Henry countered that a healthier, growing population would more than make up for the loss. "The Planters are more careful in preserving the Lives of their Negro-slaves, who are their Riches, than we are of preserving our Manufactures, tho' they are Part of ourselves, and Free-born Britons," he contended.[84] While his claim about the care for enslaved people in the Caribbean was not at all true, it spoke to Henry's concern for gin's effects not only on individuals but also on the health and morals of the entire working population. Weighing further the profits and losses incurred by gin, he concluded, "What is wantonly consumed by the Distillery may bring Gain to a few individuals: But cannot possibly add a single Penny to the public Wealth. . . . It is like Gaming," he continued, "wherein People rook each other, Money shifts from Hand to Hand, but the Company in general are never the richer."[85]

Again, commentators turned away from the ethics of consumers to the ethics of suppliers. Thomas Wilson wanted to stop the distilling of spiritous liquors and likened the ending of this business, profitable though it was, to removing a limb to save the body, or pulling down houses to save an entire city from fire.[86] Another, anonymous writer described a distiller as someone "who already wallows in wealth, purchased with the blood of his fellow-creatures."[87] Yet another wrote in 1760 that he "knows many Persons, who might be very good Christians, if they were not Distillers." Not only that, but the notion that gin helped farmers was wrong; instead, distillers were "gradually sinking them into Slavery; for Slaves they must be, to them or to their stock-jobbing, engrossing Agents, if Distillers should be again permitted to go about, like roving Lions, seeking whom they may devour."[88] In a letter to a London newspaper, another anti-gin author followed the commodity chain to the farmers themselves, whom he claimed were about to be ruined both financially and morally by the increase in demand for grain: "The Farmer truly will breed his eldest Son a Gentleman; they scorn to hold the Plow: His Wife and Daughters wear Silks and Topknots, drink Tea, and lie on Down Beds: And by Extravagancies of this kind, by Drunkenness, and other Immortalities, their Substance is consum'd, and then they complain of bad Times, low Markets, and the Oppression of their Landlords."[89] *An impartial enquiry into the present state of the British distillery* scoffed at the attempts to justify gin, or rum, or any other alcoholic drink as an inevitable vice that men and the government might as well profit from, "as if the Question . . . was only this, who should Poison the People?" and not whether the government should put a stop to it.[90]

If critics like Wilson and Henry attacked the idea that distilling increased the public wealth, defenders of distillers sometimes turned the tables, countering the claim that distilling ruined the nation's working class. The Dutch poet Robert Hennebo's 1723 poem "In praise of gin" credited gin for the independence and strength of the United Provinces. Similar to the mythic tales of ancient Greek gods first planting or discovering tobacco or tea, Hennebo praised Europa's son for planting the first juniper trees and teaching men how to mix grain with malt.[91] During the revolt against Spain, the heroes who won freedom for the Dutch did so with gin; wherever there was glory there was also gin. It made the soldiers brave, aided sailors in navigating, and helped the craftsmen work and the poets write. Hennebo sited gin in Jordaan, a working-class neighborhood of Amsterdam, and discussed industrious workers fueling themselves with gin in a way that would have appalled most writers in London at the time, arguing that it strengthened the mind and kept the body healthy.[92] Alexander Blunt (a name that was perhaps a pseudonym for the distiller Elias Bockett) asserted in 1730 that the poor needed gin more than anyone, half naked and exposed to the elements as they were and unable to afford beer.[93] The real problem was ale, Blunt thought, since only the useless, unemployable poor drank gin. Meanwhile, the alehouse deprived society of active workers.[94] In Britain, too, gin could be a symbol of patriotism. An anonymous account of *The life of Mother Gin,* eulogizing her after the Gin Act of 1736, used the spirit as a metaphor for British liberties. Mother Gin allied herself with the Tory and Country parties, asserting the rights of the British people, encouraging rioters during the Sacheverell affair to ransack Dissenting chapels, and helping to defeat an excise on wine and tobacco that would have ruined the nation, among many other patriotic acts.[95] Another anonymous author, "Jack Juniper," eulogized "Queen Gin," who stood for "Liberty, Property, and Free Drinking—Huzza."[96] By defending gin against the government's attempt to quash it, these authors aligned it with patriotic British liberties, much as Hennebo did for the Netherlands. Nationalist rhetoric could play on the ambivalent views of gin in order to defend or attack it.

Most of the writing about gin's effects on society censured the industry for demoralizing the nation's working class. Defying the claims of those like Mandeville and Smith, who celebrated the virtuous cycle of spending and economic growth, they followed the chain of sale and production from the disorder in the streets to the dram shops, distillers, government revenue agents, and landowners who profited from the sale of gin. Like Rousseau, they argued that commercial society, at least when it came to the new drugs, fostered squalor and depravity, not growth and rejuvenation.

The Luxury of the Age Will Be the Ruin of the Nation

This type of nationalist rhetoric, tarring the producers of drugs with the sins of the consumers, did not begin with the Gin Craze. It appeared as soon as tobacco entered western Europe as a commodity—for example, in 1616, when John Deacon included among his many objections to tobacco its high price, alleging that men were spending their entire inheritances on it, which in turn damaged government income.[97] Tobacco's ruinous expense and its tendency to eat away at men's estates was a common theme in anti-tobacco discourse. A rhetoric of protecting the national interest appeared in writing on coffee and tea as well. In his 1728 work of moral criticism, *Augusta triumphans: Or, the way to make London the most flourishing city in the universe*, Daniel Defoe excoriated what he called "Sunday Debauches." Of course he berated gin and its effects on working-class men and women, eroding the men's ability to work and women's ability to nurse their children. But gin was not the only problem. "The Luxury of the Age will be the Ruin of the Nation," he warned. "Tea and Wine are all we seem anxious for . . . Our very Plough-Fellows drink Wine now-a-days: . . . and the wholesome Breakfast of Water-gruel and Milk-portage is chang'd for Coffee and Tea."[98] In the francophone lands, a critic calling himself "de Reynal" expressed the belief that coffee would render workers incapable of labor—workshops would have to be converted into hospitals—and soldiers, should be they given access to coffee, would become unfit for marching and even physically incapable of shouldering their weapons.[99] De Reynal echoed N. F. J. Éloy when he warned that that coffee was making women incapable of tolerating pregnancy, childbirth, or nursing, threatening the nation with depopulation.[100] The children who did survive would remain enervated by their mothers' coffee drinking: "They do not have the vigorous constitution which would have given hope of one day seeing them usefully employed in the service of the Fatherland."[101]

In England Jonas Hanway led the charge against tea drinking among the laboring classes, linking tea with gin in their mutual corrosive effect on natalism. With its origins among the effeminate Chinese, tea attacked the nervous systems of the English who, impelled by fashion, made a custom of drinking it.[102] Tea was a "slow poison," killing two thousand of the two million tea drinkers every year, Hanway estimated. The ill effects of tea were multiplied by its combination with other stimulants. "How many thousands in this nation are annually poisoned by Tea, Gin, and Wine." As the Spanish say, "England is a country where half the people are employed to fill liquor for the other half," but for every publican who earned his livelihood this way, Hanway figured that three of his fellow countrymen died premature deaths. Over time, this added up: "In twenty years the king will lose at least sixty thousand subjects. . . . This account may startle you; but as it is justly observed, that war and famine do not make such devastation as intemperance."[103] "What an Army has Gin and Tea destroyed!" Hanway exclaimed, contemplating their effects on England's population, both in its effects on the health of adults and in its creation of a population of homeless children left to die in the streets. Mothers in the middle of the eighteenth century no longer thought anything of drinking tea, and perhaps some gin, while nursing their babies, which, "generally loaded with sugar . . . gives them the spleen, or hypocondria," illnesses unknown to their grandmothers. Hanway quoted the former prime minister Henry Pelham as saying, "Tea then is become another gin!" in its menace to the nation.[104] Hanway held out special disapproval for the nonelite, the laborers, servants, and even the impoverished who all must have their tea, noting with disgust beggars sipping their tea and special carts bringing tea out to haymakers in the field. "He who should be able to drive three Frenchmen before him," he wrote, "or she who might be a breeder of such a race of men, are to be seen sipping their tea!"[105]

With a swipe at Mandeville, Hanway concluded: "We may delude ourselves into the belief, that private vices are public benefits; but this quibbling fallacy, whilst it soothes the corruption of mankind," obscured the way in which tea was ruining the British economy.[106] The labor of the poor supported Britain, and so, many of the goods they produced had to be sold abroad to maintain employment at home. But now the labor of the British working class was "exchanged for dirt, or what is the same, for tea."[107] Hanway's concern for tea's effects on Britain reached such a pitch that he called out for a savior. He promised a statue devoted to the memory of that person, inscribed:

M.DCC.LV.

To

the remembrance

of the fair guardian spirits of BRITAIN,

whose influence and example

abolished the use of

a CHINESE drug called

TEA;

the infusion of which had been for many years drank

in these realms and dominions,

injuring the health,

obstructing the industry,

wasting the fortunes,

and exporting the riches,

of his MAJESTY's liege subjects[108]

The anonymous author of "An essay on modern luxuries" added sugar to the list of stimulants that were ruining the British nation and economy. He argued that "Fine Flour, and [white] Bread and Butter, together with Tea and Sugar, to which I subjoin Spirituous Liquors . . . and Ale-house Strong beer, are the foundation of almost all the poverty, and all the evils which affect the laboring part of mankind."[109] Not only did tea and sugar change the character of their drinkers, "to peevishness, moroseness, and ill nature," but they also "inflame the poor man's expences" and waste time. He estimated that the time spent preparing tea, taking it at the tea table, and then cleaning up "will largely account for half a day in winter."[110] He connected the rise of these luxuries to the increase in Britain's national debt, and "loss of appetite, sickness, and a puny race of children, are the wretched consequences of this pernicious liquor," throwing families who should be working onto the parish relief rolls.[111] This recurring theme of the working classes constituting a reservoir of strength for the country fit the ideas of the new fields of political economy and statistics, which reconceived the poor and working classes not as individuals embedded in communities, but as a mass that made up its own swath of the nation.[112] National power depended on harnessing the poor, and the potential of putting the poor to work depended on their health, reproductive abilities, and their proclivity to work hard, all day. All the new soft drugs, not just gin, threatened this potential.

Time's Great Consumer: Idleness and Wastefulness

Not only did the new stimulants eat away at the numbers of the working class, but they also drew healthy artisans away from productive labor. Historians of the great economic take-off in Europe tend to focus on the enormous gains in productivity that occurred, starting in the late eighteenth century, thanks to coal and mechanization—the supply side of the industrial revolution. More recently Jan de Vries and others have called our attention to the demand side: to the increase in consumption beginning one hundred years earlier that helped spur the need for a greater supply and higher productivity. They call this process the "industrious revolution" because the key to greater demand was the way that families, first in the Netherlands and England, reorganized their relationship to work and time by reorienting their consumption away from autonomous subsistence and barter and turning toward the market. Essentially, northwest Europeans began working more hours per year in order to obtain new consumer goods, and these industrious habits eventually spread to the rest of the world. The goods they were working to afford included cotton clothing, furniture, and glass windows for larger and more comfortable houses, and various sundry items like clocks and candlesticks that de Vries calls "the luxuries of the poor."[113]

These goods also included drugs like coffee, tea, chocolate, sugar, alcohol, and tobacco. They fit in well with the idea of the new luxuries, which promoted economic growth instead of wasting the wealth of individual consumers and the nation. The lure of tobacco, chocolate, coffee, and tea disciplined people instead of degrading them, spurring them to work harder and longer.[114] Yet critics disagreed, blaming these new luxuries for the spread of idleness, identifying them as undermining time-discipline and economic growth. Defenders of commercial society countered that truly industrious people would not fall prey to the temptations of vice; only the idle aristocracy who consumed the old luxuries were susceptible to that kind of corruption. But the dram shops excoriated by Henry and Chandler did not figure into the thinking of the boosters for industriousness and the new luxuries like Mandeville and Smith.

Gin came under heavy scrutiny for eroding industriousness. An anonymous *Dissertation on drunkenness* from 1727 lamented that all of the arts, sciences, and trades of Britain have been lost, "and the whole Kingdom become nothing but a Brewer or Distillery, and the Inhabitants all Drunkards." Not confined to tippling houses, gin had insinuated itself into the wares of increasing numbers of shops.[115] Allowing "Chandlers, and other inferior Traders" to sell gin meant that they pressed it onto servants running errands, hurting the work force. Those who drank gin, especially among the poor, began selling it "and take delight to help others to what they love themselves, as Whores commence Bawds."[116] For those who did so, it was a terrible living. "Whoever would thrive in it," the author wrote, "must . . . with Patience and good Humour he must be able to endure the filthy Actions and vile Language of nasty Drabs, and the lewdest Rake-Hells; and without a Frown, or the least Aversion, bear with all the Stench and Squaller, Noise and Impertinence, that the utmost Indigence, Laziness, and

Ebriety can produce in the most shameless and abandoned Vulgar."[117] Another pamphlet from 1760 pointed out that the inexpensiveness of gin hurt industriousness, since it was so cheap that one only had to work one day to purchase enough gin for a week spent not working, but "in Idleness and Debauchery.—The expensive Luxuries, for the most Part, excite Labour and Industry, but the Luxury of cheap Drunkenness tends more directly to Sloth and Depopulation."[118]

The author of *An impartial enquiry into the present state of the British distillery* targeted the sites of consumption as engines of anti-capitalism. Tippling houses and alehouses, with their shuffleboards, ninepins, and other games, enticed "idle people" in "to habituate themselves to Drunkenness." They were places, he continued, "where Artificers learn by those Recreations to spend both Time and Money, leave their Families in the mean time starving or to the care of the Parish, Apprentices learn to waste their Master's Time, and from thence are taught by degrees to rob them, to defray the expence of it."[119] Note his use of the verb "learning"; dram shops were schools teaching anti-capitalist behavior. An anonymous "Country Justice of the Peace" writing in the mid-eighteenth century also identified tippling houses and alehouses as sites of anti-capitalism. Objecting to those who claimed that distilling increased tax revenue, he wrote, "I can compare it to nothing more properly than an Highway-man who robs an honest Traveller; it is true, he gets his Money, but it frequently ends in his Ruin. In this Case the publick Revenues are increased, but this Method increases the publick Disorders; publick Disorders increase the publick Expences; Mankind becomes debauched in their Manners, insult Magistracy, resist Government, and occasion double the Expence to the Publick that this Revenue brings in."[120] Not everyone agreed. Alexander Blunt wrote a poem addressed to Robert Walpole in which he depicted gin as a woman named Clara put on trial by Feculento, who represented gin's rival, ale. When Feculento accused gin of promoting "laziness" and wasting money, Clara countered that ale is much more time-consuming than gin: "The market-woman, / With basket on her head, can take a glass" of gin much more quickly and with less expense than ale.[121] Like Hennebo in the Netherlands, Blunt defended gin as a drink perfectly designed for those without enough time or money to linger in the alehouse. On the one hand, concerns that gin taught its users anti-industrious habits were not so very different from the "battle over the alehouse" during the late sixteenth and early seventeenth centuries in England.[122] On the other, the panic over gin and debauchery focused on London, not the entire country, and it was intensified by the growth in printed material and of a sensationalist press in the eighteenth century. Also in the eighteenth century, gin (or perhaps its drinkers) seemed to flow out of the tippling houses and into the streets—where gin was also sold—bringing their debauchery with them, in a way that ale drinkers did not a century and a half earlier.[123]

The anonymous author of the *Dissertation on drunkenness* blamed the producers and sellers of gin for promoting idleness and undermining capitalism. He likened "Taverns, Ale-houses, Coffee-Houses, and Brandy-Shops" to the "Harlot" in Proverbs 5:3–22 who led men to their doom. "Can a Man drink and squander away almost his whole Substance, in one of these Houses, by which a poor Family is reduced to Beggary, and are the Owners of those Houses no way instrumental to their Ruin?" he inquired. "Can a Neighbour be almost every Day overtaken in Drink, and can he that supplies him with it, be altogether innocent? Can he, who feeds and cherishes his extravagant Humour, and is subservient to his Vices, and Excesses, wash his Hands of all Guilt?"[124] Here the seller of gin has perverted commerce, using it to spread sin and vice, ruin his neighbors, and is degraded in turn. Meanwhile, gin spread throughout London, ensnaring not only its drinkers but also its sellers. Adding insult to injury, the author alleged that tippling housekeepers loaned out money to their customers, ruining their credit and their good name in their neighborhoods when they could not pay.[125] The vendors of gin produced the antithesis of thriving commerce and civility. Even the argument that distilling helped landowners and farmers could be used to blame gin for encouraging idleness. According to *The occasional monitor*, the high prices sapped the discipline of farmers who lived near enough to London to sell their grain to distillers. Because distillers would take low-quality wheat that bakers would reject, farmers could maintain their income while working less: "This is a downright Argument for idleness."[126]

Concerns about drugs and industriousness began long before the Gin Craze. Like gin, tobacco gathered the workers together and taught them idleness and improvident spending. In 1617 Richard Braithwaite created a character representing "Time" who complained that gentlemen used to spend their time making foreign conquests and serving the public good, but now they spent their hours indulging in "smoake and vapour, the lightest and trivialst of all things."[127] Around the same time, Joshua Sylvester likened tobacco users to oxen put to work at a mill, trudging "in the same Circle, on the selfe same ground; / Forgetting how, Dayes, Months, and Yeeres do passe." Sites of tobacco smoking encouraged vices, like "Vain Words, vain Oathes, Dice, Daring, Drunkenness" as well as "Sloath, jesting, scoffing, turning Night to Day, / And Day to Night," attended by "the Losse of precious houres" and money alike.[128] In a satirical broadsheet from 1683, a writer named A. Marsh advised newly married husbands against tobacco, taverns, and coffeehouses, lest they become entrapped by these stimulants and the good fellowship that came with it, neglecting their wives, becoming enfeebled and unable to have sex, and wasting away their family's time and money.[129] The mercantilist projector Thomas Mun, while comparing the wealth, power, and potential of England and the Netherlands, lamented that England's great bounty of natural resources paradoxically made his countrymen wasteful and idle, unlike "the industrious Dutch," who were prodded by the poverty and small size of their country to work constantly. Worse, while Dutch merchants were roaming the seas to enrich themselves, the English spent their time "sucking smoak, and drinking healths." (Mun claimed falsely that the Dutch had largely given up tobacco and alcohol.) Tobacco also weakened English bodies, disabling those men who still did want to work hard.[130]

This was the first moral concern about the new psychotropic drugs, even before gin and sugar were tied to debauchery and slavery: their tendency to encourage indolence and sloth. This pattern began with tobacco. In 1663 Sir William Berkeley, the governor of Virginia, bemoaned the way that the colony "laid the Foundation of our wealth and industry on the vices of men."[131] The Italian Capuchin friar Eusebio da Monte Santo complained that tobacco makes the rich richer by planting it, and the poor poorer by the taxes placed on its consumption.[132] In 1608 Richard West published a collection of epigraphs, among them an acrostic for tobacco in which the first line, for "T," read: "Times great consumer, cause of idlenesse."[133] The Puritan controversialist and politician William Prynne took a swipe at tobacco in a screed against Cromwell's readmission of Jews to England. To help the English economy, he proposed, better than granting Jews legal status would be inhibiting the use of tobacco, which created "such a prodigal expence of money, time, and hindring more necessary, usefull, staple merchandizes and plantations."[134] The Dutch physician J. I. W. Beintema van Peima, who saw tobacco as another form of drunkenness, also declared that smoking was a waste of money and time.[135]

Tobacco's connection with idleness and wasting money continued into the eighteenth century, as Methodist theologian Adam Clarke called it sinful, "vilely squandering away the Time and Money which God has given for other purposes." Clarke especially targeted the poor for wasting their money on tobacco, people "scarcely able to procure the necessaries of life, and yet by sacrificing health and decency, have made a shift to procure the daily *quantum sufficit* of Tobacco." Clarke calculated that a poor family might spend £200, a hefty sum, in the course of fifty years—and this not counting the alcohol and "neglect of business" that would accompany the smoking.[136] An author calling himself "R. T.," who published a book about efficiency in 1675, warned coffee drinkers that, although they might not spend much ready money in the coffeehouse, "in Smoaking and Talking, consumes at least an Hour" in the morning, and then four hours more in the evening. Adding up the value of the lost time, R. T. reckoned that it cost over £36 per year—"a great deal of Money in a poor Tradesmans Pocket."[137] Another anonymous author, "M. P.," castigated the coffeehouses for encouraging idleness via lingering over coffee and tobacco: "At this place a man is cheated of what is, by far more valuable than Mony, that is, Time."[138] Once again, it is the site where the drug is consumed, and the purveyors, more than the drug itself that was the problem.

England was not the only place where these fears arose. The Dutch author R. V. N. explained in 1701 that hard work and frugality led to the emergence of the Netherlands as a wealthy power. As the local saying went, "Man and dog, get out; woman and cat, stay home," but since the introduction of tobacco, coffee, and tea, men left the house not to work but to idle their hours away, women spent less time at the spinning wheel, and all the good habits that led to Dutch independence and prosperity were in decline.[139] The author of the *Debauched and enchanted coffee and tea world*, published that same year, admitted that there was nothing so useful as the worldwide commerce instituted by western Europeans, especially the Dutch, but even the best gifts of heaven could bring death through misuse. Men spent their hours at the coffeehouse, where some were led into the arms of prostitutes. Women not only spent their hours idly meeting with other women and gossiping, but they also wasted their money on all the things that went with coffee and tea, including the porcelain tea service, buying new sets every time the fashion changes.[140] Even Cornelis Bontekoe, as part of his late-in-life hesitation about tea when not used strictly for health reasons, complained that people wasted time and lost their livelihoods thanks to tea. It was not really tea's fault, but tea was the pretext for leaving home to shop, as well as a cover for drinking brandy or going from drinking tea for hours to going to the tavern to gamble.[141]

While tobacco drew the most attention for encouraging anti-industriousness, the money and time that women spent on tea alarmed many observers. Godfrey McCalman moderately suggested that women be more frugal, making do with three-quarters of the amount of tea they would normally purchase in a year, but most critics were more harsh.[142] There was, however, a backlash, defending women's consumption of tea by contrasting it with men's drinking habits. James Bland criticized men who returned home at teatime, finding his wife taking a much-needed break from working all day with inexpensive tea, sometimes without even adding sugar, and respond by criticizing them for wasting money. "She has spent Five-Farthings," Bland wrote, while who knows how many pounds he has spent at the tavern in idle socializing.[143] In 1735 a writer called "J. B." published a poem praising tea, which was cheap enough even for the poor to drink, although a half pint of ale with a roll and cheese might be a better use of their money, as long as "their day's work thereby is not prevented."[144] He, too, defended wives whose husbands arrived at home to witness them drinking tea with a neighbor: "When he, perhaps has drank a quart of wine, and they an ounce of Tea. . . . The tradesman swears his wife has been his ruin, / By drinking Tea, when he's in debt for brewing."[145] A song published in 1749, "The tea drinking wife, and drunken husband," took this trope as its theme: the husband admonished his wife for preferring gossip over tea to getting his noontime dinner ready, and for wanting fine, fashionable things to match the neighboring women while he worked all day long. She retorted that he spent his evenings getting drunk in the alehouse and committing adultery.[146]

The growth of capitalism depended on the global flow of soft drugs and alcohol to western Europe as well as on the increase in industriousness among consumers of those ingestibles. Yet consuming the new psychotropic substances encouraged the waste of time and money. This tension sat at the heart of the growth of the new luxuries, and observers disagreed as to whether gin and its sister drugs made Europeans richer or poorer.

Daniel Lord Smail has remarked on the role of the state in enforcing debts in medieval Marseille and Lucca. Of all the myriad ways western Europeans might have done so, they chose the coercive and spectacularly public humiliation of having agents of the government enter into debtors' homes, seize their personal goods, and remove them in full view of their neighbors. Shame was the point of this exercise as much as the sum owed, as the creditors wanted to exact an emotional toll on the debtors in order to make a moral point about the importance of paying one's debts. Smail has also explored how medieval courts grew in power and importance not so much from delivering justice but from satisfying the emotional needs of litigants. People who brought their pleas to the courts wanted not so much to win their cases but to have them be heard and to rally their friends and allies around them in a public demonstration of support. In both of these cases, medieval governments collected fees, and the state grew larger and more powerful thanks to its ability to profit the emotional needs of their subjects.[147] A few centuries later, the early modern state was still profiting from the emotional needs of their subjects, this time by taxing the gin, sugar, tobacco, opium, tea, coffee, and chocolate that formed part of the wellness industry, soothing the nerves and anxiety of those who consumed them. Like the medieval state, the early modern European state profited from regulating the emotional well-being of its subjects. But by the eighteenth century, not just the government but the entire economy depended on western Europeans soothing their minds with psychotropic drugs, gathered to European markets by the global trade in which helped spark economic growth and greater industriousness in Europe. Gerhard Oestreich argued that the state expanded its reach and scope by discipling its subjects, teaching and coercing them into regulating their behavior and emotions along Neostoic lines, while Max Weber contended that capitalism expanded its reach and scope through the self-denial of its workers. But the rapid expansion in the market for psychotropic drugs teaches that capitalism and the state grew due, at least in part, to the actions of pleasure-seeking consumers.

Western Europeans found that as the new soft drugs became increasingly central to their economic lives, they were forced to confront questions about the nature of commercial society. From the introduction of chocolate and tobacco in the early seventeenth century through the anti-sugar boycotts of the late eighteenth century, stimulants presented western Europeans with questions about the ethics of the market, for both consumers and producers. The result was a profound ambivalence about the morality of selling gin and its sister drugs. While this unease saw its most conspicuous expression in the boycott of slave sugar, it began with the introduction of tobacco two centuries earlier and played a part in the first drug panic, the English Gin Craze. Was it ethical to profit from the cheap liquor gushing into the poor neighborhoods of

London? Might there be a better use for the grain that went into the distillers' vats than increasing vice, idleness, and poverty? Did these new products promote economic growth by inducing consumers to spend more of their hours and days working in order to afford them? Or did they seduce the working classes away from the industrious new working habits that were so crucial to capitalism? Did increasing influence of the market on people's behavior encourage civility or corruption?

Conclusion

An English Opium-Eater

Thomas De Quincey published *Confessions of an English opium-eater* in two installments of the *London Magazine* in 1821. Here he publicly chronicled his use of opium, which he began taking to counteract pain. Immediately after his first dose, however, he also began using it "for the sake of creating an artificial state of pleasurable excitement."[1] Although opium was a widely used medicine throughout early modern Europe and well known since antiquity, De Quincey showed that there still something new to say about it. He published his *Confessions* anonymously, but very quickly the British literary establishment discovered who wrote the narrative. In it he detailed his entire life up until 1821, partly to put into context both his decision to use opium and the dreams that it gave him, and partly to emphasize his unique sensibility in the style of a true Romantic writer like his idol William Wordsworth. As a young boy he suffered the twin shocks of the death of his father in 1793 and the death of his older sister, Elizabeth, which he depicted as the founding trauma of his emotional life. Running away from his grammar school, De Quincey spent several months tramping around Wales and then London, where he suffered another heartbreak when he lost touch with a young prostitute, Anne, whom he had befriended in Soho. After returning to his family, he attended Oxford University, and while visiting London in 1804 he first used opium in order to combat rheumatic pains in the face and head. Two years later, aged twenty-one, he sought out Wordsworth, and soon De Quincey had abandoned Oxford to live with Wordsworth and his sister, Dorothy. By 1818 he had used up all of his inheritance, and Wordsworth arranged for him to edit a local newspaper; three years later the *Confessions* set him up as a celebrated and somewhat scandalous writer.[2] His autobiographical tale serves as a useful hinge, summing up early modern western Europeans' relationship with drugs and alcohol while pointing to changes that would occur in the nineteenth and twentieth centuries.

De Quincey was part of a small but noticeable number of opium addicts among Britain's elite, of whom he helpfully included a list in the *Confessions,* including the poet Samuel Taylor Coleridge and the antislavery activist William Wilberforce.[3] While physicians had been writing for at least a hundred years about patients of theirs becoming dependent on opium, this group was new for the social standing of its members and also because some of them took opium not as a medicine but for pleasure. De Quincey was one of these, and he wanted to emphasize that for him opium was not so much a physical but an intellectual pleasure, and this points to a shift in modern ideas of drug use, stressing their mental and social effects over the physical. Romanticism also influenced De Quincey's portrayal of his opium use, encouraging him to emphasize its emotional, irrational, and sensational effects. Before him, writers on opium tended to be physicians who tried to explain the effects and dangers of opium scientifically, or travelers to the Middle East who highlighted the exotic behavior of opium-using Turks and Arabs.

These changes in emphasis pointed to the future, when scientific breakthroughs and the invention of hypodermic needles led to morphine replacing opium as the most popular and effective painkiller. Further technical advances plus the increasingly global nature of trade then led to the incorporation of cocaine into the western European pharmacopeia in the late nineteenth century, followed by the Bayer Company's production of heroin for retail sale in 1895. The incorporation of cannabis, amphetamines, and hallucinogens in the twentieth century completed the mix of drugs that constitutes the global regime of recreational drug use today. But De Quincey was also firmly a part of early modern European drug culture, wrestling with issues of pleasure and the senses, exoticism, luxury, custom, and slavery as metaphors for dependence, wellness culture, and sociability. Mike Jay has claimed that since opium was so well known to early nineteenth-century Europeans,

De Quincey did not so much explore a taboo but create one when he spoke of the pleasures of recreational opium use, but perhaps it is better to say that De Quincey was the first to grapple with the problem of opium, pleasure, and self-discipline, and with the intense ambivalence that it caused him and his contemporaries.[4]

Humans first domesticated opium-producing poppies in prehistoric Europe, but by the early modern period western Europe was importing its opium from the Middle East and India. Ancient Greece associated opium with fertility cults and the goddesses Demeter and Persephone, probably as a psychoactive ingredient in religious practice. The Greek physicians who created the medical corpus of knowledge that Romans, Arabs, and medieval Europeans adopted as their own wrote of opium's use as a painkiller and a sleep aid, as well as for its help against diarrhea, and they were also aware that large quantities might kill the user.[5] During the European Renaissance, the idiosyncratic German physician Paracelsus promoted the use of laudanum, a mixture of opium with some spices like cinnamon that he then infused into distilled spirits. This was a simpler version of medicines like mithridatum that had combined opium with exotic ingredients like frankincense, saffron, and cardamom, and an even more stripped-down version of laudanum consisting of just opium and alcohol became the standard method of taking opium in western Europe by 1700.[6] Other ways to consume opium were simply to eat it, and by the seventeenth century users in Southeast Asia were smoking it, first with tobacco and then later in a purified form that could be smoked in pipes on its own.[7] A standard ingredient in every printed guide of materia medica in early modern western Europe, opium could be found in any well-stocked apothecary. Although writers warned against dependence and overdose, and the growing influx of opium into Europe attracted increasing scientific attention, not until De Quincey published his *Confessions* did opium become controversial.[8]

De Quincey broke with the tradition on European writing on opium by emphasizing what he called "The Pleasures of Opium," a phrase he used as a title for a section of the *Confessions*. "If opium-eating be a sensual pleasure," he wrote, "I am bound to confess that I have indulged in it to an excess, not yet recorded of any other man" (although in a footnote he accused Coleridge of consuming even more opium than he did, albeit secretly, so unrecorded).[9] De Quincey also accused opium of causing pain—of withdrawal, as well as the distress of disordered dreaming and visions, some while awake and others while asleep. But his rapturous celebration of the pleasure of using opium, which he described as "unimaginable pleasure" and "celestial pleasure," set him apart from writers before him.[10] The attention he paid to opium's pleasure and physicality, however, certainly put him squarely in the tradition of early modern Europeans writing about drugs. Like Andrew Burn (discussed in the first chapter of this book) detailing the filthy process by which enslaved Africans in the Caribbean produced sugar in an effort to make his listeners repulsed by the idea of ingesting it into their bodies, De Quincey lingered on the physical and sensory aspects of opium.

De Quincey did not seem to feel any repulsion toward opium; indeed he prided himself as a man without disgust.[11] But the consequences of opium use were plainly visible on De Quincey's body, including agitated sleeplessness and lips "parched and baked with fever."[12] Coleridge's addiction was even more visible—for example, as he struggled, feverish and with blackened lips, through a speaking tour in 1801, barely able to move his mouth to speak, and at other times a sweat-sheened, brooding look on his face. These corporeal alterations, however, were not so much the consequence of taking opium as from Coleridge's attempts to stop.[13] As for the sensory properties of opium itself, certainly medical experts like Angelo Sala and George Young used its color, taste, and consistency to judge its quality. De Quincey had little to say on this besides mocking men like them, whom he considered to be limited by sticking to what was rationally knowable rather than the true inner nature of opium's powers. He facetiously agreed with their observation that, yes, it was "dusky brown in colour."[14] What the physicians did not understand was the "abyss of divine enjoyment" that opium gave him, causing "an apocalypse of the world within me!"[15] For De Quincey, opium was different from sugar and the other drugs because its pleasure overrode any concerns one might have with its effects on the body, impact on the senses, or disgusting qualities.

This was not the case with its exotic racial aspects, which De Quincey personified in the form of "the Malay." Like John Chamberlayne (discussed in the second chapter of this book), who was careful to set chocolate in the cultural geography of global drugs and alcohol, De Quincey was highly aware of opium's connections to Asia. De Quincey did not explicitly address the anxieties that opium, like chocolate, caused among western Europeans about gender and class, although he did like to go slumming in the poor neighborhoods of London on his Saturday opium sessions, mixing and talking with working-class families.[16] Nevertheless, the Malay was a prominent character in *Confessions of an English opium-eater*, speaking to De Quincey's intense religious, gendered, and racial anxieties. He claimed that one evening while he was living in the remote Lake District of England a Malaysian man appeared at his door, a "tiger-cat" seeming to want something but unable to speak English. De Quincey noted the surprise and apprehension that his serving woman and the local people expressed toward the turban-wearing, dark-skinned, "ferocious looking" visitor. De Quincey made some polite, mutually unintelligible conversation with the Malaysian traveler, let him rest on the floor of his cottage, and then offered him some opium, of which he ate a dangerously large amount before leaving. It is unclear whether there truly was a man from Southeast Asia passing through northwest England, or if De Quincey dreamed or invented his visit. Real or imagined, the Malay certainly embodied all the racialized fears that western Europeans harbored about the new stimulants. Like "The Marriage of the Turk," De Quincey portrayed the Malay as lewd, standing too close to De Quincey's female servant. Later, when De Quincey was using opium every day, he described his troubled dreams by claiming, "The Malay has been a fearful enemy for months." He then recounted recurring nightmares about being transported "through his means . . . into Asiatic scenes." He dreamt he was in China and then other Asian locales, where he was "terrified by the modes of life, by the manners, and the barrier of utter abhorrence, and want of sympathy, placed between us by feelings deeper than I can analyze." He would rather live with "lunatics, or brute animals" than Asians, and the dreams gave him "unimaginable horror" as he contemplated the swarming masses of people and the incomprehensibly ancient civilizations that he imagined characterized China and the rest of Asia. He elided the difference between Asian people and Asian animals such as monkeys, snakes, and crocodiles. His fears were religious as well as racial: "I was the idol; I was the priest; I was worshipped; I was sacrificed." De Quincey dreamt of being pursued by Hindu and ancient Egyptian gods, then being entombed under pyramids for thousands of years, and, finally, "laid, confounded with all unutterable slimy things, amongst reeds and Nilotic mud." Waking from the dreams into the domestic setting of his home, surrounded by his children, was so jarring it caused him to weep.[17] Eating opium meant eating Asia and becoming Asian, although in this case it threatened De Quincey's mind more than his body. While antislavery activists struggled to make sugar consumers mindful of the global sweep of slavery and misery that produced the sweetener for their hot drinks, for De Quincey opium's connections with the regions where it was produced came unbidden. Opium threatened to dissolve the self-discipline of a scholarly, elite, Anglican Englishman over his mind, body, and behavior, and these fears were common among the western Europeans who used the new exotic drugs.

If addiction puzzled early modern observers of tobacco and other drugs, it was central to the *Confessions*, which is considered the first memoir of addiction, and that De Quincey wrote to explain why he took opium. "How came any reasonable being to subject himself to such a yoke of misery, voluntarily to incur a captivity so servile, and knowingly to fetter himself with such a seven-fold chain?" he asked toward the beginning of the text, straightaway employing the metaphor of slavery and bondage to explain his compulsive use of opium.[18] De Quincey first tried opium when a friend in London recommended it for the excruciating rheumatic pains he was experiencing.[19] As demonstrated in the third chapter of this book, the stamp of approval by medical experts for tobacco and the other new stimulants paved the way for their use, and of course opium had been part of the European pharmacopoeia since the time of the ancient Greeks. Following the broad patterns of tobacco and other soft drugs, as soon as he began taking opium as a medicine, De Quincey also began using it for the pursuit of pleasure. He claimed that he carefully decided when and where he would take opium, reserving it for about one in every three Saturdays.[20]

> I have often been asked, how I first came to be a regular opium-eater; and have suffered, very unjustly . . . from being reputed to have brought upon myself all the sufferings which I shall have to record, by a long course of indulgence in this practice purely for the sake of creating an artificial state of pleasurable excitement. . . . True it is, that for nearly ten years I did occasionally take opium, for the sake of the exquisite pleasure it gave me: but, so long as I took it with this view, I was effectually protected from all material bad consequences, by the . . . long intervals between the several acts of indulgence, in order to renew the pleasurable sensations.[21]

This control ended in 1813, when De Quincey began using opium daily. He blamed the stomach pains he began experiencing the previous year as well as his grief after the death of Wordsworth's young daughter Catherine, with whom he was close.[22] Eight years later, when he published the *Confessions*, De Quincey claimed to have quit opium altogether. If he was guilty of indulging in opium for pleasure, he nevertheless maintained that "it is no less true, that I have struggled against this fascinating enthrallment with a religious zeal" and succeeded. De Quincey claimed to "have untwisted, almost to the final links, the accursed chain which fettered me." This was almost certainly a lie, and, in any event, he was addicted to opium again later in his life and perhaps never quite stopped until his death. (In his defense, as he was taking opium in the form of laudanum, every time De Quincey tried to quit opium he also experienced withdrawal from alcohol.)[23] He continued with the metaphors of mastery and bondage, using the phrase "self-conquest" to describe his getting free of opium.[24] Regardless of whether he was abstaining from opium when he published the *Confessions*, De Quincey wrestled with self-discipline his entire life. By the time he published the *Confessions* he wrote that the pleasure of opium had abandoned him, and only the pains of withdrawal kept him using it. His description of trying to stop taking opium would seem familiar to any dopesick sufferer in the twenty-first century.[25] And yet he seemed proud of his pioneering exploration of the pleasures of opium. He justified writing the memoir by claiming that his dreams, suffused with grief and loss from earlier episodes in his life, would be more exquisite and noteworthy to readers than that of other opium addicts such as Manchester laborers thanks to his status as "a philosopher" endowed with "a superb intellect" and "moral faculties." He still managed to look down on his friend Coleridge for being more hopelessly addicted than he was.[26] For his part Coleridge loathed his own dependence on opium and despaired over the way De Quincey glorified its recreational use.[27] De Quincey's mixed feelings about his opium dependency, and the mix of titillation and condemnation that greeted the publication of the *Confessions*, exemplifies the ambivalence that western Europeans had about opium, and psychotropic drugs in general.

Opium was certainly used by many for nervous ailments in the late eighteenth and early nineteenth centuries, like the coffee that N. F. J. Éloy deplored (as shown in chapter 4), although De Quincey did not refer much to his nerves. His use of opium did fit into the idea of early modern wellness culture in several ways, however—for example, into the new category of cheap luxuries meant to be consumed and repurchased. Opium use was a regimen for him; he dosed himself with laudanum every three weeks or so for years, and, later, daily. His main purpose was the regulation of his mental state, and opium became both the cause of ill mental health for De Quincey and its solution. When he shifted to daily use, he claimed that, because of his stomach ailments and the recent death of Catherine Woodsworth, "I could not have done otherwise." He explained "that I am too much of a Eudaemonist: I hanker too much after a state of happiness. . . . I cannot face misery."[28] In the initial period of his use, then, opium staved off not just physical pain but mental anguish, giving him relief from grief—of Catherine's death, the loss of Anne, and the death of his sister—and stabilizing his mood. Certainly this relief came in the form of an easily purchased commodity. "Here was the secret of happiness," he reflected. "Happiness might now be bought for a penny, and carried in the waistcoat pocket: portable ecstasies might be had corked up in a pint bottle: and peace of mind could be sent down in gallons by the mail coach."[29] Here was a perfect description of the logic behind the early wellness industry.

For De Quincey, titrating the dosage of laudanum was also a form of regimen—and mood regulation. In 1816, after three years of daily use, he found himself "insulated, in the gloom and cloudy melancholy of opium." He cut his use by three-quarters and reported that "instantaneously, and as if by magic, the cloud of profoundest melancholy which rested upon my brain . . . drew off in one day."[30] When he increased the dosage later, he found himself beset by an "intellectual torpor," unable to write scarcely even a letter, and attacked "by deep-seated anxiety and gloomy melancholy, such as are wholly incommunicable by words."[31] This he tried to end by tapering off from opium altogether, and so, through trial and error, De Quincy searched for exact amount of laudanum that would maintain his mental equilibrium. Opium held for De Quincey an indefinite position between medicine and something pleasurable, something he used to solve his emotional and mental problems all the while suspecting that it was making them worse. For all the suffering that opium brought De Quincey, still, when he devoted a section of the *Confessions* to paint an image of perfect happiness, he did so by evoking a cottage, deep in a valley, far from town, and surrounded by mountains. In this cottage De Quincey would be found during a winter storm sitting by a fire with hearth rugs, candles, bookshelves, tea, "a fair tea-maker," and, to top it off, "a quart of ruby-coloured laudanum" placed beside him on a table.[32] As Robert Morrison argues, opium was both a blessing and a curse to De Quincey, giving him the subject matter that launched him as a celebrated writer while at the same time delivering real suffering and preventing him from the kind of steady effort at writing that would have given him a more successful career.[33]

Opium was a solitary pleasure for De Quincey, but it did rearrange his sociability to some degree, similar to the way that *The debauched and enchanted coffee- and tea-world* depicted tea and the other intoxicants of early modern western Europe. There was no coffeehouse, tea table, or dram shop that served as a site of disorder where De Quincey could take his laudanum, but his stay as a runaway schoolboy in Soho, then in decline, and the slumming he did on Saturdays after dosing himself were analogous. On his Saturday wanderings he felt that opium, "like wine, gives an expansion to the heart and the benevolent affections," but not in the superficial way that alcohol did. Instead, by taking away all irritations of the mind it put the user in a state where he was ready to greet any fellow human with true empathy.[34] At the same time, crowds and other sensations created too much stimulus while he was using, so he shied away from his normal Saturday recreation of attending the opera.[35] There were hints of sexual impropriety in his behavior, especially his friendship with the streetwalking Anne, but De Quincey denied any such bad behavior, and, anyway, opium would not have been the direct cause in the way that critics accused tea, coffee, and gin to led women into sexual misbehavior.

Opium use disordered De Quincey's social life by connecting him to people with whom a man of letters would normally not consort, such as the poor, prostitutes, and the Malaysian visitor. On the other hand, a trend had emerged by the Regency period for elite English men to prowl around unsuitable parts of the city in the pursuit of transgressive pleasures, and De Quincey's adventures in Soho as a youth and afterward certainly fit into this pattern.[36] Because the recreational use of opium was relatively new in western Europe, and there were so few who indulged in it, there were no rituals or social ties to govern and restrain De Quincey's use of opium. Nor was there any broader movement to make opium use "polite" as there was for coffee and tea, and indeed other addicts like Coleridge and Wilberforce did not publicize their opium use or get together as a group. On the other hand, neither did his social connections draw him into opium use as was so often the case for tea and other drugs. De Quincey claimed that opium did not produce the "torpid state of self-involution" that he said occurred to other users, especially "the Turks," whom he accused of sitting like statues while taking opium. Partly, De Quincey argued, this is because he timed his dose so that the "torpor" would descend on him at the normal time of sleeping, leaving him free to spend his earlier evening hours to wander about, enjoying the effects of his laudanum.[37] This careful planning, plus his insistence that he spaced out opium-taking over three week intervals, suggests that De Quincey himself came up with some rituals to help govern his drug use, at least until he began dosing himself every day. Despite his deliberate habits, opium certainly did cut him off from normal life in the broader sense, in that it hindered his career, denying him the prosperity that should have come to him as a talented man of letters. Nevertheless, the *Confessions* brought opium-taking out into the open, moving it from a secretive, solitary activity to a public one, an important move on the way to conceiving of opiate use as a social problem.

De Quincey's ironic comments about purchasing happiness, carrying it around on his person, and knowing that large quantities were pulsing through the commercial arteries of England demonstrate that he was aware of opium's status as a commodity, and he was certainly apprehensive about the supply chain of opium production connecting him to East Asia, as evidenced by his obsession with "the Malay" and orientalist dreaming. But he did not worry about the morality of opium production or sale like the clergymen made anxious by the sale of gin, Willian Henry and Edward Chandler (featured in chapter 6). While he was aware of how opium use hamstrung his own productivity and financial success, De Quincey made no generalizing conclusions about it. Although he dreamt of China, India, and Egypt, most opium consumed in Britain during De Quincey's day came from Asia Minor in the Ottoman Empire.[38] However, British merchants and officials in India were wresting control of the opium trade to Southeast Asia from the Dutch and spreading it to southern China. Opium became the centerpiece of British prosperity and power in Asia, stopping the flow of bullion from Europe and the European-controlled Americas into China, subsidizing British control of India and creating enormous wealth for the East India Company. Two decades after the publication of De Quincey's *Confessions*, the opium trade from British India to China led to the First Opium War, which both symbolized and contributed to the ebbing of Chinese power, and eventually the carving up of China into zones of influence exercised by foreign governments. The opium trade and its enormous revenues made possible both the growth of the British Empire and the fall of the Qing dynasty.[39] All of this happened at the time that antislavery activists scored two important victories in Britain: the end of the slave trade in 1807, and the end of slavery in the British Empire in 1833. But the end of one immoral commodity chain in the Americas occurred at the same time that another was growing in Asia, fostering the entanglement of opium with commerce, power, coercion, profit, taxes, and imperialism. Ironically, the changes in the opium trade worked to reinforce exoticizing, racializing stereotypes among Westerners in the form of Chinese "coolies" emigrating to work in mines and port cities around the world, bringing "opium dens" to cities like London, San Francisco, and Sydney.

For all that De Quincey's opium use fit into familiar patterns for early modern European drug and alcohol use, his *Confessions* also pointed to a future for drugs in Europe. If previous commentators had tended to focus on the physical effects of drugs and alcohol over their emotional, moral, or social effects, De Quincey was the opposite. He insisted that, for him, the pleasure of opium was emotional, a refined, intellectual sensation that he likened to listening to the opera, a pleasure that no Turk, "of all that ever entered the Paradise of opium-eaters," could ever experience. "By greatly increasing the activity of the mind," De Quincey explained, opium turned sound into "an elaborate intellectual pleasure."[40] Here he differentiated his experience with the drug from previous Western scholars who tried to explain its effects. In *The mysteries of opium reveal'd* from 1700, for example, the London physician John Jones tried to describe the "agreeable, pleasant, and charming Sensation" that the drug created: "It has been compar'd (not without good cause) to a permanent gentle Degree of that Pleasure, which Modesty forbids the naming of."[41] De Quincey would never compare opium to sex. Opium also helped him write his breakthrough piece of his career—similar to Coleridge, inspired by opium to write "Kubla Khan." The pains were mental as well as physical. Indeed De Quincey emphasized the dreams and night phantoms far more than the bodily effects of withdrawal, as "the whole burthen of horrors which lies up on my brain."[42] Even his anxiety about racialization manifested itself in dreams, not physical changes, unlike previous critics' treatment of chocolate and the other drugs. De Quincey's description of opium's pleasures and pains marked a transition between the early modern drug regime of physicality and the modern regime that emphasized moral and mental degeneration. The nineteenth-century temperance movement saw alcohol as a severe ethical and social problem, and attitudes about morphine were essentially the same.[43] *Confessions of an English opium-eater* prefigured the nineteenth-century categories of "inebriety," a mental illness that caused people to lose control over their drinking, and "morphinomania," which drove people who were not in physical pain to crave morphine nonetheless.

Opium, like its sister psychoactive drugs, was a catalyst for change while serving as a salient symbol of those changes. It forced western Europeans to confront their position in a society and culture beset by developments in global commerce, power, and knowledge. The ambivalence that De Quincey felt about his opium habit can serve as a microcosm of western Europe's ambivalence about all of the soft drugs that had become so common during the early modern period. De Quincey's struggle with self-constraint can also stand in for the increased scrutiny on the discipline that Weber, Elias, Oestreich, Habermas, and Foucault claim to have characterized the period. Weber believed that austerity fueled capitalism, but in truth commerce in stimulants fueled the growing economy even while threatening to enmesh workers in time- and money-wasting habits. Elias and Oestreich thought that modernity meant the discipline of one's emotions, but early modern drugs were a key element of wellness culture's regime maintaining emotional stability. Elias also thought that modernity depended on distancing oneself from bodily functions, but instead drugs made their users focus on both bodily filth and bodily pleasure. Habermas held the view that modern information relied on opening up new spaces of public discourse like the coffeehouse, but the new drugs created new sites and spaces of unpoliced speech, celebrated by some and condemned by others. Foucault argued that institutions like the prison and the clinic fostered self-discipline among modern Europeans, but the at the same time the new stimulants caused their users to lose control over their own bodies, social position, and wills. Perhaps modernity did not bring more discipline so much as it brought a new age of anxiety over discipline in an age where new pleasurable temptations rose alongside new efforts to restrain one's self.

The landscape of drugs and alcohol would shift during the nineteenth century due to scientific changes, the advent of big business, and modern advertising. Morphine, cocaine, heroin, cannabis, and amphetamines would all become available in Europe within a hundred years of the publication of the *Confessions*. The middle of the twentieth century saw the enormous cultural changes that led to the permissive society and also the popularity of hallucinogens in the West. But six constants would remain from the seventeenth century through the twenty-first. First, despite the increased emphasis on the mental and social aspects of drug use, critics of drug use emphasize their filthiness. The archetype of the "junkie," the effects of cocaine use on the nose, and "meth mouth" are all ways to shame drug takers by emphasizing the foul consequences that can be read on the users' bodies. The immense pleasure that drugs and alcohol provide are, of course, the reason why so many people use them. Although the neuroscientist Carl Hart is a vocal defender of the pleasures of using illicit drugs, normally people do not defend their use so much as simply use them, silently testifying to their power to make users—at least in the short term—feel good.[44] With legal drugs, of course, there is plenty of everyday testimony to the pleasures of chocolate, coffee, tea, sugar, and alcohol in all their various forms. Even tobacco, beleaguered by health concerns, has its aficionados. For both opponents and users, drugs and alcohol have retained their strong effects on the senses.

Second, drugs continue to be judged by who is imagined to use them. The nineteenth-century temperance movement in the anglophone countries emphasized class, religion, race, and ethnicity in its characterization of the effects of demon rum. Later nineteenth-century observers linked opium with east Asians even more strongly than did De Quincey. In the United States, morphine was strongly associated with elite white women, cocaine with Black men, and cannabis with Mexican Americans and African Americans. In the twentieth century the shift from powder cocaine to crack was also a shift from a drug associated with wealthy whites to one associated with the Black urban poor. All of these associations dragged these stereotypes held by the press, government, and society to the drugs themselves. The stereotyping could work to the benefit of drug users, too. The reputation that cannabis gained as a medicine that helped middle-class white cancer patients aided in rehabilitating that drug, and the imagined links between oxycontin and middle-class white America helped shield the addicts of today's opioid epidemic from some of the prejudices suffered by heroin users in the past. The biological and chemical effects of drugs and alcohol cannot be separated from the gender, class, racial, and religious cultural markers that society gives them.

Third, notwithstanding the triumph of the "brain disease" model that holds sway in substance abuse research, the understanding of addiction today seems to be as much of a complicated array of competing, overlapping metaphors as it was in early modern Europe. As medical experts continued to try to understand the compulsive use of drug and alcohol, the labels they used changed, from "habitual drunkard," "morphinomaniac," and "inebriate" to "alcoholic" and "addict," and, later, shifting the label from the people to the problem: "substance use disorder." Throughout these changes, the idea of addiction remained a mix of medical and moral judgment, with medicine never quite inventing a convincing explanation for compulsive drug use that could remain stable more than a few decades, and moral judgment waxing and waning, subject to changes in drug use as well as broader social change. Blame for addiction has continued to shift from the substance to the user and back again, depending on the drug, the imagined users, and the attitude of the observer. Medicine continues to be able to describe and categorize these drugs, just like Galenic and iatrochemical medicine centuries earlier, but it seems to be no closer to comprehending, or fixing, the hold that drugs and alcohol have over a compulsive subset of their users. Fourth, drugs and alcohol have remained entrenched in the practice of wellness. Opiates were common ingredients in nineteenth-century patent medicines like "nerve tonics," and cocaine could be found in many drinks, from Vin Mariani to Coca-Cola as part of a healthy dietary regime, often as alternatives to alcohol. The mid-twentieth-century saw hallucinogens briefly become popular as a means of mind expansion as well as antidotes to alcoholism, and today they are making a recurrence as mental health tools and productivity hacks. New drugs like ayahuasca have joined older ones like cannabis as staples of the wellness industry. These drugs have sometimes had the blessing of physicians, but more often they have simply been available in the market for consumers to choose for themselves. Freed from the watchful physician's oversight, the use of drugs for regulating one's mood has been an exercise in self-discipline and self-indulgence.

Fifth, drugs and alcohol have remained catalysts for changes in sociability. The saloon, the opium den, the discotheque, Amsterdam's coffeeshops, and entire neighborhoods like Soho in London have all been excoriated as sites of disorder that threaten old sites of sociability and are feared by some but viewed as liberating to others. Social relations have continued to pull people into drug use, and, once begun, drugs start bending users' social lives around their use. The tea table and coffeehouse were new and exciting for many people in the early modern period, allowing them access to a community that would have been impossible without them. The same has been true for pool halls, hippie communes, gay bars, Ken Kesey's Merry Pranksters on the Magic Bus, and Timothy Leary and Ram Dass's League for Spiritual Discovery at Millbrook.

Lastly, as commodities, drugs have remained sources of ambivalence. Europe and the West are even more comfortable with capitalism and the market than in the eighteenth century, but, with the great expansion in power, the modern state has been able to make some drugs illegal. The drug dealer has become a public villain, and conservative thinkers—the same people who valorize the economic freedoms of the market—view the purchase and consumption of illegal drugs as a cause and a sign of national degeneracy. Commodity chains are still worrisome, thanks to the persistence of corporate oppression, child labor, and even slavery in the production of soft drugs like coffee and chocolate, leading to efforts by the fair trade movement to create ethical commerce of these commodities. Other troubling commodity chains seem to be invisible to consumers: the corruption, lawlessness, and violence in Latin America are largely absent in the debates in Europe and North America about illegal drug use. Instead of blaming drug use at home for encouraging chaos abroad, conservatives—forgetting how the laws of supply and demand work—tend to blame Latin Americans for bringing drugs and violence into Europe and North America. Anti-industriousness, too, is still a problem. Heroin, cocaine, and alcohol are all coded as encouraging or rewarding laziness and welfare dependency, a view that is inextricable from ideas about class and race. However, some drugs have emerged since De Quincey's day that are viewed as as industrious helpers, notably coffee, cigarettes in the early twentieth century, and, today, micro-dosing with hallucinogens as well as the "study drugs" Adderall and Ritalin. The prohibition of alcohol in the United States, the hesitant legalization of cannabis throughout the West, and experiments with decriminalization in places like Portugal all testify to the continuing ambivalence with profiting from drug use. And while the state is no longer so dependent on taxing drugs to fill its coffers, heavy taxes on tobacco and alcohol remain, with unclear intentions: Are they taxed to decrease use, or simply to take advantage of a commodity with an inelastic demand? This becomes even more confusing in light of the settlements from the lawsuits that US state governments made with cigarette companies leading to dependency on those companies to balance their budgets. Are the states trying to decrease tobacco use to preserve the health of their citizens, or to protect the profits of tobacco companies in order to keep the settlement money coming? Will the lawsuits against the pharmaceutical companies in light of the recent opioid epidemic follow the same pattern, keeping the Sackler family in business after all? The triumph of capitalism still leaves policy makers with few easy answers when it comes to profiting from the sale of drugs and alcohol.

Why have these patterns persisted? Were they "invented" in the early modern period and simply continue to linger on? I suspect they persist because they emerged from broad, tectonic forces in human culture and society that remain constant over centuries and can change only incrementally slowly. They persist because drugs remain a catalyst for, and a symbol of, ambivalent changes taking place in society and culture. Immigration, race, gender, and religion remain as fluid and as subject to disagreement in the twenty-first century as in the sixteenth. Global capitalism is as problematic now as it was when it began. Self-discipline remains difficult, and it is not always clear when, or whether, discipline is desirable or represents an unhealthy repression of natural desires. Impulsive and compulsive behavior remains as mysterious now as it did even before 1492, when the only mood-altering drugs that Europeans were accustomed to were wine, beer, and ale. Thus, psychotropic drugs remain powerful markers of discipline, objects and symbols for control over one's body, mind, and behavior.

Notes

Introduction

1. For nervous disorders, see Michael Stolberg, *Experiencing Illness and the Sick Body in Early Modern Europe*, trans. Leonhard Unglaub and Logan Kennedy (Houndmills: Palgrave Macmillan, 2011), 170–73; and Heather R. Beatty, *Nervous Disease in Late Eighteenth-Century Britain: The Reality of a Fashionable Disorder* (London: Pickering & Chatto, 2012).

2. Thomas Trotter, *A view of the nervous temperament*, 2nd ed. (Newcastle: Edw. Walker, and London: Longman, Hurst, Rees, and Orme, 1807), viii.

3. Trotter, *View of the nervous temperament*, xvii--xviii; Beatty, *Nervous Disease*, 141–73.

4. Thomas Trotter, *An essay medical, philosophical, and chemical on drunkenness and its effects on the human body*, ed. Roy Porter (1804; London: Routledge, 1988), 172.

5. Trotter, *View of the nervous temperament*, 285.

6. Trotter, 74.

7. Trotter, 137–39.

8. Trotter, 146.

9. Sidney W. Mintz, *Sweetness and Power: The Place of Sugar in Modern History* (New York: Penguin, 1985), 73.

10. Irene Fattacciu, "Cacao: From an Exotic Curiosity to a Spanish Commodity. The Diffusion of New Patterns of Consumption in Eighteenth-Century Spain," *Food & History* 7, no. 1 (2009): 53–78; Jordan Goodman, *Tobacco in History: The Cultures of Dependence* (London: Routledge, 1993), 134–48.

11. S. D. Smith, "Accounting for Taste: British Coffee Consumption in Historical Perspective," *Journal of Interdisciplinary History* 27, no. 2 (1996): 183–214; Jan de Vries, *The Industrious Revolution: Consumer Behavior and the Household Economy, 1650 to the Present* (Cambridge: Cambridge University Press, 2008), 156.

12. The great diversity in types of distilled liquor and in the places where it was made make the volume somewhat unknowable, but by 1743 England was producing 8.2 million gallons of gin per year, and this was just one country and one type of alcohol. Rod Phillips, *Alcohol: A History* (Chapel Hill: University of North Carolina Press, 2014), 127.

13. In *Forces of Habit*, David Courtwright calls them "failed drugs" for the failure of Europeans to adopt them and take over their distribution and production, at least until the late nineteenth centuries.

14. Cornelis Bontekoe, *Tractaat van het excellenste kruyd thee: 't welk vertoond het regte gebruyk, en de groote kragten van 't selve in gesondheyd, en siekten* (The Hague:

Pieter Hagen, 1678), from *Opuscula selecta Neerlandicorum de arte medica*, trans. anon. (Amsterdam, 1937); https://www.dbnl.org/tekst/_opu001193701_01/_opu001193701_01_0014.php, 459.

15. David T. Courtwright, *Forces of Habit: Drugs and the Making of the Modern World* (Cambridge, MA: Harvard University Press, 2001). More recently, Benjamin Breen has labeled it "the Age of Intoxication." See Benjamin Breen, *The Age of Intoxication: Origins of the Global Drug Trade* (Philadelphia: University of Pennsylvania Press, 2019).

16. Daniel Lord Smail, *On Deep History and the Brain* (Berkeley: University of California Press, 2008).

17. Alison Games, "Atlantic History: Definitions, Challenges, and Opportunities," *American Historical Review* 111, no. 3 (2006): 741.

18. For Weber and discipline, see Robert van Krieken, "Social Discipline and State Formation: Weber and Oestreich on the Historical Sociology of Subjectivity," *Amsterdams Sociologisch Tijdschrift* 17, no. 1 (1990): 3–38.

19. For Elias and discipline, see Robert van Krieken, "The Organisation of the Soul: Elias and Foucault on Discipline and the Self," *European Journal of Sociology/Archives Européennes de Sociologie* 31 (1990): 353–71.

20. For Oestreich and discipline, see Peter N. Miller, "Nazis and Neo-Stoics: Otto Brunner and Gerhard Oestreich before and after the Second World War," *Past and Present* 176 (2002): 144–86; and van Krieken, "Social Discipline and State Formation."

21. Michel Foucault, *Discipline and Punish: The Birth of the Prison*, trans. Alan Sheridan, 2nd ed. (New York: Vintage, 1995).

22. The literature on sugar plantations is vast. For sugar's impact on Europe, see Charlotte Sussman, *Consuming Anxieties: Consumer Protest, Gender, and British Slavery, 1713–1833* (Stanford, CA: Stanford University Press, 2000); Clare Midgley, *Women against Slavery: The British Campaigns, 1780–1870* (New York: Routledge, 1992); and of course Mintz, *Sweetness and Power*. For tobacco and chocolate, see Marcy Norton, *Sacred Gifts, Profane Pleasures: A History of Tobacco and Chocolate in the Atlantic World* (Ithaca, NY: Cornell University Press, 2008). For tea, see Erika Rappaport, *A Thirst for Empire: How Tea Shaped the Modern World* (Princeton, NJ: Princeton University Press, 2017). For coffee, see Brian Cowan, *The Social Life of Coffee: The Emergence of the British Coffeehouse* (New Haven, CT: Yale University Press, 2005); and Markman Ellis, *The Coffee House: A Cultural History* (London: Weidenfeld & Nicolson, 2004). For gin, see Jessica Warner, *Craze: Gin and Debauchery in an Age of Reason* (New York: Basic Books, 2002); and Patrick Dillon, *Gin: The Much-Lamented Death of Madam Geneva* (Boston: Justin, Charles, 2002). For opium, see Martin Booth, *Opium: A History* (New York: St. Martin's, 1996).

23. There are a few exceptions for Latin works translated and published in vernacular languages.

24. No doubt there are practical reasons, too: this author's greater familiarity with English and the fact that Britain has the best research tools available for early modern printed material. Early English Books Online and Eighteenth Century Collections Online were essential tools for the research of this book. Google Books and the development of online research tools like Gallica, from

the Bibliotèque nationale de France, are allowing other nations to catch up. Material printed in German and Portuguese could have been included, but I already had to learn Italian and Dutch for this project; learning two more languages would have further lengthened the time it took to complete it.

25. For both of these points, see Courtwright, *Forces of Habit.*

26. Norton, *Sacred Gifts.*

27. Jessica Warner, "'Resolv'd to Drink No More': Addiction as a Preindustrial Construct," *Journal of Studies on Alcohol* 55, no. 6 (1994): 685–91.

1. Stained with Spots of Human Blood

1. For a good overview of the history of sugar, see Elizabeth Abbott, *Sugar: A Bittersweet History* (London: Duckworth Overlook, 2009); see also the landmark Mintz, *Sweetness and Power.*

2. *Atlas of the Transatlantic Slave Trade*, ed. David Eltis and David Richardson (New Haven, CT: Yale University Press, 2010), 2.

3. Mintz, *Sweetness and Power*, 73.

4. Andrew Burn, *Second address to the people of Great Britain: containing a new, and most powerful argument to abstain from the use of West India sugar*, 2nd ed. (Rochester: W. Gillman, 1792), 2. For another analysis of Burn's *Second address*, see Charlotte Sussman, *Consuming Anxieties: Consumer Protest, Gender, and British Slavery, 1713–1833* (Stanford, CA: Stanford University Press, 2000), 119–21.

5. Burn, *Second address*, 3–6.

6. Burn, 7–9.

7. Burn, 9–11.

8. This is not the first time this has been pointed out. See, for example, Sussman, *Consuming Anxieties*; and Julie L. Holcomb, *Moral Commerce: Quakers and the Transatlantic Boycott of the Slave Labor Economy* (Ithaca, NY: Cornell University Press, 2016).

9. Andrew Kettler, *The Smell of Slavery: Olfactory Racism and the Atlantic World* (Cambridge: Cambridge University Press, 2020). See also Mark M. Smith, *How Race Is Made: Slavery, Segregation, and the Senses* (Chapel Hill: University of North Carolina Press, 2006); and William Tullett, "Grease and Sweat: Race and Smell in Eighteenth-Century English Culture," *Cultural and Social History* 13, no. 3 (2016): 307–22.

10. Norton, *Sacred Gifts*, 47–62.

11. For a review of the history of the senses, see William Tullett, "State of the Field: Sensory History," *History* 10, no. 373 (2021): 804–20.

12. Norbert Elias, *The Civilizing Process: Sociogenetic and Psychogenetic Investigations*, rev. ed., ed. Eric Dunning, Johan Goudsblom, and Stephen Mennell, trans. Edmund Jephcott (Malden, MA: Blackwell, 2000); see also Robert van Krieken, "The Organization of the Soul: Elias and Foucault on Discipline and the Self," *European Journal of Sociology/Archives Européennes de Sociologie* 31 (1990): 353–71.

13. Marcy Norton, "Tasting Empire: Chocolate and the European Internalization of Mesoamerican Aesthetics," *American Historical Review* 111, no. 3 (2006): 660–91.

14. Norton, *Sacred Gifts*, 47–62.

15. Kristen G. Brookes, "Inhaling the Alien: Race and Tobacco in Early Modern England," in *Global Traffic: Discourses and Practices of Trade in English Literature and Culture from 1550 to 1700*, ed. Barbara Sebek and Stephen Deng (New York: Palgrave Macmillan, 2008), 157–78.

16. Philaretes, *Work for chimney-sweepers: or a warning for tabacconists* (London: T. Este, 1602), fol. Bivr.

17. Philaretes, *Work for chimney-sweepers*, fols. Civ–Ciir.

18. Philaretes, fols. Ciiir–Ciiiv.

19. Barnabe Rich, *My ladies looking glasse* (London: Thomas Adams, 1616), 24–25.

20. Samuel Rowlands, *A crew of kind gossips, all met to be merrie complayning of their husbands, with their husbands answeres in their owne defence* (London: John Deane, 1613), fols. Dv–D2r.

21. Bartolomé Jiménez Patón, *Reforma de trages. Doctrina de frai Hernando de Talavera primera arçobispo de Granada* (Baeza: Juan de la Cuesta, 1638), fol. 61v.

22. John Philips, *Sportive wit the muses merriment, a new spring of lusty drollery, joviall fancies, and a la mode lamponnes* (London: Nath. Brook, 1656), 6. Phillips was the nephew and godson of John Milton.

23. Philips, *Sportive wit*, 6–9.

24. Adam Clarke, *A dissertation on the use and abuse of tobacco* (London: G. Whitfield, 1797), 7, 18–19, 24.

25. *Tobaco-mastix or thee common use of that weed in all the wayes of preparing it, taxed by arguments from reason and experience, with all the vulgar objections discust and answered* (Scotland[?]: n.p., 1677), 6, 8–9.

26. *Tobaco-mastix*, 19–20.

27. Anthony Chute, *Tabacco: the distinct and severall opinions of the late and best phisitions that have written of the divers natures and qualities thereof* (London: William Barlow, 1595), 19–21. Soldiers began removing church furnishing from Westminster Abbey in 1644. J. F. Merritt, "Reinventing Westminster Abbey, 1642–1660: A House of Kings from Revolution to Restoration," *Journal of Ecclesiastical History* 64, no. 1 (2016): 122–38.

28. Philaretes, *Work for chimney-sweepers*, fols. Ev–E2r.

29. Samuel Rowlands, *More knaves yet? The knaves of spades and diamonds. With new additions* (London: n.p., 1613).

30. Ben Jonson, "A ballad called cooklorrel," in J.[John Playford?], *An antidote against melancholy made up in pills. Compounded of witty ballads, jovial songs, and merry catches* (London: John Playford, 1669), 97–98.

31. Jonson, "Ballad called cooklorrel," 3.

32. Jonson, 26.

33. Rich, *My ladies looking glasse*, 24–25.

34. Francisco de Leiva y Aguilar, *Desengaño contra el mal uso del tabaco* (Córdoba: Salvador de Cea Tesa, 1634), fol. 12v.

35. William Tullett, *Smell in Eighteenth-Century England: A Social Sense* (Oxford: Oxford University Press, 2019).

36. Francesco Arisi, *Il tabaco masticato, e fumato* (Milan: n.p., 1725), 15.

37. *Of the use of tobacco, tea, coffee, chocolate, and drams* (London[?]: H. Parker, 1722), 9.

38. *Whipping-Tom: or, a rod for a proud lady, bundled up in four feeling discourses, both serious and merry*, 4th ed. (London: Sam. Briscoe, 1722), 7; Caroline Grigson, *Menagerie: The History of Exotic Animals in England, 1100–1837* (Oxford: Oxford University Press, 2016), 53.

39. *A cup of coffee, or coffee in its colours* (London: n.p., 1663). For this broadside, see also Gitanjali G. Shahani, *Tasting Differences: Food, Race, and Cultural Encounters in Early Modern Literature* (Ithaca, NY: Cornell University Press, 2020), 99–100.

40. One notable exception here is Emily Cockayne, *Hubbub: Filth, Noise and Stench in England, 1600–1770* (New Haven, CT: Yale University Press, 2007). For scent-scapes, see Tullett, "State of the Field," 11.

41. Tullett, *Smell in Eighteenth-Century England*, 136–37.

42. *The maidens complaint against coffee* (London: J. Jones, 1663), 4.

43. Don Bollicosgo Armuhaz, *The coffee-mans granado discharged upon the maidens complaint against coffee* (London: J. Johnson, 1663), 7–8.

44. Isidro Fernández Matienzo, *Discurso medico y phisico agradable a los medicos ancianos y despertador para los modernos contra el medicamento caphè* (Madrid: Melchor Alvarez, 1693), fol. ¶¶¶¶r.

45. Edward Ward, *The school of politicks or, the humours of a coffee-house a poem* (London: Richard Baldwin, 1690), 2.

46. Alexandro de Moya, *El café*, vol. 1. (Madrid: Imprenta de Gonzalez, 1792), 19.

47. Joseph M. Lequinio, *Préjugés déstruits* (Paris: l'Imprimerie Nationale, 1792), 151.

48. *De gedebaucheerde en betoverde koffy en theewereld, behelzende een meenigte van aardige voorvallen, welke zich sedert weinig tijds te Amsterdam, Rotterdam, en Den Haag, te Utrecht en de bijgelegene Plaatsen, op de Koffy en Theegezelschapijes* (Amsterdam: Timotheus ten Hoorn, 1701), 475–76.

49. *De gedebaucheerde*, 35–36.

50. R. V. N., *Natuur-kundige verhandelin van de theé, koffeé, tabak en snufpoeders.* (Amsterdam: J. ten Hoorn, 1701), 6.

51. John Waldron, *A satyr against tea* (Dublin: Sylvanus Pepyat, 1733), 4, 11–12. Nothing is known of Waldron; *Tea and the Tea-Table in Eighteenth-Century England*, vol. 1, *Literary Representations of Tea and the Tea-Table*, ed. Markman Ellis (London: Pickering & Chatto, 2020), 109.

52. Waldron, *Satyr against tea*, 12.

53. Thomas Lodge, *Wits miserie, and the worlds madnesse discovering the devils incarnate of this age* (London: Adam Islip, 1596), 82.

54. *A dissertation upon drunkenness* (London: T. Warner, 1727), 8–9.

55. Burn, *Second address*, 9–11.

56. *Considerations to professors of Christianity of every denomination, on the impropriety of consuming West-Indian sugar and rum, as produced by the oppressive labour of slaves* (London[?]: n.p., 1792), 2–3.

57. William Henry, *An earnest address to the people of Ireland, against the drinking of spirituous liquors* (Dublin: Peter Wilson, 1753), 10, 14–15.

58. William Fox, *An address to the people of Great Britain on the propriety of abstaining from West India sugar and rum* (London: James Phillips, 1791), 4.

59. Fox, *Address*, 4–5.

60. Fox, 14.

61. "De oozraak der slaaverny," *De vaderlander*, October 23, 1775, 343.

62. Holcomb, *Moral Commerce*, 13.

63. Holcomb, 52–57.

64. Sussman, *Consuming Anxieties*, 118–22.

65. William Naish, *Reasons for using East India sugar* (London: Howlett and Brimmer, 1828), 14–15.

66. Michel Foucault, *Discipline and Punish: The Birth of the Prison*, trans. Alan Sheridan (New York: Pantheon, 1977); see also Tullett, "State of the Field," 8.

67. Gallobelgicus, *Wine, beere, ale, and tobacco. Contending for superiority a dialogue*, 2nd ed. (London: John Grove, 1630), fol. Bv; James Hart, *Klinike, or the diet of the diseased* (London: Robert Allot, 1633), 96–97.

68. Cornelis Bontekoe, *Tractaat van het excellenste kruyd thee*, trans. anon., in *Opuscula Selecta Nederlandicorum de arte medica*, vol. 14 (Amsterdam, 1937; originally published: The Hague: Pieter Hagan, 1678), 317, accessed March 27, 2019, https://www.dbnl.org/tekst/_opu001193701_01/_opu001193701_01_0014.php (accessed March 27, 2019).

69. Daniel N. Sennert and Abdiah Cole, *The sixth book of pratical physick of occult or hidden diseases* (London: Peter Cole, 1662), 56.

70. Thomas Willis, *Two discourses concerning the souls of brutes which is that of the vital and sensitive of man*, trans. S. Pordage (London: Thomas Drink, Ch. Harper, and John Leigh, 1683), 135.

71. "A satyr upon brandy," in *Directions for brewing malt liquors* (London: J. Nutt, 1700), 26–27.

72. *Disseratation upon drunkenness*, 21.

73. *An epistle to the fair-sex on the subject of drinking* (London: T. Gardner, 1744), 9–11. Some have attributed the work to Eliza Fowler Haywood, following the *British Museum Catalogue* of 1956, but Patrick Spedding rejects the attribution. Patrick Spedding, *A Bibliography of Eliza Haywood* (London: Pickering & Chatto, 2004), 634–35. Later editions of the book appear under the title *A present for women addicted to drinking.*

74. Saynought Slyboots, *The tavern scuffle: or the club in an uproar; occasion'd by a hot dispute, between Mr. Swell-Gut, a brewer, and Mr. Scorch-Gut, a distiller, concerning geneva, the reigning liquor now in vogue among the common people* (London: T. Warner, 1726), 14–15.

75. Slyboots, *Tavern scuffle*, 20–21.

76. For hair, see Isaac Maddox, *The expediency of preventive wisdom* (London: H. Woodfall, 1750), 30; for skin and teeth, see James Yates, *The effects of drinking spiritous, and other intoxicating liquors, described in four sermons, preached at the chapel in Union-Place, Glasgow* (Glasgow: James Hedderwick, 1818), 24, 54; for legs and feet, see John Coakley Lettsom, *History of some of the effects of hard drinking*, 6th ed. (London: W. Darton, 1791), 5, 7.

77. See also Tobias Smollett, *A dissertation on Mr. Hogarth's six prints lately publish'd, viz. Gin-Lane, Beer-Street, and the Four Stages of Cruelty* (London: B. Dickinson, 1751), 11–12. For Smollett's authorship of this anonymous publication, see Donald C. Shelton, "A Satire, Not a Sermon: Four Stages of Cruelty and Murder," *Athens Journal of History* 6, no. 3 (2020): 233–86.

78. Daniel Duncan, *Wholesome advice against the abuse of hot liquors, particularly of coffee, chocolate, tea, brandy, and strong-waters*, trans. anon. (London: H. Rhodes and A. Bell, 1706), 102–16. I have not been able to find a copy of the original book in the original French.

79. *The women's petition against coffee representing to publick consideration the grand inconveniences accruing to their sex from the excessive use of that drying, enfeebling liquor* (London: n.p., 1674), 3.

80. Nicolas François Joseph Éloy, *Reflexions sur l'usage du thé dans lequelles, après avoir fait l'histoire de cette boisson étrangerie, on donne les précautions nécessaires pour la prendre avec avantage* (Mons: Chez Plon, 1750), 41–43.

81. *Whipping-Tom*, 17.

82. Tobias Venner, *A briefe and accurate treatise, concerning, the taking of the fume of tobacco which very many, in these days, doe too too licentiously use* (London: Richard Moore, 1621), fol. B4v.

83. Thomas Short, *Discourses on tea, sugar, milk, made-wines, spirits, punch, tobacco, &c., with plain and useful rules for gouty people* (London: T. Longman and A. Millar, 1750), 250–51.

84. *A treatise upon the herb tobacco, pointing out its deleterious pernicious quality, and its fatal effects upon the human constitution, by the great variety of disorders it occasions* (London: Charles Stalker, 1789), 25–28.

85. Hugh Smythson, *The compleat family physician; or, universal medical repository* (London: Harrison, 1785), 753–59.

86. Tomás Ramón, *Nueva prematica de reformacion contra los abusos de afeytes, calçado, guedejas, guardainfantes, lenguaje critic, moños, trajes; y excess en el uso del tabaco* (Zaragoza: Diego Dormer, 1635), 361–62.

87. For entrails, see Richard West, *Wits A.B.C. or a centurie of epigrams* (London: Thomas Thorp, 1608), fols. E2v–E3r; for herring, see Joshua Sylvester, *Tobacco battered; & the pipes shattered (about their eares that idely idolize so base & barbarous a weed; or at least-wise over-love so loathsome vanitie)* (London: H. Lownes, 1616 or 1617), 101–2.

88. Sylvester, *Tobacco battered*, 115.

89. Leiva y Aguilar, *Desengaño contra el mal uso del tabaco*, fols. 158r–179r.

90. *Tabaco-mastix*, 3.

91. See Richard Carr, *Dr. Carr's medicinal epistles upon several occasions*, trans. John Quincy (London: William Newton and J. Phillips, 1714) 5; John Hill, *Cautions against the immoderate use of snuff* (London: R. Baldwin and J. Jackson, 1761), 10; Short, *Discourses*, 20; Smythson, *Compleat family physician*, 754.

92. *A dissertation on the use and abuses of tobacco* (London: J. Roberts, 1720), 20.

93. Antonio Lavedán, *Tratado de los usos, abusos, propiedades y virtudes del tabaco, café, té y chocolate* (Madrid: Imprenta Real, 1796), 85.

94. Venner, *Briefe and accurate treatise*, fols. B1v–B2r.

95. Henry Butts, *Dyets dry dinner consisting of eight severall courses* (London: Tho. Creede for William Wood, 1599), fols. P3, Aiv–P3Aivr; Benedetto Stella, *Il tabacco* (Rome: F. M. Mancini, 1669), 253.

96. J. B. Sassenus, *De voortreffelijkheid van de thee, en hare bewonderenswaardige verdienste in de geneeskunde* (Rotterdam: T.J. Wijnhoven Hendriksen, 1828), 11–13.

97. Duncan, *Wholesome advice*, 58–59.

98. Frederick Slare, "A vindication of sugars against the charge of Dr. Willis, other physicians, and common prejudices: dedicated to the ladies," in *Experiments and observations upon oriental and other bezoar-stones, which prove them to be of no use in physick* (London: Tim Goodwin, 1715), 2–5.

99. *An essay on sugar* (London: E. Comyns, 1752), 4, 8–9.

100. Butts, *Dyets dry dinner*, fols. O4iir–Oiiir.

101. Walter Rumsey, Organon salutis, *an instrument to cleanse the stomach, as also divers new experiments of the virtue of tobacco and coffee: how much they conduce to preserve humane health* (London: D. Pakeman, 1657).

102. Cornelis Bontekoe and Stephan Blankaart, *Gebruik en misbruik van de thee, mitsgaders een erhandelinge wegens de deugden en kragten van de tabak. Hier nevens een verhandelingevan de coffee, met des zelfs krachten in gezonde, en ongezonde, door Stephanus Blankaart* (The Hague: Pieter Hagen and Amsterdam: Jan ten Hoorn, 1686), 17, 176–77.

103. *Carta que escrivió un medico christiano, que estava curando en Antiberi, a un cardenal de Roma, sobre la bebeda del cahuè o café* (n.p.); and *The vertues of chocolate East-India drink* (n.p., 1660).

104. Thomas Tomkis, *Lingua: or the combat of the tongue, and the five senses for superiority a pleasant comoedie* (London: Simon Waterson, 1607), fol. H4r.

105. West, *Wits A.B.C.*, fols. E2v–E3r.

106. A foul taste and odor had been a sign of effective medicine, although this idea as passing in the eighteenth century. Tullett, *Smell in the Eighteenth Century*; Edmund Gardiner, *The trial of tabacco* (London: Mathew Lownes, 1610), fol. 22v.

107. Gardiner, *Trial of tabacco*, fols. 50v–52r.

108. Gardiner, fols. 54r–54v.

109. Gardiner, fols. 14v–15v, 22r.

110. Nicolás Monardes, *Primera y seguna y tercera partes de la historia medicinal: de las cosas que se traen de nuestras Indias Occidentales, que se sirven en medicina* (Seville: Alonso Escrivano, 1574), see also Norton, *Sacred Gifts*, 110–14.

111. Short, *Discourses*, 250–52.

112. Short, 253–56.

113. Lavedán, *Tratado*, 85.

114. Juan de Castro y Medinilla, *Historia de las virtudes y propiedades del tabaco, i de los modos de tomarle para las partes intrinsecas i de aplicarle as las extrinsecas* (Córdoba: Salvador de Cea Tesa, 1620), fols. 39v–40r.

115. Bontekoe and Blankaart, *Gebruik en misbruik*, 120.

116. John Taylor, *The nipping and snipping of abuses* (London: Nathaniel Butler, 1614), fol. D1r.

117. *Essay on sugar*, 6–7.

118. Kim F. Hall, "Culinary Spaces, Colonial Spaces: The Gendering of Sugar in the Seventeenth Century," in *Feminist Readings of Early Modern Culture: Emerging Subjects*, ed. Valerie Traub, M. Lindsay Kaplan, and Dympna Callaghan (Cambridge: Cambridge University Press, 1996), 168–90.

119. Michael Kwass, "Ordering the World of Goods: Consumer Revolution and the Classification of Objects in Eighteenth-Century France," *Representations* 82, no. 1 (2003): 87–116.

120. Catherine Wilson, *Epicureanism at the Origins of Modernity* (Oxford: Clarendon, 2008).

121. Girolamo Giuntini, "Scherzo ditirambico in lode della cioccolata," in *Altro parere intorno alla natura, ed all' uso della cioccolata* by Francesco Zeti (Florence, 1728), 27–31.

122. Giambattista Sbalbi, *La cioccolata, versione dal latin rime toscane del Canonico Giambattista Sbalbi* (Piacenza: Niccolò Orcesi, 1789), 11.

123. Vincenzo Corrado, *Il credenziere di buno gusto*, 6th ed. (Napoli: Torchi di Saverio Giordano, 1820), 10.

124. Giacomo Sanvitale, *Memorie veridiche contrapposte alle memorie istoriche sull' uso del cioccolato in giorno di digiuno* (n.p., 1748), 49–50.

125. Gregorio Mayáns, "Elegía al chocolate," trans. from Latin by José María Estellés i González, "Una pincelada frívola en la obra de Mayans: Elegía al chocolate," in *Estudios dedicados a Juan Peset Aleixandre*, vol. 1 (Valencia: Universidad de Valencia, 1982), 581–600.

126. De Castro y Medinilla, *Historia*, fols. 19r–20r.

127. Francisco Maria della Volpe, *Pulvis nicotianus vulgo tabacco ad Leodocum Sofidium acclamatum* (Rome: Antonius de Rubeis Romae, 1722).

128. Francis Beaumont, *Poems: by Francis Beaumont, gent. viz. the hermaphrodite* (London: Laurence Blaiklock, 1653), fols. N5r–N6v.

129. Luigi Zorzi Prete, "In lode del tabacco," in *In lode del fico, in lode del tabacco, di ringraziamento, capitoli tre* (Verona: Pietro Bisesti, 1822), 12.

130. Michele Nicolò Chiazzari, *Osservazione sull' uso ed abuso del tabacco in istato di sanitá e di malattia* (Genoa: S. Matteo, 1819), 7–9.

131. Girolamo Baruffaldi, *La tabaccheide* (Ferrera: Eredi di B. Pometelli, 1714), 11–12.

132. Anton-Maria Borga da Rasa, *Gli arcani di venere, poemetto. La pipa, ditirambo* (Venice[?]: n.p., 1750), 39.

133. Nahum Tate, *Panacea, a poem upon tea in two canto's* (London: J. Roberts, 1700), 3–4.

134. Peter Motteux, *A poem in praise of tea* (London: J. Tonson, 1712), 6.

135. Bontekoe, *Traactat*, 303.

136. *The art of making tea, a poem, in two cantos* (Cambridge: Printed by B. Flower, 1797), 7–8.

137. For example, Nicolas Blégny, *Le bon usage du thé, du caffé et du chocolat pour la preservation & pour la guerison des maladies* (Paris: Estienne Michalet, 1687), 95–98; and Henry Carey, *Poems on several occasions* (London: J. Kent, 1713), fol. D2r.

138. Alexander Blunt, *Geneva: A Poem. Address'd To the Right Honourable Sir R- W-.* (London: Printed for T. Payne, 1729), 29.

139. *Iets over den opium* (Rotterdam: J. J. Thompson, 1800s), para. 2.

140. *Iets over den opium*, para. 2

141. James Handley, *Mechanical essays on the animal oeconomy* (London: n.p, 1721), 160–61.

142. Handley, *Mechanical essays*, 4.

143. Viktoria von Hoffman, *From Gluttony to Enlightenment: The World of Taste in Early Modern Europe* (Urbana: University of Illinois Press, 2016). For an

exploration of how taste and smell could lead to scientific knowledge, see Clare Hickman, *The Doctor's Garden: Medicine, Science, and Horticulture in Britain* (New Haven, CT: Yale University Press, 2021).

144. James I of England, *A counterblaste to tobacco* (n.p., 1604), fol. B4r.

145. De Castro y Medinilla, *Historia*, fol. 37r.

146. Lorenzo Serafini, *Lettera in cui si esaminato le ragioni addotte dall' autore del primo parere intorno all' uso della cioccolata dedicate all' illustriss. Sig. Ca. Cosimo degli Albizzi* (Florence: n.p., 1728).

147. Antoine-Augustin Parmentier, "Abus dans la fabrication du chocolat," in *Bibliothèque physique oeconomique* (Paris: Chez Buisson, 1786), 178–79.

148. Bontekoe, *Tractaat*, 303, 443, 445. Coffee's quality, too, could be judged by the senses: see Tullett, *Smell in Eighteenth-Century England*, 137.

149. John Ovington, *An essay upon the nature and qualities of tea* (London: R. Roberts, 1699), 13.

150. *De gedebaucheerde*, 25.

151. Short, *Discourses*, 30.

152. Short, 31–32.

153. Short, 164–65.

154. Robert Dossie, *An essay on spirituous liquors, with regard to their effects on health* (London: Printed for J. Ridley, 1770[?]), 37.

155. Dossie, *Essay on spirituous liquors*, 19–22.

156. For an exploration of the way that the senses could reinforce or contradict chemical analysis as science was changing, see Saskia Klerk, "The Trouble with Opium: Taste, Reason, and Experience in Late Galenic Pharmacology with Special Regard to the University of Leiden (1575–1625)," *Early Science and Medicine* 19, no. 4 (2014): 287–316.

157. M. de Reynal, *Opuscule médico-politique sur le café* (Évreux: Imprimerie de J. J. L. Ancelle, 1813), 17.

158. Thomas Short, *The Natural, Experimental, and Medicinal History of the Mineral Waters of Derbyshire, Lincolnshire, and Yorkshire* (London: F. Gyles, 1734), 317.

159. Sarah Besky, *Tasting Qualities: The Past and Future of Tea* (Oakland: University of California Press, 2020).

2. Chocolate, or an Indian Drink

1. John Chamberlayne, *The natural history of coffee, chocolate, thee, tobacco* (London: Christopher Wilkinson, 1682), 38. This might be the John Chamberlayne who became a natural historian and linguist, but, if so, that would put him at no older than fourteen years old when this book was published. See Reavley Gair, "Chamberlayne, John (1668/9–1723)," *Oxford Dictionary of National Biography*, accessed September 10, 2023 https://www.oxforddnb.com/display/10.1093/ref:odnb/9780198614128.001.0001/odnb-9780198614128-e-5060.

2. Chamberlayne, *Natural history*, 13–19.

3. For Columbus, see Inga Clendinnen, *Ambivalent Conquests: Maya and Spaniard in Yucatan, 1517–1570* (Cambridge: Cambridge University Press, 1987), 3; for Hernández, see Norton, *Sacred Gifts*, 121–27.

4. Norton, 138-40; Fattacciu, "Cacao." For the original—in a French translation because I could not find the original Spanish—see Barthelemy [Bartolomé] Marradón, *Du chocolate, dialogue entre un medicin, un indien, & un bourgeois*, trans. René Moreau (Lyon: Jean Girin and Barthelemy Riviere, 1670).

5. Norton, *Sacred Gifts*.

6. Fattacciu, "Cacao," 71.

7. Norton, *Sacred Gifts*, 141–42.

8. James Walvin, *Fruits of Empire: Exotic Produce and British Taste, 1660–1800* (New York: New York University Press, 1997), 94.

9. Jordan Goodman, "Excitantia, or, How Enlightenment Europe Took to Soft Drugs," in *Consuming Habits: Drugs in History and Anthropology*, ed. Jordan Goodman, Paul E. Lovejoy, and Andrew Sherratt (London: Routledge, 1995), 129.

10. Walvin, *Fruits of Empire*, 92-96. Much of the new production was aimed at the American markets; for example, Eduardo Arcila Farias found that 80 percent of the cacao exports from Venezuela went to New Spain. Eduardo Arcila Farias, *Haciendo y comercio de Venezuela en el siglo XVII: 1601–1650* (Caracas: Banco Central de Venezuela, 1985).

11. Fattacciu, "Cacao," 65–67.

12. Irene Fattacciu, "The Resilience and Boomerang Effect of Chocolate: A Product's Globalization and Commodification," in *Global Goods and the Spanish Empire, 1492–1824: Circulation, Resistance and Diversity*, ed. Bethany Aram and Bartolomé Yun-Casalilla (New York: Palgrave Macmillan, 2014), 255–73.

13. Fattacciu, "Resilience and Boomerang Effect," 72–76.

14. William Gervase Clarence-Smith, *Cocoa and Chocolate, 1765–1914* (London: Routledge, 2000), 14–15.

15. Norton, *Sacred Gifts*, 33–35, 68–77, 129–40.

16. William Hughes, *The American physitian* (London: William Crook, 1672), 144–46.

17. Duncan, *Wholesome advice*, 75, 127. For insight into how and why the three hot drinks were conceived of as a group, see Christine A. Jones, "Exotic Edibles: Coffee, Tea, Chocolate, and the Early Modern French How-to," *Journal of Medieval and Early Modern Studies* 43, no. 3 (2013): 623–53. For more on Duncan, see *Tea and the Tea-Table in Eighteenth-Century England*, vol. 2, *Tea in Natural History and Medical Writing*, ed. Richard Coulton (London: Pickering & Chatto, 2010), 33–34.

18. Duncan, 157–58; 171–80. Duncan thought coffee was more pernicious, because it was consumed more than chocolate in England and France (277).

19. Martin Lister, *A journey to Paris in the year 1698* (London: Jacob Tonson, 1699), 164–68.

20. For an overview of the history of thinking about race, see Ivan Hannaford, *Race: The History of an Idea in the West* (Washington, DC: Woodrow Wilson Center/Baltimore, MD: Johns Hopkins University Press, 1996); see also Andrew S. Curran, *The Anatomy of Blackness: Science and Slavery in an Age of Enlightenment* (Baltimore, MD: Johns Hopkins University Press, 2011).

21. See Roxann Wheeler, *The Complexion of Race: Categories of Difference in Eighteenth-Century British Culture* (Philadelphia: University of Pennsylvania Press, 2000); David Nirenberg, "Was There Race before Modernity? The Example of

'Jewish' Blood in Late Medieval Spain," in *Neighboring Faiths: Christianity, Islam, and Judaism in the Middle Ages and Today* (Chicago: University of Chicago Press, 2014), 169–90; Kimberly Anne Coles, *Bad Humor: Race and Religious Essentialism in Early Modern England* (Philadelphia: University of Pennsylvania Press, 2022); and María Elena Martínez, *Genealogical Fictions: Limpieza de Sangre, Religion, and Gender in Colonial Mexico* (Stanford, CA: Stanford University Press, 2008).

22. Rebecca Earle, "Diet, Travel, and Colonialism in the Early Modern World," in *Global Goods and the Spanish Empire, 1492–1824: Circulation, Resistance, and Diversity*, ed. Bethany Aram and Bartolomé Yun-Casalilla (New York: Palgrave Macmillan, 2014), 137–52.

23. Rebecca Earle, *The Body of the Conquistador: Food, Race, and the Colonial Experience in Spanish America, 1492–1700* (Cambridge: Cambridge University Press, 2012); Jorge Cañizares Esguerra, "New World, New Stars: Patriotic Astrology and the Invention of Indian and Creole Bodies in Colonial Spanish America, 1600–1650," *American Historical Review* 104, no. 1 (1999): 33–68.

24. James C. Riley, *The Eighteenth-Century Campaign to Avoid Disease* (New York: St. Martin's, 1987); Mark Harrison, *Medicine in an Age of Commerce and Empire: Britain and Its Tropical Colonies, 1660–1830* (Oxford: Oxford University Press, 2010); Suman Seth, *Difference and Disease: Medicine, Race, and the Eighteenth-Century British Empire* (Cambridge: University of Cambridge Press, 2018); Andrew Wear, "Place, Health, and Disease: The *Airs, Waters, Places* Tradition in Early Modern England and North America," *Journal of Medieval and Early Modern Studies* 38, no. 3 (2008): 443–65.

25. Norton, *Sacred Gifts*, 27–30; for its spread among all levels of society, see Robert Ferry, "Trading Cacao: A View from Veracruz, 1629–1645," *Nuevo Mundo, Mundos Nuevos*, accessed September 10, 2023, https://journals.openedition.org/nuevomundo/1430.

26. Antonio Colmenero de Ledesma, *Curioso tratado de naturaleza y calidad del chocolate* (Madrid: Francisco Martínez, 1631), fol. 1r.

27. Fattacciu, "Resilience and Boomerang Effect"; Norton, *Sacred Gifts*, 173–79.

28. Edward Ward, *The school of politicks, or, the humours of a coffee-house a poem* (London: Richard Baldwin, 1690), 3. Ellis doubts that Ward was truly the author; *Eighteenth-Century Coffee-House Culture*, vol. 1, *Restoration Satire*, ed. Markman Ellis (London: Pickering & Chatto, 2006), 205–6.

29. François-Guislier du Verger, *Traité des liqueurs, esprits ou essences, et la maniere de s'en server utilement* (Louvain: Guillaime Stryckwant, 1728), 129–31.

30. José Vicente Díaz Bravo, *El ayuno reformado, segun practica de la primitive iglesia, por los cinco breves de nuestro santissimo Padre Benedicto XIV . . . Y una disertacion historica, medico-chymica, physico-moral de el chocolate, y su uso, despues de los nuevos preceptos* (Pamplona: Pasqual Ibañez, 1753), 313.

31. Díaz Bravo, *El ayuno reformado*, 313.

32. Norton, *Sacred Gifts*, 179–81.

33. El Capitán Castro de Torres, *Panegírico al chocolate*, ed. Manuel Pérez de Guzmán, 2nd ed. (Seville: E. Rasco, 1887), 6–25.

34. Fernando Cardoso, *Utilidades del agua i de la nieve, del bever frío i caliente*, ed. Jacobo Israel Garzon (Madrid: Hebraica, 2003), fol. 107v. For more on

Cardoso, see Jon Arrizabalaga, "The World of Iberian *converso* Practitioners, from Lluís Alcanyís to Isaac Cardoso," in *Más allá de la Leyendera Negra: España y la Revolución Cientifica/ Beyond the Black Legend: Spain and the Scientific Revolution*, ed. Víctor Navarro Brotóns and William Eamon (Valencia: Publicaciones de la Universitat de Valencia, 2007), 307–22; and Yosef Hayim Yerushalmi, *From Spanish Court to Italian Ghetto. Isaac Cardosó: A Study in Seventeenth-Century Marranism and Jewish Apologetics* (New York: Columbia University Press, 1971).

35. Anon, *Vertues of chocolate East-India drink.*

36. Stephan Blankaart, *De kartesiaanse academie ofte institute der medicine* (Amsterdam: Johannes ten Hoorn, 1683), 194.

37. For more on how ingesting chocolate could alter the bodies of European drinkers, see Enrique García Santo-Tomás, "El dogma placentero: políticas de consume en chocolate y tabaco. Ayuno eclesiástico y natural (1645) de Tomás Hurtado," in *En Buena Compañía: Estudios en Honor de Luciano García Lorenzo,* ed. Joaquín Álvarez Barrientos, Óscar Cornago Bernal, Abraham Madroñal Durán, and Carmen Menéndez Onrubia (Madrid: Consejo Superior de Investigaciones Científicas, 2009), 311–17.

38. David T. Courtwright, "The Rise and Fall and Rise of Cocaine in the United States," in *Consuming Habits: Drugs in History and Anthropology*, ed. Jordan Goodman, Paul E. Lovejoy, and Andrew Sherratt (London: Routledge, 1995), 206.

39. Charles Estienne and Jean Liebault, *L'agriculture et maison rustique* (Paris: Jacques de Puys, 1574), fol. 101r. I was not able to access the original 1567 edition.

40. Juan de Fragoso, *Discursos de las cosas aromáticas, arboles y frutales, y de otras muchas medicinas simples que se traen de la India Oriental, y sirven al uso de medicina* (Madrid: Francisco Sánchez, 1572), fols. 41v–43f.

41. Butts, *Dyets dry dinner*, fols. P3Aiv–P3Aivr.

42. Brookes, "Inhaling the Alien."

43. Philaretes, *Work for chimney-sweepers*, fol. Bv.

44. Rich, *My ladies looking glasse*, 22–23.

45. Sylvester, *Tobacco battered*, 91.

46. Taylor, *Nipping and snipping of abuses*, fol. D1r.

47. Pier Luigi Origoni, *Discorso contro l'abuso del tabacco* (Milan: Filippo Ghisolfi, 1643), 13–14; Matteo Pinelli [Alessandro Sanlorini da Prunalbeta], *La polvere schernita, overo invettiva contr'al tabacco* (Florence: Francesco Onofri, 1654).

48. Roger Marbecke, *A defence of tabacco: with a friendly answer to the late printed booke called worke for chimney-sweepers, etc.* (London: Richard Field, 1602), 60–61.

49. Leiva y Aguilar, *Desengaño contra el mal uso del tabaco*, fol. 5r. See also Tomás Hurtado, *Chocolate y tabaco: ayuno eclesíastico y natural: si este le quebrante el chocolate: y el tobaco el natural, para la Sagrada Comunion* (Madrid: Francisco García, Impressor del Reyno, 1645), fols. 35v–41r.

50. Norton, *Sacred Gifts*, 118–21.

51. Thomas White, *The middle state of souls from the hour of death to the day of judgment* (n.p., 1659), 191–93.

52. James I, *Counterblaste to tobacco*, fols. B1v–B2r. For an analysis of James's *Counterblaste*, see Lauren Working, *The Making of an Imperial Polity: Civility and*

America in the Jacobean Metropolis (Cambridge: Cambridge University Press, 2020), 144-467.

53. Tomkis, *Lingua*, fols. H4r–H4v.

54. Laura Working, "Tobacco and the Social Life of Conquest in London, 1580-1625," in "Intoxicants and Early Modern European Globalization," special issue, *Historical Journal* 65 (2022): 30–48.

55. James I, *Counterblaste to tobacco*, fol. B2r. Also quoted in Lauren Working, "Locating Colonization at the Jacobean Inns of Court," *Historical Journal* 61, no. 1 (2018): 29–51, 38; and Working, "Tobacco and the Social Life of Conquest."

56. John Deacon, *Tobacco tortured; or, The filthie fume of tabacco refined* (London: Richard Field, 1616), 10.

57. Working, "Locating Colonization"; Working, *Making of an Imperial Polity*. For more on masques, theater, and tobacco, see Edward McClean Test, *Sacred Seeds: New World Plants in Early Modern English Literature* (Lincoln: University of Nebraska Press, 2019).

58. Catherine Molineux, *Faces of Perfect Ebony: Encountering Atlantic Slavery in Imperial Britain* (Cambridge MA: Harvard University Press, 2012), 148–75. See also Brookes, "Inhaling the Alien."

59. Richard Brathwaite [Blasius Multibibus], *The smoaking age, or, the man in the mist: with the life and death of tobacco* (London: E. Griffin, 1617), 155–56.

60. Rowlands, "The fifth gossips complaint," in *Crew of kind gossips*, 16–19; Rowlands, "To smokey noses, and stinking nostrils," in *More knaves yet?,* fols. D1r–v. See also Samuel Rowlands, "The Devils health-drinker," in *The knave of clubbs* (London: W. Ferebrand, 1609), fols. Eivv–Fir.

61. Ramón, *Nueva prematica*, 358–60.

62. Monardes, *Primera y segunda y tercera partes*, fols. 48v–49r; Lavedán, *Tratado*.

63. Brookes, "Inhaling the Alien," 160.

64. Butts, *Dyets dry dinner*, fol. P3Av.

65. Norton, *Sacred Gifts*, 156–61.

66. Taylor, *Nipping and snipping of abuses*, fol. D1r.

67. West, *Wits A.B.C.*, fol. B2r.

68. Working, *Making of an Imperial Polity*.

69. Samuel Rowlands, *Looke to it: for, ile stabbe ye* (London: W. Ferbrand and George Loftes, 1604), fols. D2r and D4r.

70. Samuel Rowlands, "Epigram 32," in *Humors ordinarie where a man may be verie merrie, and exceedingly well used for his sixe-pence* (London: William Firebrand, 1605), fols. C4v–D1r.

71. For more on this disruptive, "anti-patriarchal" masculinity, see Alexandra Shepard, *Meanings of Manhood in Early Modern England* (Oxford: Oxford University Press, 2003).

72. James I, *Counterblaste to tobacco*, fol. C4v.

73. Deacon, *Tobacco tortured*, 9.

74. Deacon, 4.

75. Deacon, 17–18, 39, 55, 64–65.

76. John Philips, *Sportive wit the muses merriment, a new spring of lusty drollery, joviall fancies, and* a la mode *lamponnes* (London: Nath. Brook, 1656), 47.

77. Luis Antonio, *Nuevo plato de varios manjares*, ed. Antonio Pérez Goméz (Valencia: Cieza, 1968). See also Norton, *Sacred Gifts*, 183–84, 191–92.

78. *Dissertation on the use and abuses of tobacco*, 24.

79. "The tobacco-takers song," in *An antidote against melancholy made up in pills*, ed. John Playford (London: John Playford, 1669), 125–26.

80. A. Marsh, *The confession of the new married couple, being the second part of the ten pleasures of marriage* (London: n.p., 1683), 28–33.

81. Humphrey Mill, *The second part of the nights search, discovering the condition of the various fowles of the night* (London: Henry Shepheard and William Lay, 1646), 71–72.

82. *Whipping-Tom*, 8.

83. Raphael Thorius, Hymnus tabaci; *A poem in honour of tabaco*, trans. Peter Hausted (London: Humphrey Moseley, 1650 [originally 1651, but crossed out and replaced by 1650]).

84. Richard Head, *The floating island, or, A new discovery* (London: n.p., 1673), 15–16.

85. Duncan, *Wholesome advice*, 58–62.

86. Philaretes, *Work for chimney-sweepers*, fols. Ev–E2r; Sylvester, *Tobacco battered*, 101; "Dr. Maynwaring's serious cautions against tobacco, collected out of his treatise of the scurvy," in *Two broad-sides against tobacco*, ed. John Hancock (London: John Hancock, 1672), 18.

87. Lavedán, *Tratado*, 63–64, Giovanni Piccino, *Il petopiccino, overo eccelenza, e dote del tabacco* (Viterbo: li Diotallevi, 1635), 55–56; Sebastiano Laghi, *Neve, tabacco, et acqua vita: otiose discorsi* (Milan: Filippo Ghisolfi, 1647), 69–71.

88. *A broad-side against coffee; or, the marriage of the Turk* (London: J. L., 1672). For a discussion of this poem that emphasizes English perception of the Ottoman Empire as powerful and dangerous when English merchants and travelers began venturing into the Mediterranean in the seventeenth century, see Emily M. N. Kugler, *Sway of the Ottoman Empire on English Identity in the Long Eighteenth Century* (Leiden: Brill, 2012), 29–30. For a guide to early English satires against coffee, see *Eighteenth-Century Coffee-House Culture*, vol. 1, *Restoration Satire*, ed. Markman Ellis (London: Pickering & Chatto, 2006). For this particular broadside, see also Gitanjali G. Shahani, *Tasting Differences: Food, Race, and Cultural Encounters in Early Modern Literature* (Ithaca, NY: Cornell University Press, 2020), 80–106.

89. For an overview of western European attitudes toward Ottoman sexuality, see Leslie Peirce, "Writing Histories of Sexuality in the Middle East," *American Historical Review* 114, no. 5 (2009): 1325–39. While this broadside seems to match Edward Said's idea of orientalism very well, Said was writing about the nineteenth century, when western Europe was much more powerful than the Ottoman Empire; western Europeans feared the Turks in the seventeenth century. Gerald MacLean, *Looking East: English Writing and the Ottoman Empire before 1800* (Houndmills: Palgrave Macmillan, 2007).

90. *Broad-side against coffee*.

91. *The character of a coffee-house with the symptomes of a town-wit* (London: Jonathan Edwin, 1673).

92. *A satyr against coffee* (n.p., 1674).

93. Mercurius Democritus, *The maidens complaint against coffee* (London: J. Jones, 1663), 6.

94. Mercurius Democritus, *Maidens complaint*, 3–5.

95. Philippe Sylvestre Dufour, *De l'usage du caphé, du thé et du chocolate* (Lyon: Jean Girin & Barthelemy Riviere, 1671), 28–29. On Dufour and the publishing history of *De l'usage du caphé*, see E. C. Spary, *Eating the Enlightenment: Food and the Sciences in Paris* (Chicago: University of Chicago Press, 2012), 62–67.

96. Angelo Rambaldi, *Ambrosia arabica, overo della salutare bevanda café* (Bologna: per il Longhi stampatore Arcivescogale, 1691), 61–69.

97. Francesco Merli, *Guida medica intorno all'uso del the, caffé, e cioccolata* (Naples: Vincenzo Flauto, 1768), 37.

98. Cowan, *Social Life of Coffee.*

99. *Character of a coffee-house*, 2–3.

100. Ward, *School of politicks*, 3–5.

101. Lavedán, *Tratado*, 105–6.

102. Lavedán, 185–86. Here he was repeating stereotypes that had existed for print for years; see John Coakley Lettsom, *The natural history of the tea-tree* (London: Edward and Charles Dilly, 1772), 57.

103. Markman Ellis, Richard Coulton, and Matthew Mauger, *Empire of Tea: The Asian Leaf that Conquered the World* (London: Reaktion, 2015), 73–88.

104. Erika Rappaport, *A Thirst for Empire: How Tea Shaped the Modern World* (Princeton, NJ: Princeton University Press, 2017), 52–53. Another scholar who complicates the triumphalist view of tea's easy acceptance into western Europe is David Porter; see his *Ideographia: The Chinese Cipher in Early Modern Europe* (Stanford, CA: Stanford University Press, 2001).

105. Simon Paulli, *A treatise on tobacco, tea, coffee, and chocolate*, trans. Dr. James (1665; London: T. Osborn, 1746), 118–19, 125, 132.

106. Jonas Hanway, "An essay on tea," in *A journal of eight days journey from Portsmouth to Kingston upon Thames* (London: H. Woodfall, 1756), 213.

107. Hanway, "Essay on tea," 243–45. See also Kowaleski-Wallace, *Consuming Subjects*, 31–34.

108. Lettsom, *Natural history*, 58.

109. Waldron, *Satyr against tea*, 4–5.

110. Godfrey McCalman, *A natural, commercial, and medicinal treatise on tea* (Glasgow: David Niven, 1787), 82–83.

111. Simon Mason, *The good and bad effects of tea consider'd* (London: M. Cooper, 1745), 42–45.

112. [Richard Helsham?], *An essay on the nature, use, and abuse, of tea, in a letter to a lady; With an account of its mechanical operation* (London: J. Bettenham, 1722), 4–6, 15–16, 43–49.

113. Giovanni Agostino and Morison Scozzese, *Soccinto raguaglio delle stupendi e maravivgliose virtù del cordial liquore o sia balsam potabile de i chinesi: estratto in più modi dall' erba thé* (Rome: Dom. Ant. Ercole, 1720), 18–21.

114. Thomas Tryon, *The good housewife made doctor, or, health's device and sure friend*, 2nd ed. (London: H. N. and T. S., 1692), 103–4. See Kim F. Hall, "'Extravagant Viciousness': Slavery and Gluttony in the Works of Thomas Tryon,"

in *Writing Race across the Atlantic World: Medieval to Modern*, ed. Philip D. Beidler and Gary Taylor (New York: Palgrave Macmillan, 2005), 93–111.

115. Thomas Tryon, *Healths grand preservative: or the womens best doctor* (London: printed for the author, 1682), 2–3.

116. Edward Whitaker, "A satyr upon brandy," in *Directions for brewing malt liquors* (London: J. Nutt, 1700), 25–28.

117. Slyboots, *Tavern scuffle*, 20–21.

118. Jack Juniper, *The deposing and death of Queen Gin, with the ruin of the Duke of Rum, Marquee de Nantz, and the Lord Sugarcane, &c.* (London: John Millan, 1736), 12.

119. Quoted in Dillon, *Gin*, 18.

120. Nicolas de Nicolay, *The navigations, peregrinations, and voyages, made into Turkie by Nicolas Nicholay Daulphinois, Lord of Arfeuile, chamberlaine and geographer ordinarie to the King of Fraunce*, trans. T. Washington (London: Thomas Dawsom, 1585), fol. 91r–v. The French original described opium-takers less colorfully than Washington's translation but included "vont hurland par la ville comme chiens." Nicolas de Nicolay, *Les navigations peregrinations et voyages, faicts en la turquie, par Nicolas de Nicolay Daulphinoys Seigeur d'Arfeville, valet de chamber & geographe ordinaire du Roy de France, contenants plusieurs singularitez que l'Autheur y a veu & observe* (Antwerp: Guillaume Silvius, Imprimeur du Roy, 1577), 158. See also "Nicolas de Nicolay," in *Christian-Muslim Relations: A Bibliographic History*, vol. 6, *Western Europe (1500–1600)*, ed. David Thomas and John Chesworth, with John Azumah, Stanislaw Grodz, Andrew Newman, and Douglas Pratt (Brill: Leiden: 2014), 752–61.

121. *Hactenus inaudita, or, animadversions upon the new found way of curing the small pox* (London: Io. Martin and Ia. Allestry, 1663), 72–73.

122. *Proposizione sulla necessità d'introdurre in Toscana la coltivazione dei papaveri in grande per estrarne l'oppio* (Firenze: Guglielmo Piatti, 1807), 5–7.

123. *Iets over den opium*, para. 4.

124. Timothie Bright, *A treatise, wherein is declared the sufficiencie of English medicines, for cure of all diseases, cured with medicines* (1580; London: Humphrey Lownes for Tho. Man, 1615), 17–19.

125. Nicaise Le Fèvre, *A Compendious Body of Chymystry*, trans. P. D. C. (London: Octavian Pulleyn Jr., 1664), 37–38.

126. Henry Stubbe, *Indian nectar, or a discourse concerning chocolata* (London: Andrew Crook, 1662), 137–39.

127. John Jones, *The mysteries of opium reveal'd* (London: Richard Smith, 1700), 17–18, 24.

128. Jones, *Mysteries of opium*, 25–26; N. Brooke, "An account of very many extraordinary cures produced by a preparation of opium, in a variety of obstinate cases, according to the practice in Asia," in *Observations on the manners and customs of Italy* (Bath: R. Cruttwell, 1798), 38–39.

129. Norton, *Sacred Gifts*, 107–28.

130. Fattacciu, "Cacao," 62.

131. Antonio de León Pinelo, *Questión moral: si el chocolate quebranta el ayuno eclesiástico* (Madrid: Viuda de Juan Gonçalez, 1636), fol. 36v.

132. Da'ud ibn Ùmar Antaki, *The nature of the drink kauhi, or coffe, and the berry from which it is made described by an Arabian phisitian* (Oxford: Henry Hall, 1659).

133. Luigi Ferdinando, Conte di Marsigli, *Bevanda asiatica istoria medica del cave* (Vienna: n.p., 1685). See also Duygu Yıldırım, "*Bevanda asiatica*: Scholarly Exchange between the Ottomans and Europeans on Coffee," *Osmanlı Araştırmaları/The Journal of Ottoman Studies* 56 (2020): 25–47.

134. Stephen Blankaart, "*Verhandelinge van de coffee, aangaande des selfs kragten in gesonde luiden en alle ziekten*," in Cornelis Bontekoe, *Gebruik en mis-bruik van de thee* (The Hague: Pieter Hagen, 1686), 174.

135. Johan Nieuhof, *Gezantschap der Neerlandtsche Oost-Indische Compagnie, aan den grooten Tartarischen cham, den tegenwoordigen kaizer van China* (Amsterdam: Jokob van Meurs, 1665).

136. Tate, *Panacea*, 4–14.

137. Lettsom, *Natural history of the tea-tree.*

138. Angelo Sala, *Opiologia: or, a treatise concerning the nature, properties, true preparation and safe use and administration of opium*, trans. Thomas Bretnor (London: Nicholas Okes, 1618), 4–12.

139. Jones, *Mysteries of opium;* George Young, *A treatise upon opium* (London: A. Millar, 1753).

140. Julie Landweber, "Furnishing the Taste for Coffee in Early Modern France," in *The Mobility of People and Things in the Early Modern Mediterranean*, ed. Elisabeth A. Fraser (New York: Routledge, 2019), 49–70.

3. Who from Excess Is Free?

1. Estienne and Liebault, *L'agriculture et maison rustique*, fols. 97v–98r. There were several editions of this work, adding new material over time. The first edition appeared in 1553.

2. Lawrence Spooner, *A looking-glass for smoakers* (London: A. Baldwin, 1703), 19–30.

3. Spooner, *Looking-glass for smoakers*, 32, 37–38, 44, 48, 71, 77, 88, 91.

4. In *Forces of Habit* David T. Courtwright argues that the typical course for newly adapted drugs is to start as a medicine and then move to recreational use (85).

5. Material on the failure of early modern medical language to explain addiction, in this chapter and others, draws on Scott K. Taylor, "'A Miserable Captivity' or 'Happily Redeemed from Captivity to Liberty': Tobacco, Addiction, and Early Modern Bodies and Minds," in *A Linking of Heaven and Earth: Studies in Religious and Cultural History in Honor of Carlos M. N. Eire*, ed. Emily Michelson, Scott K. Taylor, and Mary Noll Venables (Farnham: Ashgate, 2012), 191–203. Phil Withington has recently reached similar conclusions, focusing on custom and the writing of Thomas Tryon. Phil Withington, "Addiction, Intoxicants, and the Humoral Body," in "Intoxicants and Early Modern Globalization," special issue, *Historical Journal* 64, no. 1: (2022): 68–90.

6. Benjamin Rush, *An inquiry into the effects of ardent spirits upon the human body and mind: with an account of the means of preventing, and of the remedies for curing them*, 2nd ed. (Philadelphia: Thomas Dobson, 1787[?]). Jessica Warner puts the publication of the first edition as "in or around 1784" in Warner, "'Resolv'd

to Drink No More': Addiction as a Preindustrial Construct," *Journal of Studies on Alcohol* 55 (1994): 685–91. Pinning Rush's work as the origins of the idea of alcoholism-as-disease dates back to Harry G. Levine, "The Discovery of Addiction: Changing Conceptions of Habitual Drunkenness in America," *Journal of Studies on Alcohol* 39 (1978): 143–74.

7. Warner, "Resolv'd to Drink No More,"; Roy Porter, "The Drinking Man's Disease: The 'Pre-History' of Alcoholism in Georgian Britain," *British Journal of Addiction* 80 (1985): 385–96.

8. Warner, 685–86.

9. Jose Murgatroyd Cree, "Protestant Evangelicals and Addiction in Early Modern English," *Renaissance Studies* 32, no. 3 (2018): 446–62. See also Rebecca Lemon, *Addiction and Devotion in Early Modern England* (Philadelphia: University of Pennsylvania Press, 2018).

10. Norton, *Sacred Gifts*, 142–43, 50–51.

11. Norton, 153–56.

12. Norton, 163.

13. Norton, 201.

14. Jordan Goodman, *Tobacco in History: The Cultures of Dependence* (New York: Routledge, 1993), 134–48.

15. Goodman, *Tobacco in History*, 154; Matthew Romaniello and Tricia Starks, "*Tabak*: An Introduction," in *Tobacco in Russian History and Culture: From the Seventeenth Century to the Present*, ed. Matthew Romaniello and Tricia Starks (New York: Routledge, 2009), 1–8.

16. Carol Benedict, *Golden-Silk Smoke: A History of Tobacco in China, 1550–2020* (Berkeley: University of California Press, 2011), 1–2.

17. Nicolás Monardes, *Dos libros. El uno trata de todos las cosas que traen de nuestras Indias Occidentales que sirven al uso de medicina* (Seville: Sebastián Trujillo, 1565). The second book dealt with bezoar stones and scorzonera grass. The discussion of Monardes is taken from Norton, *Sacred Gifts*, 110–21.

18. Nicolás Monardes, *Segunda parte del libro, de los cosas que se traen de nuestras Indias Occidentales, que sirven al uso del medicina* (Seville: Alonso Escrivano, 1571).

19. Monardes, *Segunda parte*, fols. 41r–42r.

20. Monardes, fols. 42v–50r.

21. Norton, *Sacred Gifts*, 116–17.

22. For the role of humoral theory in the early modern period, see Stolberg, *Illness and the Sick Body*, 85–89.

23. Chute, *Tabacco*, fols. Aiiiv–Aivv, 4–5. For Chute's self-description, see Robert J. Kane, "Anthony Chute, Thomas Nashe, and the First English Work on Tobacco," *Review of English Studies* 7, no. 26 (1931): 151–59.

24. Chute, *Tabacco*, 9–10.

25. Chute, 11.

26. Chute, 19.

27. See Philaretes, *Work for chimney-sweepers*; and Marbecke, *Defence of tabacco*.

28. Paul S. Lloyd, "Dietary Advice and Fruit-Eating in Late Tudor and Early Stuart England," *Journal of the History of Medicine and Allied Sciences* 67, no. 4 (2011): 553–86, 575.

29. Butts, "Tabacco," *Dyets dry dinner*, para. 1–2.

30. William Barclay, *Nepenthes, or the vertues of tabacco* (Edinburgh: Andro Hart, 1614), fols. A3r–A3v.

31. Barclay, *Nepenthes*, fols. A6r–A6v.

32. Barclay, fol. A7r.

33. James Hart, *Klinike, or The diet of the diseased* (London: Robert Allot, 1633), 317–18.

34. Laghi, *Neve, tabacco, et acqua vita*, 69–73.

35. Piccino, *Il petopiccino*.

36. Jiménez Patón, *Reforma de trages*, fols. 63r–64v.

37. De Castro y Medinilla, *Historia*, fols. 40v–44r.

38. Ramón, *Nueva prematica*.

39. For a description of using tobacco to induce the Duke of Buckingham to vomit, see George Bate, *The regall apology, or, the declaration of the Commons, Feb. 11, 1647, canvassed wherein every objection to their whole charge against His Majesty is cleared, and for the most part, retorted* (1648), 21–22; for the eyes and worms, see Rumsey, *Organon salutis*, 28–29, 48–49; for lice, see Beaumont, *Poems*, fols. N5r–N6v; as a lambitive, see Stella, *Il tabacco*; for tobacco smoke as an enema, see H. V. Nokken, *Beschryving van een nieuw werktuig, om den rook van tabak in de darmen te brengen* in *Uitgegeeven door de Hollandsche maatschappye der weetenschappen, te Haarlem* (Haarlem: J. Bosch, 1765), 252.

40. John Archer, *Every man his own doctor in two parts* (London: Printed by Peter Lillicrap for the author, 1671), 92–95.

41. Johannes Ignatius Worp Beintema van Peima, *Tabacologia, ofte korte verhandelinge over de tabak, deselvs deugd, gebruik, ende kennisse: waar door aangeweesen word teen wegh om lang, vroolijk, ende gesond te leeven* (The Hague: Levyn van Dyck, 1690), 1–9.

42. De Leiva y Aguilar, *Desengaño contra el mal vso del tabaco*, fols. 12v–13r.

43. James I, *Counterblaste to tobacco*, fols. B3r, B4r.

44. See Hill, *Cautions*; and Smythson, *Compleat family physician*, 755–56.

45. Philaretes, *Work for chimney-sweepers*, fol. E5v.

46. P. van R., *Nieuwe en naauwkeurige verhandeling van den tabak* (Amsterdam: Gerrit Bom, 1785), 38.

47. Sophie D. Coe and Michael D. Coe, *The True History of Chocolate* (London: Thames & Hudson, 1996), 81–84; Norton, *Sacred Gifts*, 121–28. See also *Searching for the Secrets of Nature: The Life and Works of Dr. Francisco Hernández*, ed. Simon Varey, Rafael Chabrán, and Dora B. Weiner (Stanford, CA: Stanford University Press, 2002).

48. Marradón, *Du chocolate*, 172, 178–79, 182–83. See also Norton, *Sacred Gifts*, 139.

49. Santiago de Valverde Turices, *Un discurso de chocolate* (Seville: Juan de Cabrera, 1624), fols. A4v–A4r, B3v–B4r (mislabeled as fol. A instead of B); see also Norton 124–25.

50. Giovanni Batista Felici, *Parere intorno all'uso della cioccolata* (Florence: Giusepep Manni, 1728), 17–18; see also Giovanni Batista Gudenfridi, *Differenza tra' il cibo e il cioccolate* (Florence: Condotta, 1680); Lorenzo Serafini, *Lettera in cui si esaminano le ragioni addotte dall'Autore del primo parere intorno all'uso della cioccolata dedicata all'illustriss. sig. Ca. Cosimo degli Albizzi* (Florence: n.p., 1728), and

Giacomo Sanvitale, *Memorie veridiche contrapposte alle memorie istoriche sull'uso del cioccolato in giorno di digiuno* (n.p.: 1748).

51. Chamberlayn, *Natural history*, 18.

52. Fattacciu, "Cacao," 53–78.

53. Rappaport, *Thirst for Empire*; Cowan, *Social Life of Coffee.*

54. Agostino and Scozzese, *Soccinto raguaglio*, 11.

55. For more on Bontekoe, see Christoph Schweikardt, "More than Just a Propagandist for Tea: Religious Argument and Advice on a Healthy Life in the Work of the Dutch Physician Cornelis Bontekoe (1647–1685)," *Medical History* 47, no. 3 (2003): 357–68.

56. For iatrochemistry, see Roy Porter, *The Greatest Benefit to Mankind: A Medical History of Humanity* (New York: W. W. Norton, 1997), 201–11; Mary Lindemann, *Medicine and Society in Early Modern Europe*, 2nd ed. (Cambridge: Cambridge University Press, 2010), 102–3; and Alan G. Debus, *The Chemical Philosophy: Paracelsian Science and Medicine in the Sixteenth and Seventeenth Centuries*, 2 vols. (New York: Science History Publications, 1977).

57. Blegny, *Le bon usage*, 105–6.

58. Giuseppe Galeano, *Il caffè con piu diligenza esaminato* (Palermo: Domenico d'Anselmo, 1674), 3.

59. *Dichiarazione della virtù della bevanda del caffè* (Rome: A. Bernabò, 1683).

60. Readers of English could have consulted Hollandus in *A hundred and fourtene experiments and cures of the famous physition Philippus Aureolus Theophrastus Paracelsus . . . Also certaine secrets of Isacke Hollandus concerning the vegetal and animall worke*, trans. John Hester (London: Vallentine Sims, 1596), 32–36.

61. Hughes, *American physitian*, 142–43.

62. Thomas Short, *Vinum Britannicum: or, An essay on the properties and effects of malt liquors* (London: D. Midwinter, 1727), i–ii.

63. Thomas Newton, *Approoved medicines and cordiall receiptes with the natures, qualities, and operations of sundry samples* (London: Thomas Marshe, 1580), 11–12.

64. Benjamin Moseley, *Medical tracts*, 2nd ed. (London: John Nichols, 1800), 82, 98–99. See also Norman Moore, "Moseley, Benjamin (1742–1819)" *Oxford Dictionary of National Biography*, accessed November 10, 2023, https://www.oxforddnb.com/display/10.1093/ref:odnb/9780198614128.001.0001/odnb-9780198614128-e-19387.

65. Estienne and Liebault, *L'agriculture et maison rustique*, fols 222v, 329r. For an overview of opium as a medicine in early modern Europe, see Andreas-Holger Maehle, *Drugs on Trial: Experimental Pharmacology and Therapeutic Innovation in the Eighteenth Century* (Amsterdam: Rodopi, 1999).

66. Conrad Gesner, *The newe iewell of health wherein is contayned the most excellent secretes of phiscike and philosophie*, trans. George Baker (London: Henrie Denham, 1576), fols. 83v–84r.

67. Gesner, *Newe iewell of health*, fol. 83v.

68. Monardes, *Dos libros*, fols. 48v–49r.

69. Willis, *Dr. Willis's practice of physick*, 137–43.

70. Slyboots, *Tavern scuffle*, 14.

71. Stolberg, *Experiencing Illness*, 85–89.

72. For an insightful look at melancholy's place in early modern culture, see Timothy Barr, "Without Apparent Occasion: Recent Research on Melancholy," *Journal of the History of Ideas* 80, no. 2 (2019): 313–32.

73. Erik H. C. Midelfort, *Mad Princes of Renaissance Germany* (Charlottesville: University Press of Virginia, 1992), 4–5.

74. Philaretes, *Work for chimney-sweepers*, fols. G4r–G4v.

75. Cardoso, *Utilidades del agua*, fol. 107v.

76. Bontekoe, *Tractaat*, 269, 399–401.

77. Leonard Biet, *Le bon usage du caffé volatile* (Paris: n.p., 1687–1700), 24.

78. Duncan, *Wholesome advice*, 58–59.

79. Thomas Wilson, *Distilled spirits the bane of the nation* (London: J. Roberts, 1736), 28, 30–31, 48.

80. Andrew Boorde, *A compendyous regiment or a dyetary of healthe made in Mountpyllyer* (London: Wyllyam Powell, 1547); see also Patricia E. S. Fletcher, "The Life of Andrew Boorde, c. 1490–1549," *Adverse Drug Reactions and Toxicological Reviews* 21, no. 4 (2002): 243–52.

81. Thomas Brugis, *Vade mecum, or a companion for a chyrurgion* (London: Thomas William, 1652), 104–7; Nicaise Le Fèvre, *A compendious body of chymystry*, trans. P. D. C. (London: Octavian Pulleyn Jr., 1664), 37–38; see also Paul Dorveaux, "Les grand pharmaciens: XVII. L'apothicaire Le Febvre Nicaise dit Nicolas," *Revue d'Histoire de la Pharmacie* 42 (1924), 345–56.

82. Jones, *Mysteries of opium*, 235–37.

83. De Castro y Medinilla, *Historia*, fols. 19r–21r.

84. De Castro y Medinilla, fols. 19r–20r.

85. Sylvester, *Tobacco battered*, fol. F3r.

86. Sylvester, 92.

87. Sylvester, 95–98.

88. Sylvester, 83, 100–101.

89. Sylvester, 88–91.

90. Sylvester, 102–3.

91. Sylvester, 103–4, 108–9.

92. Hurtado, *Chocolate y tabaco*, fol. 40v.

93. Hurtado, fols. 35v–36r.

94. Hurtado, fols. 35v–36r.

95. Gardiner, *Triall of tabacco*, fol. 16v.

96. Humphrey Brooke, *ΥΓΙΕΙΝΗ or A conservatory of health* (London: G. Whittington, 1650), 35–39.

97. James Primrose, *Popular errours, or the errours of the people in physick* (London: Nicholas Bourne, 1651), 332; see also Hall, *Practical and polemical commentary*, fols. 99–101.

98. Carr, *Medical epistles*, 12.

99. Steven Shapin, "Why Was 'Custom a Second Nature' in Early Modern Medicine?," *Bulletin of Medical History* 93, no. 1 (2019): 1–26.

100. Nicolas François Joseph Éloy, *Examen de la question médico-politique: si l'usage habituel du caffé est avantageux ou doit être mis au rang des choses indifférentes à la conservation de la santé* (Mons: H. Hoyois, [late eighteenth century]), 47.

101. Edward Chandler, *A sermon preached to the Societies for Reformation of Manners, at St. Mary-le-Bow, on Monday January the 4th, 1724* (London: James Knapton, 1724), 15.

102. Carr, *Medicinal epistles*, 34, 36–37.

103. See, for example, de Fragoso, *Discursos*, fols. 179r–179v, Richard Younge, *The victory of patience and benefit of affliction, and how to husband it so, that the weakest Christian (with blessing from above) may bee able to support himselfe in his most miserable exigents* (London: R. B., 1636), 92–93; and Primrose, *Popular errours*, 328–29.

104. For an overview of premodern views of gluttony, see William Ian Miller, "Gluttony," *Representations* 60 (1997): 92–112; and Jodi Campbell, *At the First Table: Food and Social Identity in Early Modern Spain* (Lincoln: University of Nebraska Press, 2017), 160–72.

105. See Jessica Warner, "Before There Was Alcoholism: Lessons from the Medieval Experience with Alcohol," *Contemporary Drug Problems* 19, no. 3 (1992): 409–29; and A. Lynn Martin, *Alcohol, Violence, and Disorder in Traditional Europe* (Kirksville, MO: Truman State University Press, 2009), 15–26, 30–34.

106. James I, *Counterblaste*, fol. C3v.

107. Deacon, *Tobacco tortured*, fols. **2r–**2v, 17–18.

108. Dirck Pieterszoon Pers and Gillis van Scheyndel, *Bacchus wonderwercken: Waer in het recht gebruyck en misbruyck des wijns door verscheyden vermaecklijcke eerlijcke en leerlijcke historien wort afgebeeld ende lasteringe der dronckenschap met levende verwen afgemaelt* (Amsterdam: Dirck Pieterzsoon Pers, 1628), 68; Benedetto Stella, *Il tabacco*, 223–24.

109. Leonard Lessius, Jan Hendrik Glazemaker, and Cornaro Luigi, *De schat de soberheit; or, Bequame middle tot onderhouding der gezonheit, en bewaring van de volkomenheit der zinnen, van't verstant, en van de geheugenis aan d'uitterste ouderdom* (Middelburg: Johannes Meertens, 1678).

110. Johannes Ignatius Worp Beintema van Peima, *Nuttelyke consideration of sedige aanmerkingen over het heedendaags tabak-suigen, of, en hoe verre het selve geoolofd zy, of niet* (Amsterdam: Cornelis van Hogenhuisen, 1692), fol. *4v.

111. De León Pinelo, *Questión moral*, fols. 21v–22r.

112. Henry Ramsden, *A gleaning in gods harvest foure choyce handfuls; the gate to happinesse, wounded savior* (London: J. D. and R. M., 1639), 191–93.

113. *Le bon usage du tabac en poudre* (Paris: La veuve de G. Quinet, 1700), 10–16.

114. *Le bon usage*, 10–16.

115. André Thevet, *The new found world, or Antarctike wherin is contained wonderful and strange things*, trans. anonymous (London: Henrie Bynneman for Thomas Hacket, 1568), fols. 8r–8v.

116. Bontekoe, *Tractaat*, 303–5.

117. Duncan, *Wholesome advice*, 138.

118. Duncan, 105.

119. De Reynal, *Opuscule médico-politique sur le café*, 36.

120. Yates, *Effects of drinking spirituous*, 6–7.

121. Gardiner, *Trial of tobacco*, fols. 16v–17r.

122. Venner, *Brief and accurate treatise*, fol. B4v.

123. Shapin, "Why Was 'Custom a Second Nature?'"

124. Maxine Berg and Elizabeth Eger, "The Rise and Fall of the Luxury Debates," *in Luxury in the Eighteenth Century: Debates, Desires and Delectable Goods*, ed. Maxine Berg and Elizabeth Eger (Houndmills: Palgrave Macmillan, 2003), 7–27; for a full exploration of luxury, see Maxine Berg, *Luxury and Pleasure in Eighteenth-Century Britain* (Oxford: Oxford University Press, 2005).

125. James I, *Counterblaste*, fols B1r–v.

126. George Wither, *Abuses stript, and whipt* (London: Francis Burton, 1613), fol. M8r.

127. Rich, *My ladies looking glasse*, 22–23.

128. Edward Chamberlayne, *Englands wants, or, Several proposals probably beneficial for England humbly offered to the considerations of all good patriots in both houses of Parliament* (London: Jo. Martin, 1667), 4.

129. Burlot de Campaña, "*Sátira contra el tabaco*," in *Romance del burlador Burlot de Campaña, fabricado, y destruihido en la Rambla, dia de la Natividad de nuestra Señora, Año 1642* (Barcelona: Gabriel Nogues, 1643), fols. A2r–A2v.

130. R. V. N., *Natuur-kundige verhandelin*, 8.

131. Lister, *Journey to Paris*, 33, 164–68.

132. Stubbe, *Indian nectar*, 6–7.

133. Joseph Browne, *An account of the wonderful cures perform'd by the cold baths*, 2nd ed. (London: A. Bettesworth, 1707[?]), 5–6.

134. Chamberlayne, *Natural history*, 26–31.

135. *The occasional monitor* (London: H. Cooke and E. Cooke, 1731), 5.

136. He called it both a vice and a habit. Gaetano Maria da Bergamo, "*Pratico esame sopra il vizio detto volgarmente dell'osteria*," in *Opera del padre Fr. Gaetano Maria da Bergamo Cappuccino*, vol. 2 (Rome; Arangelo Casaletti, 1776), 67.

137. Smythson, *Compleat family physician*, 745, 764.

138. *Strictures on an address to the people of Great Britain, on the propriety of abstaining from West-India sugar and rum*, 2nd ed. (London: T. Boosey, 1792), 6.

139. *A vindication of the use of sugar, the produce of the West-India islands* (London: T. Boosey, 1792), 20.

140. *Answers to the queries, in defence of the malt distillery* (London: T. Payne, 1760), 7.

141. Bellamy, Dr., *A new and short defense of tabacco: with the effects of the same: and of the right use* (London: n.p., 1602), fols. Cv–C3v.

142. See D. Bruce Hindmarsh, *The Evangelical Conversion Narrative: Spiritual Autobiography in Early Modern England* (Oxford: Oxford University Press, 2005); Roger M. Payne, *The Self and the Sacred: Conversion and Autobiography in Early American Protestantism* (Knoxville: University of Tennessee Press, 1980); and Michael C. Questier, *Conversion, Politics, and Religion in England, 1580–1625* (Cambridge: Cambridge University Press, 1997).

143. Risto Saarinen, *Weakness of Will in Renaissance and Reformation Thought* (Oxford: Oxford University Press, 2011); *Erasmus and Luther: The Battle over Free Will*, ed. Clarence H. Miller (Indianapolis: Hackett, 2012).

144. Ben Agar, *King James, his apophthegms, or table-talke as they were by him delivered occasionally and by the publisher (his quondam servant) carefully received, and*

now humbly offered to publique view, as not impertinent to the present times (London: B. W., 1643), 5.

145. Henry Burton, *A replie to a relation, of the conference between William Laude and Mr. Fisher the Jesuite* (n.p., 1640).

146. Warner, "Resolv'd to Drink No More."

147. Thomas Hooker, *The application of redemption by the effectual work of the word, and spirit of Christ, for the bringing home of lost sinners to God* (London: Peter Cole, 1656), 68–69.

148. Thomas Goddard, *Miscellanea, or, serious, useful considerations, moral, historical, theological together with the characters of a true believer, in paradoxes and seeming contradictions, an essay* (London: Tho. William, 1661), 27–29.

149. Duncan, *Wholesome advice*, 12–13, 24.

150. Duncan, 61–62.

151. Joan Baptista van Helmont, *A ternary of paradoxes the magnetick cure of wounds, nativity of tartar in wine, image of God in man*, translated and "amplified" by Walter Charlteon (London: William Lee, 1650), 58–60.

152. Thomas Adams, *The devills blanket described in foure sermons* (London: Thomas Snodham, 1614), 255.

153. Stephen Jerome, *The haughty heard humbled* (London: Richard More, 1628), 98–99; see Kevin Killeen, "Powder for Padlocks: The Rhetoric of Thanksgiving and the Politics of Flight in Caroline Plague," in *Literature and Popular Culture in Early Modern England*, ed. Matthew Dimmock and Andrew Hatfield (Farnham: Ashgate, 2009), 197.

154. Samuel Rolle, Shlohavot, *or, the burning of London in the year 1666 commemorated and improved in a CX discourses, meditations, and contemplations, divided into four parts* (London: Nathaniel Ranew and Jonathan Robinson, 1667).

155. Pinelli, *La polvere schernita*, 20.

156. James I, *Counterblaste* fol. C4r.

157. Tomás, *Nueva prematica*, 358–60.

158. David Papillon, *The vanity of the lives and passions of men* (London: Robert White, 1651), 69–70; Agar, *King James*, 5.

159. *Tobaco-mastix*, 8–9, 12–13, 20, 26.

160. Short, *Discourses*, 240–41, 248–52.

161. Díaz Bravo, *El ayuno reformado*, 346–47.

162. For coffee, see *The women's petition against coffee*, 2; for tea, see *An effectual remedy totally to prevent smuggling, and to bring into the revenue 195,000 pounds yearly* (London: G. Woodfall, C. Corbet, J. Collier, and J. Jolliffe, 1765[?]), vi. For gin, see Saynought, *Tavern scuffle*, 20–21; and Philanthropos, *The trial of the spirits: or some considerations upon the pernicious consequences of the gin-trade to Great Britain* (London: T. Cooper, 1736), 22.

163. Bontekoe, *Tractaat*, 197.

164. Eliza Fowler Haywood, *A present for women addicted to drinking* (London: W. Own, 1750), 65, chap. 1.

165. Stephen Hales, *A friendly admonition to the drinkers of brandy, and other distilled spirituous liquors* (London: Joseph Downing, 1733), 8.

166. Hales, *Friendly admonition*, 18.

167. Charles Lamb, "Confessions of a Drunkard," in *The Works of Charles and Mary Lamb*, vol. 1, *Miscellaneous Prose (1798–1834)*, ed. E. V. Lucas (London: Methuen, 1903) 135–36. The print is probably of Correggio's *Allegory of Vice* from the studiolo of Isabella d'Este in Mantua, now in the Musée de Louvre. David Eskerdjian, *Correggio* (New Haven, CT: Yale University Press, 1997), 281.

168. David Clemis, "Medical Expertise and the Understandings of Intoxication in Britain, 1660 to 1830," in *Intoxication and Society: Problematic Pleasures of Drugs and Alcohol*, ed. Jonathan Herring, Ciaran Regan, Darin Weinberg, and Phil Withington (London: Palgrave Macmillan, 2013).

4. Do We Take Physick Every Day?

1. For Éloy's life, see *Technologia* 10, no. 1 (1987) from the Belgian Nationaal Centrum voor de Geschiedenis van de Wetenschappen/Centre National d'Histoire des Sciences. Work on Éloy, coffee, and wellness in this and other chapters draws on Scott K. Taylor, "Coffee and the Body: From Exoticism to Wellness in Eighteenth-Century Europe," *Eighteenth Century Studies* 54, no. 3 (2021).

2. Éloy, *Examen de la question médico-politique.*

3. There is a vast literature on Habermas's idea of the public sphere, but for a reassessment of how it compares with the actual institutions of early modern coffeehouses and salons, see David Zaret, "Religion, Science, and Printing in the Public Spheres in Seventeenth-Century England"; and Keith Michael Baker, "Defining the Public Sphere in Eighteenth-Century France: Variations on a Theme by Habermas," both in *Habermas and the Public Sphere*, ed. Craig Calhoun (Cambridge, MA: MIT Press, 1992).

4. Steven Pincus, "'Coffee Politicians Does Create': Coffeehouses and Restoration Political Culture," *Journal of Modern History* 67, no. 4 (1995): 807–34; Markman Ellis, *The Coffee House: A Cultural History* (London: Weidenfeld & Nicolson, 2004); Cowan, *Social Life of Coffee.*

5. For an overview of changes in the social history of medicine, see David Gentilcore, *Food and Health in Early Modern Europe: Diet, Medicine, and Society, 1450–1800* (London: Bloomsbury Academic, 2016); for an overview of the historiography of the consumer revolution, see Bruno Blondé and Wouter Ryckbosch, "Material Cultures," in *Interpreting Early Modern Europe*, ed. C. Scott Dixon and Beat Kümin (New York: Routledge, 2019) 183–214.

6. For coffee in France, see Spary, *Eating the Enlightenment.* For Venice, see Larry Wolff, *Paolina's Innocence: Child Abuse in Casanova's Venice* (Stanford, CA: Stanford University Press, 2012).

7. Duncan, *Wholesome advice,* 28–32.

8. Duncan, 41–42.

9. Merli, *Guida medical*, 47–48.

10. *Klaar en naakt bewijs van het groot misbruyk vande vreemdelantse en uytheemse thee en coffy, waar in onwedersprekelijk wort bewesen, dat deselve niet en dienen tot gesontheit, maar veel meer tot ongesontheit, ja tot afkortinge van het leven der menschen; en at dienvolgens dit gebruik tot groot nadeel van dese onse natie is aangenomen.* (The Hague: Engelbrecht Boucquet, 1695), 9–11, 13–14.

11. *Klaar en naakt bewijs*, 23–24.
12. *De gedebaucheerde*, 35–36.
13. Courtwright, *Forces of Habit*, 69–90; Norton, *Sacred Gifts*.
14. Edward Kellet, Tricoenium Christi in nocte proditionis suae, *the threefold supper of Christ in the night that he was betrayed* (London: Andrew Crooke, 1641), 7–8.
15. Tryon, *Healths grand preservative*, 1.
16. A British Freeholder, *The true state of the British malt-distillery* (London: R. Stevens, 1670), 20.
17. Chute, *Tabacco*, 4–5.
18. Piccino, *Il petopiccino*, 32–42.
19. Thomas Hall, *A practical and polemical commentary, or, exposition upon the third and fourth chapters of the latter epistle of Saint Paul to Timothy* (London: John Starkey, 1658), 99–100.
20. Beintema van Peyma, *Nuttelyke consideratien*, fols. *3r–v, 4–8.
21. Venner, *A briefe and accurate treatise* (London: Richard Moore, 1621).
22. De Leiva y Aguilar, *Desengaño*, fols. 12r–12v.
23. De Leiva y Aguilar, fols. 12v–13r.
24. Ramón, *Nueva prematica*, 354–55.
25. Ramón, 366.
26. Santiago de Valverde Turices, *Un discurso de chocolate* (Seville: Juan de Cabrera, 1624), fol. C3r.
27. Valverde Turices, *Un discurso de chocolate*, 152.
28. Merli, *Guida medica*, 73–74, 76–77, 95–96.
29. De Valverde Turices, *Un discurso de chocolate*, fols. Cr–Cv.
30. De León Pinelo, *Questión moral*, fol. 8v.
31. Cardoso, *Utilidades*, fols. 106r–106v.
32. Vicente Lardizabal, *Memoria sobre las utiladades del chocolate* (Pamplona: Antonio Castilla, 1788).
33. Pierre-Hippolyte Boutigny, *Du chocolat, de sa fabrication, des moyens de reconnaître sa falsification, et de ses propriétés alimentaires et médicales* (Évreaux: Ancelle fils, 1825).
34. Bontekoe, *Tractaat*, 459.
35. Bontekoe, 333.
36. Bontekoe, 303–11.
37. Handley, *Mechanical essays*, 370–72.
38. R. V. N., *Natuur-kundige verhandelin*, 31–32, 86–90.
39. Lavedán, *Tratado*, 158–59. Lavedán also mentioned a "Te de Paraguay," used by miners in Peru, which might mean yerba mate.
40. Lavedán, 171.
41. Lavedán, 195.
42. Lavedán, 148–49, 169–70.
43. J. B., *In praise of tea. A poem. Dedicated to the ladies of Great Britain* (Canterbury: printed for the author, 1736), 11.
44. Tobias Venner, Via recta ad vitam longam, *or a plaine philosophical discourse of the nature, faculties, and effects, of all such things, as by way of nourishments, and dieteticall observations, make for the preservation of health with their just applications into every age, constitution of bodie, and time of yeare* (London: Edward Griffin, 1620).

45. Alexander Philip Wilson, *An experimental essay, on the manner in which opium acts on the living animal body* (London: J. Johnson and G. G. & J. Robinson, 1795), 3–4.

46. *An impartial enquiry into the present state of the British distillery* (London: J. Roberts, 1736), 13–14.

47. Elaine Leong, *Recipes and Everyday Knowledge: Medicine, Science, and the Household in Early Modern England* (Chicago: University of Chicago Press, 2018).

48. Phil Withington, "Where Was the Coffee in Early Modern England?," *Journal of Modern History* 92, no. 1 (2020): 40–75.

49. Gentilcore, *Food and Health*. See also Sandra Cavallo and Tessa Storey, *Healthy Living in Late Renaissance Italy* (Oxford: Oxford University Press, 2014); and Sandra Cavallo, *Artisans of the Body in Early Modern Italy: Identities, Families, and Masculinities* (Manchester: Manchester University Press, 2007).

50. *Lifestyle and Medicine: The Six Non-Naturals in the Long Eighteenth Century*, ed. James Kennaway and Rina Knoeff (New York: Routledge, 2020).

51. For more on the combination of the consumer revolution and eighteenth-century medicine and drugs, see Patrick Wallis, "Consumption, Retailing, and Medicine in Early-Modern London," *Economic History Review* 61, no. 1 (2008): 26–53; Patrick Wallis, "Exotic Drugs and English Medicine: England's Drug Trade, c. 1550–c.1800" (Economic History Working Papers 143/10, Department of Economic History, London School of Economics and Political Science, 2010, accessed September 12, 2023, http://eprints.lse.ac.uk/28577/); Harold J. Cook and Timothy D. Walker, "Circulation of Medicine in the Early Modern Atlantic World," *Social History of Medicine* 26, no. 3 (2013): 337–51; and Pratik Chakrabarti, *Medicine and Empire, 1600–1960* (Basingstoke: Palgrave Macmillan, 2014).

52. McCalman, *Treatise on tea*, 83–84.

53. Albert G. Nicholls, "Nicolas de Blegny and the first medical periodical," *Canadian Medical Association Journal* 31, no. 2 (1934): 198–202.

54. Blégny, *Le bon usage du thé, du caffé et du chocolat* (Lyon: n.p., 1687), 183–84, 280–81.

55. Gudenfridi, *Differenza tra' il cibo e il cioccolate* (Florence: Condotta, 1680), 47. See also Sanvitale, *Memorie veridiche*, 21–22.

56. Smythson, *Compleat family physician*, 745.

57. Smythson, 750.

58. Smythson, 763–64.

59. Steven Shapin, "How to Eat Like a Gentleman: Dietetics and Ethics in Early Modern England," in *Right Living: An Anglo-American Tradition of Self-Help Medicine and Hygiene*, ed. Charles E. Rosenberg (Baltimore, MD: Johns Hopkins University Press, 2003), 21–58.

60. Thomas Willis, *Dr. Willis's practice of physick being the whole works of that renowned and famous physician wherein most of the diseases belonging to the body of man are to be treated of, with excellent methods and receipts for the cure of the same* (London: T. Dring, C. Harper, and J. Leigh, 1684), 137–43.

61. Benjamin Moseley, *Observations on the properties and effects of coffee* (London: Printed for John Stockdale, 1785), 36–38.

62. Moseley, *Medical tracts*, 157–62.

63. Moseley, 168.

64. Stubbe, *Indian nectar*, fols. A3r–A6v, 91–93.

65. Manuel Navas de Carrera, *Dissertacion historica phisico-chimica, y analysis del cacao, su uso, y dossis* (Zaragoza: Francisco Moreno, 1751), 21.

66. Navas de Carrera, *Dissertacion historica phisico-chimica*, 54–55.

67. Origoni, *Discorso contro l'abuso del tabacco*, 45.

68. Maehle, *Drugs on Trial.*

69. Spary, *Eating the Enlightenment.*

70. For a brief overview of the historiography of the medical market in early modern Europe, see Jonathan Andrews, "History of Medicine: Health, Medicine and Disease in the Eighteenth Century," *British Journal of Eighteenth Century Studies* 34, no. 4 (2011): 503–15.

71. David Gentilcore, "The 'Golden Age of Quackery' or 'Medical Enlightenment'? Licensed Charlatanism in Eighteenth-Century Italy," *Cultural and Social History* 3, no. 3 (2008): 250–63.

72. For coffeehouses as sites of dissent in the nineteenth century, see Iain McCalman, *Radical Underworld: Prophets, Revolutionaries, and Pornographers in London, 1795–1840* (Cambridge: Cambridge University Press, 1988).

73. Kevin Siena, "Pliable Bodies: The Moral Biology of Health and Disease," in *A Cultural History of the Human Body in the Age of Enlightenment*, ed. Carole Reeves (Oxford: Berg, 2010), 33–52.

74. De Vries, *Industrious Revolution*; Blondé and Ryckbosch, "Material Cultures."

75. Berg, *Luxury and Pleasure*, 20–45.

76. Christine Fertig and Ulrich Pfister, "Coffee, Mind, and Body: Global Material Culture and the Eighteenth-Century Hamburg Import Trade," in *The Global Lives of Things: The Material Culture of Connections in the Early Modern World*, ed. Anne Gerritsen and Giorgio Riello (London: Routledge, 2016), 221–40.

77. Londa Schiebinger, *Plants and Empire: Colonial Bioprospecting in the Atlantic World* (Cambridge MA: Harvard University Press, 2007); Matthew James Crawford, *The Andean Wonder Drug: Chinchona Bark and Imperial Science in the Spanish Atlantic, 1630–1800* (Pittsburgh, PA: University of Pittsburgh Press, 2016); Paula de Vos, "The Science of Spices: Empiricism and Economic Botany in the Early Spanish Empire," *Journal of World History* 17 (2006): 399–428; Breen, *Age of Intoxication*; *Drugs on the Page: Pharmacopeias and Healing Knowledge in the Early Modern Atlantic World*, ed. Matthew James Crawford and Joseph M. Gabriel (Pittsburgh, PA: University of Pittsburgh Press, 2019).

78. Lister, *Journey to Paris*, 33.

79. Antonio Valisneri, *Dell'uso e dell'abuso delle bevande, e bagnature calde o fredde* (Modena: Pel' Capponi, 1725).

80. Sassenus, *De voortreffelijkheid van de thee.*

81. See Beatty, *Nervous Disease*, 101–31.

82. Éloy, *Examen*, i–iv.

83. Éloy, *Examen*, 5.

84. Here he was at least in part citing an earlier, anonymous writer on coffee. Éloy, 17–18.

85. Éloy, 33–35, 38–40.

86. See Stolberg, *Experiencing Illness*, 170–82; Beatty, *Nervous Disease*; Clemis, "Medical Expertise," 38.

87. For physicians mixing theoretical paradigms, see Joel Shackelford, "Paracelsian Uroscopy and German Chemiatric Medicine in the *Medicina Pennsylvania* of George de Benneville," in *Medical Theory and Therapeutic Practice in the Eighteenth Century: A Transatlantic Perspective*, ed. Jürgen Helm and Renate Wilson (Stuttgart: Franz Steiner Verlag, 2008), 13–36. For the Hippocratic revival, see Andrew Wear, "Place, Health, and Disease: The *Airs, Waters, Places* Tradition in Early Modern England and North America," *Journal of Medieval and Early Modern Studies* 38, no. 3 (2008): 443–65; Seth, *Difference and Disease*; and Kennaway and Knoeff, *Lifestyle and Medicine*.

88. Éloy, *Examen*, 6–7.

89. Éloy, 26–27.

90. Éloy, 33–35.

91. Éloy, 26–27.

92. Éloy, 42–43.

93. For an overview of sensibility in the eighteenth century, see G. J. Barker-Benfield, *The Culture of Sensibility: Sex and Society in Eighteenth-Century Britain* (Chicago: University of Chicago Press, 1992); see also Beatty, *Nervous Disease*, 19–28.

94. Andrew Wilson, *Medical researches: Being an enquiry into the nature and origin of hysterics in the female constitution, and into the distinction between that disease and hypochondriac or nervous disorders* (London: S. Hooper and Robson, 1776), 103–14.

95. Beatty, *Nervous Disease*, 20–23; Stolberg, *Experiencing Illness*, 181–82.

96. For an overview of George Cheyne's contribution to nervous disorders and what we today would call mental health, see Roy Porter, "Introduction," in *George Cheyne: The English Malady (1733)* (London: Tavistock/Routledge, 1991), ix–li.

97. *The maidens complaint against coffee* (London: J. Jones, 1663), 4.

98. Thomas Curteis, *Essays on the preservation and recovery of health* (London: Richard Wilkin, 1704), 99.

99. Giovanni dalla Bona, *L'Uso, e l'abuso del caffe dissertazione storico-fisico-medica del Dottor Giovanni Dalla Bona Veronese*, 2nd ed. (Verona: Pierantonio Berno, 1751), 40.

100. Lavedán, *Tratado*, 109–15.

101. Lavedán, 108–9.

102. Lavedán, 115–17.

103. Guillaume Massieu, *Traite du café, contenant l'histoire, la description, la culture et les propriétés, de ce végetal* (Paris: n.p., 1798), 97. It is possible that the author of this treatise was in fact Olivier de Serres, and Massieu only translated the original from Latin into French.

104. Beatty, *Nervous Disease*, 8–26.

105. Gómez Arias, *Tratado physic medico, de las virtudes, qualidades, provechos, uso, y abuso, del café, del the, del chocolate, y del tabaco* (Madrid: En la Imprenta de los Herederos de Francisco del Hierro, 1752).

106. Moseley, *Observations*, 36–38.

107. De Moya, *El café*, vol. 1 (Madrid: Imprenta de Gonzales, 1792), 21–22.

108. Reynal, *Opuscule medico-politique sur le café*, 31.

109. Reynal, 31.

110. Reynal, 34.

111. Reynal, 37–38.

112. Reynal, 38–39.

113. Felici, *Parere intorno all'uso della cioccolata*, 22–24. See also Donatella Lippi, "Chocolate in History: Food, Medicine, Medi-Food," *Nutrients* 5, no. 5 (2013): 1573–84.

114. Éloy, *Reflexions sur l'usage du thé*, 25–26.

115. Éloy, 35–36.

116. Éloy, 43–48. For other soft drugs, see *Epistle to the fair-sex*; and Young, *Treatise upon opium*.

117. John Wesley, *A letter to a friend, concerning tea* (London: A. Macintosh, 1825); this later edition contains a copy of a letter dated 1748 and first printed in 1749, 3–4.

118. Wesley, *Letter to a friend*, 4

119. Wesley, 8.

120. Lettsom, *Natural history of the tea-tree*, 43. See also *Tea and the Tea-Table in Eighteenth-Century England*, vol. 2, *Tea in Natural History and Medical Writing*, ed. Richard Coulton (London: Pickering & Chatto, 2010), 137–38.

121. Lettsom, 44.

122. Lettsom, 45–48.

123. J. N. Surgeon, *Remarks on Mr. Mason's treatise upon tea* (London: J. Roberts, 1745), 18–21.

124. *An essay on tea, sugar, white bread and butter, country alehouses, strong beer and genenva, and other modern luxuries* (Salisbury: J. Hodson, 1777), 13.

125. Lavedán, *Tratado*, 179–81.

126. William Woodville, *Advice to parents on the management of their children in the natural small pox, and during inoculation; with a few cases confirming the author's opinion. To which are added, some general observations on the use of tea, and the present regimen of diet among the higher ranks of society* (Newark: S. and J. Ridge, 1797), 54.

127. Woodville, *Advice to parents*, 56–59.

128. Hugh Smith, *An essay on the nerves, illustrating their efficient, formal, material, and final causes . . . to which is added an essay on foreign teas* (London: Norman, 1780), 53–54.

129. Carr, *Medicinal epistles*, 32–33.

130. Lettsom, *History*, 1, 5–6.

131. Lamb, "Confessions of a drunkard," 133–34.

132. Young, *Treatise upon opium*, 101.

133. Young, 101.

134. Young, 112–14.

135. Samuel Crumpe, *An inquiry into the nature and properties of opium* (London: G. G. & J. Robinson, 1793).

136. Daniel Mutain, *Theses medicae. De natura, usu & abusu caffé, thé, chocolatae, & tabaci* (Besançon: Nicolai Couche, 1726), 39–40.

137. Edward Teare, *A treatise on the use and abuse of tobacco tending to shew why this plant is hurtful to the nervous system in particular, and of course to the whole human frame in general; the beneficial use of tobacco is also considered* (Doncaster: n.p., 1789[?]).

138. Hill, *Cautions*, 10, 54.

139. *Le bon usage du tabac*, 19–23.

140. Smith, *Essay on the nerves*, 38.

141. Smith, 53.

142. Smith, 45.

143. Smith, 54.

144. *Epistle to the fair-sex*, 11.

145. Lettsom, *History*, 5–6.

146. Hales, *Friendly admonition*, 9–10.

147. Hales, 5–6.

148. Hales, 11.

149. Philaretes, *Work for chimney-sweepers*, fol. Er.

150. Philaretes.

151. For an overview of the origins of today's wellness culture, see Daniela Blei, "The False Promises of Wellness Culture," JSTOR Daily, January 4, 2017, https://daily.jstor.org/the-false-promises-of-wellness-culture/. See also Rina Raphael, *The Gospel of Wellness: Gyms, Gurus, GOOP, and the False Promise of Self-Care* (New York: Henry Holt, 2022); and Pooja Lakshmin, *Real Self-Care: A Transformative Program for Redefining Wellness (Crystals, Cleanses, and Bubble Baths Not Included)* (New York: Penguin Life, 2023).

152. *The New Wellness Revolution: How to Make a Fortune in the Next Trillion Dollar Industry*, ed. Paul Zane Pilzer (Hoboken, NJ: John Wiley & Sons, 2002).

153. There are many other examples from other historians, but see William M. Reddy, *The Navigation of Feeling: A Framework for the History of Emotions* (New York: Cambridge University Press, 2001); and Barbara H. Rosenwein, *Emotional Communities in the Early Middle Ages* (Ithaca, NY: Cornell University Press, 2006).

5. And So the Game Goes Round

1. For an overview of ten Horn's career selling, among other things, pornography and the works of Spinoza, see Frank Peeters, "Leven en bedrijf van Timotheus ten Hoorn (1644–1715)," *Medelingen van de Stichting Jacob Camp Weyerman* 25 (2002): 20–28.

2. *De gedebaucheerde*, fols. *2v–*5v, 1–9.

3. *De gedebaucheerde*, 31–39.

4. *De gedebaucheerde*, 85–94.

5. *De gedebaucheerde*, 469–90.

6. Elizabeth Kowaleski-Wallace makes a similar point about sexuality and disciplining female bodies during tea time. Kowaleski-Wallace, *Consuming Subjects*, 21.

7. Cowan, *Social Life of Coffee*, 148–49.

8. Cowan, 196–202.

9. Cowan, 224–56.

10. Paul Langford, *A Polite and Commercial People: England 1727–1783* (Oxford: Oxford University Press, 1992).

11. Cowan, 237–38, 259.

12. *Character of a coffee-house*, 2–3. The author was perhaps Joseph Glanville. *Eighteenth-Century Coffee-House Culture*, vol. 1, *Restoration Satire*, ed. Markman Ellis (London: Pickering & Chatto, 2006), 81–82.

13. Thomas Brown, *Amusements serious and comical, calculated for the meridian of London* (London: n.p., 1702), 130.

14. Daniel Defoe, *Every-body's business, is no-body's business; or, private abuses, publick grievances: Exemplified in the pride, insolence, and exorbitant ages of our women-servants, footmen, &c.* (London: T. Warner, A. Dodd, and E. Nutt, 1725), 21–22.

15. Richard Steele, *Spectator* 49, April 26, 1711.

16. *The ale-wives complaint, against the coffee-houses, in a dialogue between a victuallers wife and a coffee-man, being at difference about spoiling each others trade* (London: John Tomson, 1675), 2–4.

17. *Coffee-houses vindicated in answer to the late published character of a coffee-house asserting from reason, experience, and good authours, the excellent use and physicall vertues of that liquor: with the grand conveniency of such civil places of resort and ingenious conversation* (London: I. Clarke, 1675), 2–4. For the price of beer, see Pincus, "Coffee Politicians Do Create," 817.

18. Pincus, 825–27.

19. For consensus over debate, see Cowan, *Social Life of Coffee*, 237.

20. *A brief description of the excellent vertues of that sober and wholesome drink, called coffee* (London: Paul Greenwood, 1674). The printer, Paul Greenwood, was himself a coffeehouse merchant and not a professional printer; this was the only thing he ever printed. See Markman, *Eighteenth-Century Coffee-House Culture*, 127–28.

21. *The mens answer to the womens petition against coffee, vindicating their own performances, and the vertues of that liquor, from the undeserved aspersions lately cast upon them by their scandalous pamphlet* (London: n.p., 1674), 2.

22. Andrew Marvell, "A Dialogue between Two Horses," in *The second part of the collection of poems on affairs of state* (London: n.p., 1689). The poem was written years before 1689 and included in this collection of poems by many authors.

23. Withington, "Where Was the Coffee?," 40–75.

24. Sophus A. Reinert, *The Academy of Fisticuffs: Political Economy and Commercial Society in Enlightenment Italy* (Cambridge MA: Harvard University Press, 2018).

25. Alfonso Muzzarelli, "La bottega del caffè," in *Il tempio della fedeltà* (Bologna: Ferdinando Pisarri, 1774).

26. *Le porte feuille galant, contenant les entretiens des caffez, & autres ouvrages mêlez de prose & de vers* (Paris: Jean Moreau, 1700), 3.

27. De Moya, *El café*. For the possible identity of Moya, see Joaquín Álvarez Barrientos, "Miscelánea y tertulia: El café, de Alejandro Moya," *Diechiocho: Hispanic Enlightenment* 27, no. 1 (2004): 59–74.

28. Ellis, Coulton, and Mauger, *Empire of Tea*, 14–25.

29. Ellis, Coulton, and Mauger, 23, 32–35, 39, 164.

30. Ellis, Coulton, and Mauger, 56.

31. Rappaport, *Thirst for Empire*, 41.

32. De Vries, *Industrious Revolution*, 159–60.

33. Ellis, Coulton, and Mauger, *Empire of Tea*, 174.

34. Rappaport, *Thirst for Empire*, 48–51.

35. Jane T. Merritt, *The Trouble with Tea: The Politics of Consumption in the Eighteenth-Century Global Economy* (Baltimore, MD: Johns Hopkins University Press, 2017), 25–27.

36. Ellis, Coulton, and Mauger, *Empire of Tea*, 165–82.

37. De Vries, *Industrious Revolution*, 156.

38. Peter Motteux, *A poem in praise of tea* (London: J. Tonson, 1712), fols. A2r–v. The poem was probably composed and even published a decade earlier; see *Tea and the Tea-Table in Eighteenth Century England*, vol. 1, *Literary Representations of Tea and the Tea-Table*, ed. Markman Ellis (London: Pickering & Chatto, 2010), 37–38.

39. Margaret Cavendish, Duchess of Newcastle, *Observations upon experimental philosophy to which is added the description of a blazing new world* (London: A. Maxwell, 1666).

40. A. N., *A circular letter of Christian friendship to the Honourable the late Lady Mayoress* (London: printed for the author, 1722), 2–6.

41. Woodruff D. Smith, *Consumption and the Making of Respectability, 1600–1800* (New York: Routledge, 2002).

42. Beth Kowaleski-Wallace, "Tea, Gender, and Domesticity in Eighteenth-Century England," *Studies in Eighteenth-Century Culture* 23 (1994): 131–45.

43. Bontekoe and Blankaart, *Gebruik en misbruik*, 57–60, 70–71.

44. *Whipping-tom*, 16–18.

45. "The Tea-table," in *A banquet of the muses: or, the miscellany of miscellanies* (London: Jacob Bickerstaff, 1746), 23–24.

46. *Tea, a poem. In three cantos* (London: Aaron Ward, 1743), 6, 24–31. See Ellis, Coulton, and Mauger, *Empire of Tea*, 87–88.

47. *The rise and progress of tea, &c.* (Dublin: n.p., 1729[?]).

48. Mason, *Good and bad effects*, 33, 42–45.

49. Abram di Vri, *Thee-geselschap, gehouden tusschen eenige juffrouwen klugt-spel. Gedrukt na de kopy van Groningen, in de koffi-stamper: tot kontantetement van de thee-drinkers* (Amsterdam: Sander Wybrantz, 1702), 8–20.

50. Di Vri, *Thee-geselschap*, 25–36.

51. R. V. N., *Natuur-kundige verhandelin*, 191–92.

52. Eliza Fowler Haywood, *The tea-table: or, a conversation between some polite persons of both sexes, at a lady's visiting day* (London: J. Roberts, 1725), 2.

53. Haywood, *Tea-table*, 2.

54. James Bland, *An essay in praise of women: or, a looking-glass for ladies to see their perfections in* (London: Printed by the author, 1733), 105–7. One scholar who has studied this work describes Bland as "otherwise unknown (and possibly pseudonymous)." Eve Williams, "Alexander Pope and the Tracts Advising Women of the Long Eighteenth Century" (master's thesis, Victoria University of Wellington, 2013), 27.

55. Bland, *Essay in praise of women*, 195–96.

56. Bland, 65–67.

57. Bland, 104–5.

58. Duncan Campbell, *A poem upon tea* (London: Mrs. Dodd, 1735 [actually 1734]), 23–24, 31–32.

59. *A new tea-table miscellany: or, bagatelles for the amusement of the fair sex* (London: E. Duncomb, 1750), iv–v.

60. Richard Johnson, *Tea-table dialogues, between a governess, and Mary Sensible, Eliza Thoughtful, Jane Bloom, Ann Hopeful, Dinah Sterling, Lucy Lively, and Emma Tempest* (London: Darton and Harvey, 1996). Johnson seems to have published a similar pamphlet, with grown women and men and no governess, two decades earlier: *Tea-table dialogues; between Miss Thoughtful, Miss Sterling, Miss Prattle, Mast. Thoughtful, Master Goodwill, Master Poplin* (London: T. Carnan, 1772).

61. For porcelain driving the use of tea rather than vice versa see Ellis, Coulton, and Mauger, *Empire of Tea*, 156.

62. David Hancock, "Commerce and Conversation in the Eighteenth-Century Atlantic: The Invention of Madeira Wine," *Journal of Interdisciplinary History* 29, no. 2 (1998): 197–219.

63. See, for example, *Fama: The Politics of Talk and Reputation in Medieval Europe*, ed. Thelma Fenster and Daniel Lord Smail (Ithaca, NY: Cornell University Press, 2003); Daniel Lord Smail, "Telling Tales in Angevin Courts," *French Historical Studies* 20 (1997): 18–215; Chris Wickham, "Gossip and Resistance among the Medieval Peasantry," *Past and Present* 160, no. 24 (1998): 3–24; and Scott K. Taylor, *Honor and Violence in Golden Age Castile* (New Haven, CT: Yale University Press, 2008).

64. Craig Muldrew, *The Economy of Obligation: The Culture of Credit and Social Relations in Early Modern England* (Houndmills: Palgrave Macmillan, 1998).

65. For the healthy patterns of nonelite women's sociability, see, for example, Bernard Capp, *When Gossips Meet: Women, Family, and Neighbourhood in Early Modern England* (Oxford: Oxford University Press, 2003).

66. Karen Harvey, "Barbarity in a Teacup? Punch, Domesticity, and Gender in the Eighteenth Century," *Journal of Design History* 21, no. 3 (2008): 205–21.

67. Warner, *Craze;* Dillon, *Gin*.

68. Linda Zionkowski argues that any female gathering raised suspicions of women drinking alcohol together and the dissolution of their domestic roles. Tim Reinke-Williams argues that women drinking together, even with unrelated men, was sometimes permissible, but certainly the Gin Craze was obsessed with alcohol corroding the morality of women. Linda Zionkowski, "Mother Gin, Motherhood, and the Problem of Domestic Order," *Eighteenth-Century Women: Studies in Their Lies, Works, and Culture* 4 (2006): 1–26; Tim Reinke-Williams, *Women, Work and Sociability in Early Modern London* (Houndmills: Palgrave Macmillan, 2014).

69. *Epistle to the fair-sex*, 4–5.

70. *Epistle to the fair-sex*, 14.

71. *Epistle to the fair-sex*, 15–16.

72. *Epistle to the fair-sex*, 18–19.

73. Ellen Hartigan-O'Connor, *The Ties That Buy: Women and Commerce in Revolutionary America* (Philadelphia: University of Pennsylvania Press, 2009).

74. *Epistle to the fair-sex*, 62.

75. Henry, *Earnest address*, 17–19.

76. For disorder, see Martin, *Alcohol, Violence, and Disorder*. For the importance of taverns and alehouses more generally, see Beat Kümin, *Drinking Matters: Public Houses and Social Exchange in Early Modern Central Europe* (Houndsmills: Palgrave Macmillan, 2007); and Mark Hailwood, *Alehouses and Good Fellowship in Early Modern England* (Woodbridge: Boydell, 2014).

77. Louis Sébastian Mercier, *Tableau de Paris*, ed. Jean-Claude Bonnet (Paris: Mercure de France, 1994), 186–87; Thomas Brennan, *Public Drinking and Popular Culture in Eighteenth-Century Paris* (Princeton, NJ: Princeton University Press, 1988).

78. *Dissertation upon drunkenness*, 1–2.

79. *Dissertation upon drunkenness*, 3.

80. *Dissertation upon drunkenness*, 8–9.

81. *Dissertation upon drunkenness*, 20–21.

82. *Dissertation upon drunkenness*, 25–26.

83. Hailwood, *Alehouses and Good Fellowship*.

84. *Ale-wives complaint*. For the disruption in old ways of consumption caused by new exotic drugs, see also Phil Withington, "Intoxicants and Society in Early Modern England," *Historical Journal* 54, no. 3 (2011): 631–57.

85. Philanthropos, *Trial of the spirits*, 24.

86. T. S., *A proper reply to a scandalous libel, intitulated, The trial of the spirits*, 2nd ed. (London: J. Roberts, 1736), 9.

87. Warner, *Craze*, 118–19.

88. Juniper, *Deposing and death of Queen Gin*, 12.

89. Juniper, 9.

90. A Country Justice of the Peace, *Serious thoughts in regard to the publick disorders, with several proposals for remedying the same* (London: Printed for C. Corbett and J. Barnes, 1750[?]), 9–10, 38.

91. William Henry, *A letter to the Right Honourable John Ponsonby, Esq; Speaker of the Honourable House of Commons; concerning the abuse of spirituous liquors* (Dublin: Peter Wilson, 1760), 5.

92. Nathaniel Blackerby, *The speech of Nathaniel Blackerby, Esq: at a general meeting of His Majesty's justices of the peace for the city and liberty of Westminster* (London: J. and J. Fox, 1738), 3–4.

93. Tobias Smollett, *A dissertation on Mr. Hogarth's six prints lately publish'd, viz. Gin-Lane, Beer-Street, and the Four Stages of Cruelty* (London: B. Dickerson, 1751), 9–10, 18.

94. Smollett, *Dissertation*, 12–14.

95. Smollett, 32.

96. Warner, *Craze*; see also Dillon, *Gin*.

97. Reinke-Williams, *Women, Work and Sociability*.

98. Stephen Buck, *Geneva: A poem in blank verse* (London: T. Cooper, 1734), 4–5.

99. Yates, *Effects of drinking*, 6–7.

100. Yates, 24.

101. Charles Lamb, "Confessions of a drunkard," 133–39.

102. For tobacco's place among its fellow drugs in seventeenth-century England, see Withington, "Intoxicants and Society."

103. Barclay, *Nepenthes*, fol. A4r.

104. Tomkis, *Lingua* (London: Simon Waterson, 1607), fol. H4r.

105. Barnabe Rich, *Faultes fault, and nothing else but faultes* (London: Jeffrey Chorleton, 1606), fol. 9r.

106. Working, *Making of an Imperial Polity*.

107. *Le bon usage du tabac*, 3–4.

108. Lavedán, *Tratado*, 65.

109. Piccino, *Il petopiccino*, 26–30.

110. Deacon, *Tobacco tortured*, fols. **2r–**2v.

111. Deacon, 17–18.

112. Sylvester, *Tobacco battered*, 96–97.

113. De Leiva y Aguilar, *Desengaño*, fols. 12r–v.

114. Ramón, *Nueva prematica*, 373–78.

115. *Tobaco-mastix*, 3.

116. *Tobaco-mastix*, 22.

117. Beintema van Peyma, *Nuttelyke consideration*, fol. **2r.

118. Nathaniel Mist, *A collection of miscellany letters, selected out of Mist's* Journal (London: N. Mist, 1722), 2:254.

119. Fox, *Address to the people*, 4–5.

120. Smith, *Consumption and the Making of Respectability*.

121. Midgley, *Women against Slavery*, 36.

122. Wither, *Abuses stript*, 172.

123. Spooner, *Looking-glass for smoakers*, 22–23.

124. Lavedán, *Tratado de los usos*, 80–82.

125. Norton, *Sacred Gifts*, 159.

126. *Memoirs of the Bedford Coffee-house, by a genius*, 2nd ed. (London: J. Single, 1763), 1–7.

127. Étienne-François Bazot, *Les cafés de Paris ou revue politique, critique et littéraire des moeurs du siècles, par un flaneur patenté* (Paris: Lécrivain, 1819).

128. Saynought, *Tavern scuffle*, 22–23.

129. Saynought, 20–21.

130. Warner, *Craze*, 135–78.

131. *A short history of the Gin Act: or, an impartial account of the conduct of some of those who have been instructed with the execution of it* (London: H. Goreham, 1738), 17.

132. *Short history of the Gin Act*, 19–21.

133. Short *history of the Gin Act*, 17–18.

134. Hales, *Friendly admonition*, 28–29.

135. Wesley, *Letter to a friend*.

136. Hall, *Practical and polemical commentary*, 99.

137. James Boswell, *Boswell's London Journal, 1762–1763*, ed. Frederick A. Pottle (New York: McGraw-Hill, 1950), 98.

6. Who Should Poison the People?

1. Henry, *Earnest address*, 20–21.

2. Chandler, *Sermon*, 15.

3. Chandler, 15.

4. Mark Lawrence Schrad, *Smashing the Liquor Machine: A Global History of Prohibition* (New York: Oxford University Press, 2021).

5. Dennis C. Rasmussen, *The Problems and Promise of Commercial Society: Adam Smith's Response to Rousseau* (University Park: Penn State University Press, 2008); Reinert, *Academy of Fisticuffs*, 8–15. For more on the term "commercial society," see Paul Cheney, "István Hont, the Cosmopolitan Theory of Commercial Globalization, and Twenty-First-Century Capitalism," *Modern Intellectual History* (2021): 1–29.

6. Daniel Lord Smail, *Legal Plunder: Households and Debt Collection in Late Medieval Europe* (Cambridge MA: Harvard University Press, 2016), 17.

7. Lister, *Journey to Paris*, 164–68.

8. There is a vast literature about the connections between exploration, natural history, and commerce. A good place to start would be with Richard Drayton, *Nature's Government: Science, Imperial Britain, and the "Improvement" of the World* (New Haven, CT: Yale University Press, 2000); Schiebinger, *Plants and Empire*; Harold J. Cook, *Matters of Exchange: Commerce, Medicine, and Science in the Dutch Golden Age* (New Haven, CT: Yale University Press, 2007); James Delbourgo, "Sir Hans Sloan's Milk Chocolate and the Whole History of the Cacao," *Social Text* 106, no. 1 (2011): 71–101; Daniela Bleichmar, *Visible Empire: Botanical Expeditions and Visual Culture in the Hispanic Enlightenment* (Chicago: University of Chicago Press, 2012); and Crawford, *Andean Wonder Drug*.

9. B. Ann Tlusty, "Water of Life, Water of Death: The Controversy over Brandy and Gin in Early Modern Augsburg," *Central European History* 31 no. 1–2 (1998): 1–30.

10. For a broad view of the history of gin, see Richard Barnett, *The Book of Gin* (New York: Grove, 2011). For other fortified wines, see, for example, David Hancock, *Oceans of Wine: Madeira and the Emergence of American Trade and Taste* (New Haven, CT: Yale University Press, 2009).

11. Phillips, *Alcohol*.

12. Warner, *Craze*; see also Dillon, *Gin*.

13. See, for example, Peter Clark, *The English Alehouse: A Social History 1200–1830* (London: Longman, 1983); Kümin, *Drinking Matters*; Martin, *Alcohol, Violence, and Disorder*; Phil Withington, "Intoxicants and Society in Early Modern England"; and Hailwood, *Alehouses and Good Fellowship*.

14. Giusepe Pedeliento, Valeria Pinchera, and Daniela Andreini, "Gin: A Marketplace Icon," *Consumption Markets and Culture*, 2020, accessed September 13, 2023, https://www.tandfonline.com/doi/abs/10.1080/10253866.2020.1806066?journalCode=gcmc20.

15. Pedeliento, Pinchera, and Andreini, "Gin," 71–76.

16. Rudmer Biljsma, "Alienation in Commercial Society: The Republican Critique of Jean-Jacques Rousseau and Adam Ferguson," *Southern Journal of Philosophy* 57, no. 3 (2019): 347–77.

17. Dufour, *Usage du caphé*, fols. *5r–*5v.

18. William King, *The transactioneer, with some of his philosophical fancies in two dialogues* (London: n.p., 1700), 86.

19. Bland, *Essay in praise of women*, 107–8.

20. Bernard Mandeville, *The fable of the bees or private vices public benefits* (1714; London: T. Ostell, 1806), 45–47.

21. Berg, *Luxury and Pleasure*. See also the work of Amanda Vickery—for example, "His and Hers: Gender, Consumption, and Household Accounting in Eighteenth-Century England," in "The Art of Survival: Gender and History in Europe, 1450-2000," supplementary issue, *Past and Present*, no. 1 (2006): 12–38; and "Fashioning Difference in Georgian England: Furniture for Him and for Her," in *Early Modern Things: Objects and their Histories, 1500–1800*, ed. Paula Findlen (London: Routledge: 2013), 12–38.

22. A British Freeholder, *The true state of the British malt-distillery, being a defence of Mr. M-wb-y's queries* (London: R. Stevens, 1670), 43–45.

23. Pietro Verri, "Considerazioni sul lusso," in *Scritti vari di Pietro Verri*, vol. 2, ed. Giuliu Carcano (Florence: Felice le Monnier, 1854; orig. published in *Il caffé*, 1764), 28–35. For more on Verri, see Reinert, *Academy of Fisticuffs*.

24. Chiazzari, *Osservazioni* (Genoa: Stamperia Como da S. Matteo, 1819), 8.

25. *Vindication of the use of sugar*, 20.

26. *Answers to the queries*, 7.

27. Philip J. Stern and Carl Wennerlind, "Introduction," in *Mercantilism Reimagined: Political Economy in Early Modern Britain and Its Empire*, ed. Philip J. Stern and Carl Wennerlind (Oxford: Oxford University Press, 2013), 3–5.

28. Philipp Robinson Rössner, *Freedom and Capitalism in Early Modern Europe: Mercantilism and the Making of the Modern Economic Mind* (Cham, Switzerland: Palgrave Pilot, 2020).

29. Larry Harrison, "Tobacco Battered or the Pipes Shattered: A Note on the Fate of the First British Campaign against Tobacco Smoking," *British Journal of Addiction* 81 (1986): 553–58; Fredrik Albritton Jonsson, "Natural History and Improvement: The Case of Tobacco," in *Mercantilism Reimagined: Political Economy in Early Modern Britain and Its Empire*, ed. Philip J. Stern and Carl Wennerlind (Oxford: Oxford University Press, 2013), 117–30. For more on England's dependence on tax revenues from soft drugs, see William J. Ashworth, *Customs and Excise: Trade, Production, and Consumption in England, 1640–1845* (Oxford: Oxford University Press, 2003).

30. Daniel Defoe, *A brief case of the distillers, and of the distilling trade in England* (London: n.p., 1726), v.

31. Steven Pincus, *1688: The First Modern Revolution* (New Haven, CT: Yale University Press, 2009), 366–99.

32. E. P. Thompson, "The Moral Economy of the English Crowd in the Eighteenth Century," *Past & Present* 50 (1971): 76–136. For an assessment of the legacy of Thompson's article, see Francesca Trivellato, "The Moral Economies of Early Modern Europe," *Humanity: An International Journal of Human Rights, Humanitarianism, and Development* 11, no. 2 (2020): 193–201.

33. Defoe, *Brief case of the distillers*, 11.

34. Defoe, 46–48.

35. *A letter to a friend in the country, in relation to the new law concerning spirituous liquors* (London: M. Cooper, 1743), 12, 17.

36. Slyboots, *Tavern scuffle*, 28–29.

37. Warner, "Can Legislation Prevent Debauchery?"

38. *Impartial enquiry*, 15.

39. Rössner, *Freedom and Capitalism*, 26–27.

40. C. T., *An advice how to plant tobacco in England and how to bring it to colour and perfection, to whom it may be profitable, and to whom harmful* (London: Nicholas Okes, 1615), fols. A4iir–A4iiv.

41. Edward Bennett, *A treatise divided into three parts, touching the inconveniences, that the importation of tobacco out of Spaine, hath brought to this land* (London: John Budge, 1620), 1–3. For the long history of tobacco cultivation in Great Britain, see Fredrik Albritton Jonsson, "Scottish Tobacco and Rhubarb: The Natural Order of Civil Cameralism in the Scottish Enlightenment," *Eighteenth-Century Studies* 49, no. 2 (2016): 129–47.

42. Norton, *Sacred Gifts*, 201.

43. Jacob M. Price, *France and the Chesapeake: A History of the French Tobacco Monopoly, 1674–1791, and of Its Relationship to the British and American Tobacco Trades*, vol. 1 (Ann Arbor: University of Michigan Press, 1973).

44. Niccolò Gavelli, *Storia distinta, e curiosa del tabacco* (Ferrara: F. Altieri, 1758).

45. Ellis, Coulton, and Mauger, *Empire of Tea*, 108–14.

46. Rappaport, *Thirst for Empire*, 40–46; Merritt, *Trouble with Tea.*

47. Man of Kent, *An effectual remedy totally to prevent smuggling, and bring into the revenue 195,000 pounds yearly* (London: G. Woodfall, C. Corbet, J. Collier, and J. Jolliffe, 1756[?]), v–vi.

48. Merritt, *Trouble with Tea.*

49. *Speculative Historische aanmerkingen, dewelke op de heedendaagse nieuwe belasting der coffy, thee, chocolaat en andere medicinale dranken van water, huy ofte melk, door het mengen met eenige kruiden ofte spetien (hoe ok bereid) en door ded doctorenveelmaalen als een huis-medicyn, tot voorkoming van verscheide ziekte geordineert, bescheidentlijktoegepast kunnen werden* (n.p., 1699).

50. P. J. Laborie, *The coffee planter of Saint Domingo* (London: T. Cadell and W. Davies, 1798).

51. M. C. de T., *Café Français: recette économique, analysée, d'après plusieurs savans* (Paris: Dondey-Dupré, Père et Fils, 1824), 6–21.

52. Thomas Tryon, *Tryon's letters, domestick and foreign, to several persons of quality* (London: Geo. Conyers and Eliza. Harris, 1700), 219.

53. *De vaderlander*, 1775–78, nos. 1–2 (January 2, 1775) through 209 (December 25, 1778) (Amsterdam: Erven van F. Houttuyn), 337–41.

54. Joseph-François Charpentier-Cossigny, *Moyens d'amélioration et de restauration proposes aux habitans des colonies*, 3 vols. (Paris: Je. Batilliot, 1803).

55. *L'oppio nostrale suoi effetti, e virtù* (Naples: Amato Cone, 1788).

56. *Proposizione sulla necessità d'introdurre in Toscana la coltivazione dei papaveri*; Giovanni Palmieri, *Il papavero sonnifero per far l'oppio superiore di efficacia al tebajco in commercio* (Foligno: G. Tomassini, 1808).

57. Hans Derks, *History of the Opium Problem: The Assault on the East, ca. 1600–1950* (Leiden: Brill, 2012).

58. Edward Chamberlayne, *Englands wants, or several proposals probably beneficial for England humbly offered to the consideration of all good patriots in both houses of Parliament* (London: Jo. Martin, 1667), 4.

59. See Hancock, *Oceans of Wine*; and Jennifer L. Anderson, *Mahogany: The Costs of Luxury in Early America* (Cambridge MA: Harvard University Press, 2012).

60. Christopher J. Berry, *The Idea of Commercial Society in the Scottish Enlightenment* (Edinburgh: Edinburgh University Press, 2013), 206–7.

61. Holcomb, *Moral Commerce*, 27–35.

62. Bronwen Everill, *Not Made by Slaves: Ethical Capitalism in the Age of Abolition* (Cambridge MA: Harvard University Press, 2020), 48–49, 51–53.

63. See especially Midgley, *Women against Slavery*; and Sussman, *Consuming Anxieties*.

64. Everill, *Not Made by Slaves*, 48–49.

65. William Allen, *The duty of abstaining from the use of West Indian produce* (London: n.p., 1792), 7–8.

66. Allen, *Duty of abstaining*, 10.

67. Allen, 16.

68. Philanthropos, *Trial of the spirits*, 4–7.

69. Philanthropos, 8–14.

70. Philanthropos, 14–16.

71. Philanthropos, 22.

72. Thomas Wilson, *Distilled spirituous liquors the bane of the nation* (London: J. Roberts, 1736), ii.

73. Wilson, *Distilled spirituous liquors*, iv.

74. Wilson, 8.

75. Sandra Sherman, *Imagining Poverty: Quantification and the Decline of Paternalism* (Columbus: Ohio State University Press, 2001). Sherman puts the shift at the very end of the eighteenth century, but it seems to begin earlier in the century.

76. Wilson, *Distilled spirituous liquors*, 9–10.

77. Wilson, 26.

78. Wilson, 42–43.

79. Wilson, 36–37.

80. Maddox, *Expediency of preventive wisdom*, iii–iv.

81. Maddox, 16.

82. Ted McCormick, "Population: Modes of Seventeenth-Century Demographic Thought," in *Mercantilism Reimagined: Political Economy in Early Modern Britain and Its Empire*, ed. Philip J. Stern and Carl Wennerlind (Oxford: Oxford University Press, 2013), 25–40.

83. Henry, *Letter*, 5.

84. Henry, 10–11.

85. Henry, 20.

86. Wilson, *Distilled spiritous liquors*, iv–v.

87. *Full answers to Mr. M—y's queries in defence of the malt-distillery* (London: J. Scott, 1760), 28.

88. *An oration, delivered before an audience of distillers, by Baalzebub* (London: J. Scott, 1760), 5–6.

89. *A collection of letters published in the daily papers relating to the British distillery* (London: J. Roberts, 1736), 23–24.

90. *Impartial enquiry*, 1.

91. Robert Hennebo, *Rouwklachten van den heere Jacobus Veenhuizen; beneevens de lof de jenever, eerste en tweede deel* (Amsterdam: Printed by the author, 1723), 19.

92. Hennebo, *Rouwklachten,* 18–23, 27.

93. Alexander Blunt, *Blunt to Walpole: a familiar epistle in behalf of the British distillery* (London: J. Wilford, 1730), 25–26.

94. Blunt, *Blunt to Walpole*, 24–26, 28.

95. An Impartial Hand, *The life of Mother Gin* (London: W. Webb, 1736).

96. Juniper, *Deposing and death of Queen Gin*, 12.

97. Deacon, *Tobacco tortured*, 60–61.

98. Daniel Defoe, *Augusta triumphans: or, the way to make London the most flourishing city in the universe* (London: J. Roberts, 1728), 41–44.

99. Reynal, *Opuscule*, 37–39.

100. Reynal, 39–42.

101. Reynal, 42.

102. Hanway, "Essay on tea" In *A journal of eight days journey from Portsmouth to Kingston upon Thames* (London: H. Woodfall, 1756), 213, 219. See also Ellis, Coulton, and Mauger, *Empire of Tea*, 187–91.

103. Hanway, 230–31.

104. Hanway, 235–38.

105. Hanway, 244.

106. Hanway, 273.

107. Hanway, 278.

108. Hanway, 246.

109. *An essay on tea*, 7.

110. *An essay on tea*, 13–14.

111. *An essay on tea*, 14.

112. Sherman, *Imagining Poverty*.

113. De Vries, *Industrious Revolution*.

114. István Hont, "The Early Enlightenment Debate on Commerce and Luxury," in *The Cambridge History of Eighteenth-Century Political Thought*, ed. Mark Goldie and Robert Wokler (Cambridge: University of Cambridge Press, 2006), 379–418.

115. *Dissertation upon drunkenness*, 2.

116. *Dissertation upon drunkenness*, 13–14.

117. *Dissertation upon drunkenness*, 15–16.

118. *Answers to the queries*, 9–10.

119. *Impartial enquiry*, 48–49.

120. A Country Justice of the Peace, *Serious thoughts in regard to the publick disorders, with several proposals for remedying the same* (London: C. Corbett and J. Barnes, 1750[?]), 40.

121. Blunt, *Geneva*, 24–25.
122. Hailwood, *Alehouses and Good Fellowship*.
123. See Warner, *Craze*; and Dillon, *Gin*.
124. *Dissertation on drunkenness*, 17–18.
125. *Dissertation on drunkenness*, 6–7.
126. *Occasional monitor*, 3–5.
127. Braithwaite, *Smoaking age*, 171–72.
128. Sylvester, *Tobacco battered*, 108–09.
129. Marsh, *Confession*.
130. Thomas Mun, *England's treasure by forraign trade* (London: Printed by J. G. for Thomas Clark, 1664), 178–80.
131. Sir William Berkeley, *A discourse and view of Virginia* (n.p., 1663), 5.
132. Eusebio da Monte Santo, *Lettera critica in ordine all'uso del tabacco* (Fogligno: Pompeo Campana, 1758).
133. West, *Wits A.B.C.*, fol. E2v.
134. William Prynne, *A short demurrer to the Jewes long discontinued barred remitter into England* (London: Edward Thomas, 1655), 123.
135. Beintema van Peyma, *Nuttelyke consideratien*, fol. ***2r.
136. Clarke, *Dissertation*, 19–20.
137. R. T., *Good husbandry, or the improvement of time; being a sure way to get and keep money* (London: J. G., 1675), 2–3. See also Aino Mäkikalli, *From Eternity to Time: Conceptions of Time in Daniel Defoe's Novels* (Bern: Peter Lang AG, 2007), 250–51.
138. M. P., *A character of coffee and coffee-houses by M.* (London: John Starkey, 1661), 5. For more on the author, see Ellis, *Eighteenth-Century Coffee-House Culture* (London: Pickering & Chatto, 2006), 1:1–2.
139. R. V. N., *Natuur-kundige verhandelin*, 173–74.
140. *De gedebaucheerde*, 1–2, 472–73, 481–86.
141. Bontekoe and Blankaart, *Gebruik en misbruik*, 59–60, 67–68.
142. McCalman, *Treatise on tea*, 117.
143. Bland, *Essay in praise of women*, 28–29.
144. Bland, 9.
145. Bland, 5–6.
146. *The tea drinking wife, and drunken husband. To which is added, three other songs* (Newcastle-upon-Tyne: n.p., 1749), 2–3.
147. Smail, *Legal Plunder*; Daniel Lord Smail, *The Consumption of Justice: Emotions, Publicity, and Legal Culture in Marseille, 1264–1423* (Ithaca, NY: Cornell University Press, 2003).

Conclusion

1. Thomas De Quincey, *Confessions of an English Opium-Eater and Related Writings*, ed. Joel Faflak (Peterborough, NH: Broadview, 2009), 11.
2. The two best biographies of De Quincey are Frances Wilson, *Guilty Thing: A Life of Thomas De Quincey* (New York: Farrar, Straus & Giroux, 2016); and Robert Morrison, *The English Opium-Eater: A Biography of Thomas De Quincey* (London: Weidenfeld & Nicolson, 2009).

3. De Quincey, *Confessions*, 52n1.

4. This from a review of Robert Morrison's biography of De Quincey: Mike Jay, "Drink It, Don't Eat It or Smoke It," *London Review of Books*, May 13, 2010.

5. Carl A. Trocki, *Opium, Empire, and the Global Political Economy* (London: Routledge, 1999), 17–21.

6. Booth, *Opium*, 26–27.

7. Trocki, *Opium*, 34–35.

8. E. C. Spary, "Opium, Experimentation, and Alterity in France," in "Intoxicants and Early Modern Globalization," special issue, *Historical Journal* 65 (2022): 49–67.

9. De Quincey, *Confessions*, 51.

10. De Quincey, 88.

11. De Quincey, 70.

12. De Quincey, 85–86.

13. Wilson, *Guilty Thing*, 151–52.

14. De Quincey, *Confessions*, 90.

15. De Quincey, 89.

16. De Quincey, 97–98.

17. De Quincey, 124–26.

18. De Quincey, 54.

19. De Quincey, 88.

20. De Quincey, 95.

21. De Quincey, 55–56.

22. De Quincey, 56, 103.

23. Wilson, *Guilty Thing*, 309–10; Morrison, *English Opium-Eater*, 164–65.

24. De Quincey, *Confessions*, 51–52.

25. De Quincey, 114.

26. De Quincey, 53–55; see also Joel Faflak, "Introduction," *Confessions of an English Opium-Eater*, by Thomas De Quincey, 23.

27. Wilson, *Guilty Thing*, 231.

28. De Quincey, *Confessions*, 104.

29. De Quincey, 89.

30. De Quincey, 106.

31. De Quincey, 117–19.

32. De Quincey, 109–12.

33. Morrison, *English Opium-Eater*, 165.

34. De Quincey, *Confessions*, 91–92.

35. De Quincey, 97–99.

36. See, for example, Jane Rendell, *The Pursuit of Pleasure: Gender, Space, and Architecture in Regency London* (New Brunswick, NJ: Rutgers University Press, 2002).

37. De Quincey, *Confessions*, 94–95.

38. Virginia Berridge and Griffith Edwards, *Opium and the People: Opiate Use in Nineteenth-Century England* (London: Allen Lane/St. Martin's, 1981), 3–4.

39. Trocki, *Opium*.

40. De Quincey, *Confessions*, 96.

41. Jones, *Mysteries of opium*, 20.

42. De Quincey, *Confessions*, 113.

43. Susan Zieger, *Inventing the Addict: Drugs, Race, and Sexuality in Nineteenth-Century and American Literature* (Amherst: University of Massachusetts Press, 2008).

44. Carl L. Hart, *Drug Use for Grown-Ups: Chasing Liberty in the Land of Fear* (New York: Penguin, 2021).

Bibliography

Primary Sources

A. N. *A circular letter of Christian friendship to the Honourable the late Lady Mayoress*. London: printed for the author, 1722.

Adams, Thomas. *The devills blanket described in foure sermons*. London: Thomas Snodham, 1614.

Agar, Ben. *King James, his apophthegms, or table-talke as they were by him delivered occasionally and by the publisher (his quondam servant) carefully received, and now humbly offered to publique view, as not impertinent to the present times*. London: B. W., 1643.

Agostino, Giovanni, and Morison Scozzese. *Soccinto raguaglio delle stupendi e maravivgliose virtù del cordial liquore o sia balsam potabile de i chinesi: estratto in più modi dall' erba thé*. Rome: Dom. Ant. Ercole, 1720.

The ale-wives complaint, against the coffee-houses, in a dialogue between a victuallers wife and a coffee-man, being at difference about spoiling each others trade. London: John Tomson, 1675.

Allen, William. *The duty of abstaining from the use of West Indian produce*. London: n.p., 1792.

Answers to the queries, in defence of the malt distillery. London: T. Payne, 1760.

An antidote against melancholy made up in pills. Edited by John Playford. London: John Playford, 1669.

Antonio, Luis. *Nuevo plato de varios manjares*. Edited by Antonio Pérez Goméz. Valencia: Cieza, 1968.

Arias, Gómez. *Tratado physic medico, de las virtudes, qualidades, provechos, uso, y abuso, del café, del the, del chocolate, y del tabaco*. Madrid: En la Imprenta de los Herederos de Francisco del Hierro, 1752.

Archer, John. *Every man his own doctor in two parts*. London: Printed by Peter Lillicrap for the author, 1671.

Arisi, Francesco. *Il tabaco masticato, e fumato*. Milan: n.p., 1725.

Armuhaz, Don Bollicosgo. *The coffee-mans granado discharged upon the maidens complaint against coffee*. London: J. Johnson, 1663.

The art of making tea, a poem, in two cantos. Cambridge: Printed by B. Flower, 1797.

Barclay, William. *Nepenthes, or the vertues of tabacco*. Edinburgh: Andro Hart, 1614.

Baruffaldi, Girolamo. *La tabaccheide*. Ferrera: Eredi di B. Pometelli, 1714.

Bate, George. *The regall apology, or, the declaration of the Commons, Feb. 11, 1647, canvassed wherein every objection to their whole charge against His Majesty is cleared, and for the most part, retorted*. N.p., 1648.

Bazot, Étienne-François. *Les cafés de Paris ou revue politique, critique et littéraire des moeurs du siècles, par un flaneur patenté*. Paris: Lécrivain, 1819.

Beaumont, Francis. *Poems: by Francis Beaumont, gent. viz. the hermaphrodite*. London: Laurence Blaiklock, 1653.

Beintema van Peima, Johannes Ignatius Worp. *Nuttelyke consideration of sedige aanmerkingen over het heedendaags tabak-suigen, of, en hoe verre het selve geoolofd zy, of niet*. Amsterdam: Cornelis van Hogenhuisen, 1692.

Beintema van Peima, Johannes Ignatius Worp. *Tabacologia, ofte korte verhandelinge over de tabak, deselvs deugd, gebruik, ende kennisse: waar door aangeweesen word teen wegh om lang, vroolijk, ende gesond te leeven*. The Hague: Levyn van Dyck, 1690.

Bellamy, Dr. *A new and short defense of tabacco: with the effects of the same: and of the right use*. London: n.p., 1602.

Bennett, Edward. *A treatise divided into three parts, touching the inconveniences, that the importation of tobacco out of Spaine, hath brought to this land*. London: John Budge, 1620.

Berkeley, Sir William. *A discourse and view of Virginia*. N.p., 1663.

Biet, Leonard. *Le bon usage du caffé volatile*. Paris: n.p., 1687–1700.

Blackerby, Nathaniel. *The speech of Nathaniel Blackerby, Esq: at a general meeting of His Majesty's justices of the peace for the city and liberty of Westminster*. London: J. and J. Fox, 1738.

Bland, James. *An essay in praise of women: or, a looking-glass for ladies to see their perfections in*. London: Printed by the author, 1733.

Blankaart, Stephan. *De kartesiaanse academie ofte institute der medicine*. Amsterdam: Johannes ten Hoorn, 1683.

Blankaart, Stephan. "*Verhandelinge van de coffee, aangaande des selfs kragten in gesonde luiden en alle ziekten*." In Cornelis Bontekoe, *Gebruik en mis-bruik van de thee*, 133–52. The Hague: Pieter Hagen, 1686.

Blégny, Nicolas. *Le bon usage du thé, du caffé et du chocolat pour la preservation & pour la guerison des maladies*. Paris: Estienne Michalet, 1687.

Blunt, Alexander. *Blunt to Walpole: a familiar epistle in behalf of the British distillery*. London: J. Wilford, 1730.

Blunt, Alexander. *Geneva: A Poem. Address'd To the Right Honourable Sir R- W-*. London: Printed for T. Payne, 1729.

Le bon usage du tabac en poudre. Paris: la veuve de G. Quinet, 1700.

Bontekoe, Cornelis. *Tractaat van het excellenste kruyd thee: 't welk vertoond het regte gebruyk, en de groote kragten van 't selve in gesondheyd, en siekten*. The Hague: Pieter Hagen, 1678. From *Opuscula Selecta Neerlandicorum de arte medica*, translated by anonymous. Amsterdam, 1937. Accessed September 11, 2023. https://www.dbnl.org/tekst/_opu001193701_01/_opu001193701_01_0014.php.

Bontekoe, Cornelis, and Stephan Blankaart, *Gebruik en misbruik van de thee, mitsgaders een verhandelinge wegens de deugden en kragten van de tabak. Hier nevens een verhandelingevan de coffee, met des zelfs krachten in gezonde, en ongezonde, door Stephanus Blankaart*. The Hague: Pieter Hagen and Amsterdam: Jan ten Hoorn, 1686.

Boorde, Andrew. *A compendyous regiment or a dyetary of healthe made in Mountpyllyer*. London: Wyllyam Powell, 1547.

Borga da Rasa, Anton-Maria. *Gli arcani di venere, poemetto. La pipa, ditirambo.* Venice[?]: n.p., 1750.

Boswell, James. *Boswell's London Journal, 1762–1763.* Edited by Frederick A. Pottle. New York: McGraw-Hill, 1950.

Boutigny, Pierre-Hippolyte. *Du chocolat, de sa fabrication, des moyens de reconnaître sa falsification, et de ses propriétés alimentaires et médicales.* Évreaux: Ancelle fils, 1825.

Braithwaite, Richard (Blasius Multibibus). *The smoaking age, or, the man in the mist: with the life and death of tobacco.* N.p.: "Oenox Thopolis," 1617.

A brief description of the excellent vertues of that sober and wholesome drink, called coffee. London: Paul Greenwood, 1674.

Bright, Timothie. *A treatise, wherein is declared the sufficiencie of English medicines, for cure of all diseases, cured with medicines.* London: Humphrey Lownes for Tho. Man, 1615.

A British Freeholder, *The true state of the British malt-distillery.* London: R. Stevens, 1670.

A broad-side against coffee; or, the marriage of the Turk. London: J. L., 1672.

Brooke, Humphrey. ΥΓΙΕΙΝΗ *or A conservatory of health.* London: G. Whittington, 1650.

Brooke, N. *Observations on the manners and customs of Italy.* Bath: R. Cruttwell, 1798.

Brown, Thomas. *Amusements serious and comical, calculated for the meridian of London.* London: n.p., 1702.

Browne, Joseph. *An account of the wonderful cures perform'd by the cold baths.* 2nd ed. London: A. Bettesworth, 1707[?].

Brugis, Thomas. Vade mecum, *or a companion for a chyrurgion.* London: Thomas William, 1652.

Buck, Stephen. *Geneva. A poem in blank verse.* London: T. Cooper, 1734.

Burlot de Campaña. "Sátira contra el tabaco." In *Romance del burlador Burlot de Campaña, fabricado, y destruihido en la Rambla, dia de la Natividad de nuestra Señora, Año 1642*, fols. A2r–A3v. Barcelona: Gabriel Nogues, 1643.

Burn, Andrew. *Second address to the people of Great Britain: containing a new, and most powerful argument to abstain from the use of West India sugar.* 2nd ed. Rochester: W. Gillman, 1792.

Burton, Henry. *A replie to a relation, of the conference between William Laude and Mr. Fisher the Jesuite.* N.p., 1640.

Butts, Henry. *Dyets dry dinner consisting of eight severall courses.* London: Tho. Creede for William Wood, 1599.

C. T. *An advice how to plant tobacco in England and how to bring it to colour and perfection, to whom it may be profitable, and to whom harmful.* London: Nicholas Okes, 1615.

Campbell, Duncan. *A poem upon tea.* London: Mrs. Dodd, 1735 [actually 1734].

Cardoso, Fernando. *Utilidades del agua i de la nieve, del bever frío i caliente.* Edited by Jacobo Israel Garzon. Madrid: Hebraica, 2003.

Carey, Henry. *Poems on several occasions.* London: J. Kent, 1713.

Carr, Richard. *Dr. Carr's medicinal epistles upon several occasions.* Translated by John Quincy. London: William Newton and J. Phillips, 1714.

Carta que escrivió un medico christiano, que estava curando en Antiberi, a un cardenal de Roma, sobre la bebeda del cahuè o café. N.p.

Castro de Torres, El Capitán. *Panegírico al chocolate*. Edited by Manuel Pérez de Guzmán. 2nd ed. Seville: E. Rasco, 1887.

Chamberlayne, Edward. *Englands wants, or, several proposals probably beneficial for England humbly offered to the considerations of all good patriots in both houses of Parliament*. London: Jo. Martin, 1667.

Chamberlayne, John. *The natural history of coffee, chocolate, thee, tobacco*. London: Christopher Wilkinson, 1682.

Chandler, Edward. *A sermon preached to the Societies for Reformation of Manners, at St. Mary-le-Bow, on Monday January the 4th, 1724*. London: James Knapton, 1724.

The character of a coffee-house with the symptomes of a town-wit. London: Jonathan Edwin, 1673.

Charpentier-Cossigny, Joseph-François. *Moyens d'amélioration et de restauration proposes aux habitans des colonies*. 3 vols. Paris: Je. Batilliot, 1803.

Chiazzari, Michele Nicolò. *Osservazione sull' uso ed abuso del tabacco in istato di sanitá e di malattia*. Genoa: S. Matteo, 1819.

Chute, Anthony. *Tabacco: the distinct and severall opinions of the late and best phisitions that have written of the divers natures and qualities thereof*. London: William Barlow, 1595.

Clarke, Adam. *A dissertation on the use and abuse of tobacco*. London: G. Whitfield, 1797.

Coffee-houses vindicated in answer to the late published character of a coffee-house asserting from reason, experience, and good authours, the excellent use and physicall vertues of that liquor: with the grand conveniency of such civil places of resort and ingenious conversation. London: I. Clarke, 1675.

A collection of letters published in the daily papers relating to the British distillery. London: J. Roberts, 1736.

Colmenero de Ledesma, Antonio. *Curioso tratado de naturaleza y calidad del chocolate*. Madrid: Francisco Martínez, 1631.

Considerations to professors of Christianity of every denomination, on the impropriety of consuming West-Indian sugar and rum, as produced by the oppressive labour of slaves. London[?]: n.p., 1792.

Corrado, Vincenzo. *Il credenziere di buno gusto*. 6th ed. Napoli: Torchi di Saverio Giordano, 1820.

A Country Justice of the Peace. *Serious thoughts in regard to the publick disorders, with several proposals for remedying the same*. London: Printed for C. Corbett and J. Barnes, 1750[?].

Crumpe, Samuel. *An inquiry into the nature and properties of opium*. London: G. G. and J. Robinson, 1793.

A cup of coffee, or coffee in its colours. London: n.p., 1663.

Curteis, Thomas. *Essays on the preservation and recovery of health*. London: Richard Wilkin, 1704.

Da Bergamo, Gaetano Maria. "*Pratico esame sopra il vizio detto volgarmente dell'osteria*." In *Opera del padre Fr. Gaetano Maria da Bergamo Cappuccino*. Vol. 2, 66–98. Rome; Arangelo Casaletti, 1776.

Da Monte Santo, Eusebio. *Lettera critica in ordine all'uso del tabacco*. Fogligno: Pompeo Campana, 1758.

Dalla Bona, Giovanni. *L'Uso, e l'abuso del caffe dissertazione storico-fisico-medica del Dottor Giovanni Dalla Bona Veronese*. 2nd ed. Verona: Pierantonio Berno, 1751.

De Castro y Medinilla, Juan. *Historia de las virtudes y propiedades del tabaco, i de los modos de tomarle para las partes intrinsecas i de aplicarle as las extrinsecas*. Córdoba: Salvador de Cea Tesa, 1620.

De Fragoso, Juan. *Discursos de las cosas aromáticas, arboles y frutales, y de otras muchas medicinas simples que se traen de la India Oriental, y sirven al uso de medicina*. Madrid: Francisco Sánchez, 1572.

De Leiva y Aguilar, Francisco. *Desengaño contra el mal uso del tabaco*. Córdoba: Salvador de Cea Tesa, 1634.

De León Pinelo, Antonio. *Questión moral: si el chocolate quebranta el ayuno eclesiástico*. Madrid: Viuda de Juan Gonçalez, 1636.

De Moya, Alexandro. *El café*. Vol. 1. Madrid: Imprenta de Gonzalez, 1792.

De Nicolay, Nicolas. *The navigations, peregrinations and voyages, made into Turkie by Nicolas Nicholay Daulphinois, Lord of Arfeuile, chamberlaine and geographer ordinarie to the King of Fraunce*. Translated by T. Washington. London: Thomas Dawsom, 1585.

De Nicolay, Nicolas. *Les navigations peregrinations et voyages, faicts en la turquie, par Nicolas de Nicolay Daulphinoys Seigeur d'Arfeville, valet de chamber & geographe ordinaire du Roy de France, contenants plusieurs singularitez que l'autheur y a veu & observe*. Antwerp: Guillaume Silvius, Imprimeur du Roy, 1577.

De Quincey, Thomas. *Confessions of an English Opium-Eater and Related Writings*. Edited by Joel Faflak. Peterborough, NH: Broadview, 2009.

De Reynal, M. *Opuscule médico-politique sur le café*. Évreux: Imprimerie de J. J. L. Ancelle, 1813.

De Valverde Turices, Santiago. *Un discurso de chocolate*. Seville: Juan de Cabrera, 1624.

Deacon, John. *Tobacco tortured; or, the filthie fume of tabacco refined*. London: Richard Field, 1616.

Defoe, Daniel. *Augusta triumphans: or, the way to make London the most flourishing city in the universe*. London: J. Roberts, 1728.

Defoe, Daniel. *A brief case of the distillers, and of the distilling trade in England*. London: n.p., 1726.

Defoe, Daniel. *Every-body's business, is no-body's business; or, private abuses, publick grievances: Exemplified in the pride, insolence, and exorbitant ages of our women-servants, footmen, &c*. London: T. Warner, A. Dodd, and E. Nutt, 1725.

Della Volpe, Francisco Maria. *Pulvis nicotianus vulgo tabacco ad Leodocum Sofidium acclamatum*. Rome: Antonius de Rubeis Romae, 1722.

Di Vri, Abram. *Thee-geselschap, gehouden tusschen eenige juffrouwen klugt-spel. Gedrukt na de kopy van Groningen, in de koffi-stamper: tot kontantetement van de thee-drinkers*. Amsterdam: Sander Wybrantz, 1702.

Díaz Bravo, José Vicente. *El ayuno reformado, segun practica de la primitive iglesia, por los cinco breves de nuestro santissimo Padre Benedicto XIV . . . Y una disertacion historica, medico-chymica, physico-moral de el chocolate, y su uso, despues de los nuevos preceptos*. Pamplona: Pasqual Ibañez, 1753.

Dichiarazione della virtù della bevanda del caffè. Rome: A. Bernabò, 1683.

A dissertation on the use and abuses of tobacco. In relation to smoaking, chewing, and taking of snuff. London: J. Roberts, 1720.

A dissertation upon drunkenness. London: T. Warner, 1727.

Dossie, Robert. *An essay on spirituous liquors, with regard to their effects on health*. London: Printed for J. Ridley, 1770[?].

Dufour, Philippe Sylvestre. *De l'usage du caphé, du thé et du chocolate*. Lyon: Jean Girin & Barthelemy Riviere, 1671.

Duncan, Daniel. *Wholesome advice against the abuse of hot liquors, particularly of coffee, chocolate, tea, brandy, and strong-waters*. Translated by anonymous. London: H. Rhodes and A. Bell, 1706.

Du Verger, François-Guislier. *Traité des liqueurs, esprits ou essences, et la maniere de s'en server utilement*. Louvain: Guillaime Stryckwant, 1728.

An effectual remedy totally to prevent smuggling, and to bring into the revenue 195,000 pounds yearly. London: G. Woodfall, C. Corbet, J. Collier, and J. Jolliffe, 1765[?].

Éloy, Nicolas François Joseph. *Examen de la question médico-politique: si l'usage habituel du caffé est avantageux ou doit être mis au rang des choses indifférentes à la conservation de la santé*. Mons: H. Hoyois, n.d.

Éloy, Nicolas François Joseph. *Reflexions sur l'usage du thé dans lequelles, après avoir fait l'histoire de cette boisson étrangerie, on donne les précautions nécessaires pour la prendre avec avantage*. Mons: Chez Plon, 1750.

An epistle to the fair-sex on the subject of drinking. London: T. Gardner, 1744.

An essay on sugar. London: E. Comyns, 1752.

An essay on tea, sugar, white bread and butter, country alehouses, strong beer and geneva, and other modern luxuries. Salisbury: J. Hodson, 1777.

An essay on the nature, use, and abuse, of tea, in a letter to a lady; With an account of its mechanical operation. London: J. Bettenham, 1722.

Estienne, Charles, and Jean Liebault. *L'agriculture et maison rustique*. Paris: Jacques de Puys, 1574.

Felici, Giovanni Batista. *Parere intorno all'uso della cioccolata*. Florence: Giuseppe Manni, 1728.

Fernández Matienzo, Isidro. *Discurso medico y phisico agradable a los medicos ancianos y despertador para los modernos contra el medicamento caphè*. Madrid: Melchor Alvarez, 1693.

Fox, William. *An address to the people of Great Britain on the propriety of abstaining from West India sugar and rum*. London: James Phillips, 1791.

Full answers to Mr. M—y's queries in defence of the malt-distillery. London: J. Scott, 1760.

Galeano, Giuseppe. *Il caffè con piu diligenza esaminato*. Palermo: Domenico d'Anselmo, 1674.

Gallobelgicus. *Wine, beere, ale, and tobacco. Contending for superiority a dialogue*. 2nd ed. London: John Grove, 1630.

Gardiner, Edmund. *The trial of tabacco. Wherein, his worth is most worthily expressed: as, in the name, nature, and qualitie of the sayd herb; his speciall use in all physicke, with the true and right use of taking it, as well for the seasons, and times, as also the complexions, dispositions, and constitutions, of such bodies, & persons, as are fittest: and to whom it is not profitable to take it.* London: Mathew Lownes, 1610.

Gavelli, Niccolò. *Storia distinta, e curiosa del tabacco.* Ferrara: F. Altieri, 1758.

De gedebaucheerde en betoverde koffy en theewereld, behelzende een meenigte van aardige voorvallen, welke zich sedert weinig tijds te Amsterdam, Rotterdam, en Den Haag, te Utrecht en de bijgelegene plaatsen, op de koffy en theegezelschapijes. Amsterdam: Timotheus ten Hoorn, 1701.

Gesner, Conrad. *The newe iewell of health wherein is contayned the most excellent secretes of phiscike and philosophie.* Translated by George Baker. London: Henrie Denham, 1576.

Giuntini, Girolamo. "Scherzo ditirambico in lode della cioccolata." In Francesco Zeti, *Altro parere intorno alla natura, ed all' uso della cioccolata*, 27–31. Florence: n.p., 1728.

Goddard, Thomas. *Miscellanea, or, serious, useful considerations, moral, historical, theological together with the characters of a true believer, in paradoxes and seeming contradictions, an essay.* London: Tho. William, 1661.

Gudenfridi, Giovanni Batista. *Differenza tra' il cibo e il cioccolate.* Florence: Condotta, 1680.

Hactenus inaudita, or, animadversions upon the new found way of curing the small pox. London: Io. Martin and Ia. Allestry, 1663.

Hales, Stephen. *A friendly admonition to the drinkers of brandy, and other distilled spirituous liquors.* London: Joseph Downing, 1733.

Hall, Thomas. *A practical and polemical commentary, or, exposition upon the third and fourth chapters of the latter epistle of Saint Paul to Timothy.* London: E. Tyler, 1658.

Handley, James. *Mechanical essays on the animal oeconomy.* London: n.p. 1721.

Hanway, Jonas. *A journal of eight days journey from Portsmouth to Kingston upon Thames.* London: H. Woodfall, 1756.

Hart, James. *Klinike, or the diet of the diseased.* London: Robert Allot, 1633.

Haywood, Eliza Fowler. *A present for women addicted to drinking.* London: W. Own, 1750.

Haywood, Eliza Fowler. *The tea-table: or, a conversation between some polite persons of both sexes, at a lady's visiting day.* London: J. Roberts, 1725.

Head, Richard. *The floating island, or, A new discovery.* London: n.p., 1673.

Hennebo, Robert. *Rouwklachten van den heere Jacobus Veenhuizen; beneevens de lof de jenever, eerste en tweede deel.* Amsterdam: Printed by the author, 1723.

Henry, William. *An earnest address to the people of Ireland, against the drinking of spirituous liquors.* Dublin: Peter Wilson, 1753.

Henry, William. *A letter to the Right Honourable John Ponsonby, Esq; Speaker of the Honourable House of Commons; concerning the abuse of spirituous liquors.* Dublin: Peter Wilson, 1760.

Hill, John. *Cautions against the immoderate use of snuff.* London: R. Baldwin and J. Jackson, 1761.

Hollandus, Isaac. *A hundred and fourtene experiments and cures of the famous physition Philippus Aureolus Theophrastus Paracelsus . . . Also certaine secrets of Isacke Hollandus concerning the vegetal and animall worke.* Translated by John Hester. London: Vallentine Sims, 1596.

Hooker, Thomas. *The application of redemption by the effectual work of the word, and spirit of Christ, for the bringing home of lost sinners to God.* London: Peter Cole, 1656.

Hughes, William. *The American physitian.* London: William Crook, 1672.

Hurtado, Tomás. *Chocolate y tabaco: ayuno eclesíastico y natural: si este le quebrante el chocolate: y el tobaco el natural, para la Sagrada Comunion.* Madrid: Francisco García, Impressor del Reyno, 1645.

Ibn Ùmar Antaki, Da'ud. The nature of the drink *kauhi*, or coffe, and the berry from which it is made described by an Arabian phisitian. Oxford: Henry Hall, 1659.

Iets over den opium. Rotterdam: J. J. Thompson, 1800's.

An impartial enquiry into the present state of the British distillery. London: J. Roberts, 1736.

An Impartial Hand. *The life of Mother Gin.* London: W. Webb, 1736.

J. B. *In praise of tea. A poem. Dedicated to the ladies of Great Britain.* Canterbury: printed for the author, 1736.

James I, King of England. *A counterblaste to tobacco.* N.p., 1604.

Jerome, Stephen. *The haughty heard humbled.* London: Richard More, 1628.

Jiménez Patón, Bartolomé. *Reforma de trages. Doctrina de frai Hernando de Talavera primera arçobispo de Granada.* Baeza: Juan de la Cuesta, 1638.

Johnson, Ben. "A ballad called cooklorrel." In *An antidote against melancholy made up in pills. Compounded of witty ballads, jovial songs, and merry catches*, edited by J. P., 96–98. London: John Playford, 1669.

Johnson, Richard. *Tea-table dialogues, between a governess, and Mary Sensible, Eliza Thoughtful, Jane Bloom, Ann Hopeful, Dinah Sterling, Lucy Lively, and Emma Tempest.* London: Darton and Harvey, 1796.

Johnson, Richard. *Tea-table dialogues; between Miss Thoughtful, Miss Sterling, Miss Prattle, Mast. Thoughtful, Master Goodwill, Master Poplin.* London: T. Carnan, 1772.

Jones, John. *The mysteries of opium reveal'd.* London: Richard Smith, 1700.

Juniper, Jack. *The deposing and death of Queen Gin, with the ruin of the Duke of Rum, Marquee de Nantz, and the Lord Sugarcane, &c.* London: John Millan, 1736.

Kellet, Edward. Tricoenium Christi in nocte proditionis suae, *the threefold supper of Christ in the night that he was betrayed.* London: Andrew Crooke, 1641.

King, William. *The transactioneer, with some of his philosophical fancies in two dialogues.* London: n.p., 1700.

Klaar en naakt bewijs van het groot misbruyk vande vreemdelantse en uytheemse thee en coffy, waar in onwedersprekelijk wort bewesen, dat deselve niet en dienen tot gesontheit, maar veel meer tot ongesontheit, ja tot afkortinge van het leven der menschen; end at dienvolgens dit gebruik tot groot nadeel van dese onse natie is aangenomen. The Hague: Engelbrecht Boucquet, 1695.

Laborie, P. J. *The coffee planter of Saint Domingo.* London: T. Cadell and W. Davies, 1798.

Laghi, Sebastiano. *Neve, tabacco, et acqua vita: otiose discorsi*. Milan: Filippo Ghisolfi, 1647.

Lamb, Charles. "Confessions of a Drunkard." In *The Works of Charles and Mary Lamb*, vol. 1., *Miscellaneous Prose (1798–1834)*, edited by E. V. Lucas, 155–63. London: Methuen, 1903.

Lardizabal, Vicente. *Memoria sobre las utiladades del chocolate*. Pamplona: Antonio Castilla, 1788.

Lavedán, Antonio. *Tratado de los usos, abusos, propiedades y virtudes del tabaco, café, té y chocolate*. Madrid: Imprenta Real, 1796.

Le Fèvre, Nicaise. *A compendious body of chymystry*. Translated by P. D. C. London: Octavian Pulleyn Jr., 1664.

Lequinio, Joseph M. *Préjugés déstruits*. Paris: l'Imprimerie Nationale, 1792.

Lessius, Leonardus, Jan Hendrik Glazemaker, and Cornaro Luigi. *De schat de soberheit; or, Bequame middle tot onderhouding der gezonheit, en bewaring van de volkomenheit der zinnen, van't verstant, en van de geheugenis aan d'uitterste ouderdom*. Middelburg: Johannes Meertens, 1678.

A letter to a friend in the country, in relation to the new law concerning spirituous liquors. London: M. Cooper, 1743.

Lettsom, John Coakley. *History of some of the effects of hard drinking*. 6th ed. London: W. Darton, 1791.

Lettsom, John Coakley. *The natural history of the tea-tree*. London: Edward and Charles Dilly, 1772.

Lister, Martin. *A journey to Paris in the year 1698*. London: Jacob Tonson, 1699.

Lodge, Thomas. *Wits miserie, and the worlds madnesse discovering the devils incarnate of this age*. London: Adam Islip, 1596.

M. C. de T. *Café Français: recette économique, analysée, d'après plusieurs savans*. Paris: Dondey-Dupré, Père et Fils, 1824.

M. P. *A character of coffee and coffee-houses by M. P.* London: John Starkey, 1661.

The maidens complaint against coffee. Or, the coffee-house discovered, besieged, stormed, taken, untyled, and lain open to publick view. London: J. Jones, 1663.

Maddox, Isaac. *The expediency of preventive wisdom*. London: H. Woodfall, 1750.

Man of Kent. *An effectual remedy totally to prevent smuggling, and bring into the revenue 195,000 pounds yearly*. London: G. Woodfall, C. Corbet, J. Collierand J. Jolliffe, 1756[?].

Mandeville, Bernard. *The fable of the bees or private vices public benefits*. London: T. Ostell, 1806.

Marbecke, Roger. *A defence of tabacco: with a friendly answer to the late printed booke called worke for chimney-sweepers, etc.* London: Richard Field, 1602.

Marradón, Barthelemy [Bartolomé]. *Du chocolate, dialogue entre un medicin, un indien, & un bourgeois*. Translated by René Moreau. Lyon: Jean Girin & Barthelemy Riviere, 1670.

Marsh, A. *The confession of the new married couple, being the second part of the ten pleasures of marriage*. London: n.p., 1683.

Marsigli, Conte di, Luigi Ferdinando. *Bevanda asiatica istoria medica del cave*. Vienna: n.p., 1685.

Marvell, Andrew. "A Dialogue between Two Horses." In *The second part of the collection of poems on affairs of state*, 1–6. London: n.p., 1689.

Mason, Simon. *The good and bad effects of tea consider'd*. London: M. Cooper, 1745.

Massieu, Guillaume. *Traite du café, contenant l'histoire, la description, la culture et les propriétés, de ce végetal*. Paris: n.p., 1798.

Mayáns, Gregorio. "Elegía al chocolate." Translated by José María Estellés i González. In Jose María Estellés i González, "Una pincelada frívola en la obra de Mayans: Elegía al chocolate," *Estudios dedicados a Juan Peset Aleixandre*, 581–600, vol. 1. Valencia: Universidad de Valencia, 1982.

McCalman, Godfrey. *A natural, commercial and medicinal treatise on tea*. Glasgow: David Niven, 1787.

Memoirs of the Bedford Coffee-house, by a genius. 2nd ed. London: J. Single, 1763.

The mens answer to the womens petition against coffee, vindicating their own performances, and the vertues of that liquor, from the undeserved aspersions lately cast upon them by their scandalous pamphlet. London: n.p., 1674.

Mercier, Louis Sébastian. *Tableau de Paris*. Edited by Jean-Claude Bonnet. Paris: Mercure de France, 1994.

Mercurius Democritus. *The maidens complaint against coffee*. London: J. Jones, 1663.

Merli, Francesco. *Guida medica intorno all'uso del the, caffé, e cioccolata*. Naples: Vincenzo Flauto, 1768.

Mill, Humphrey. *The second part of the nights search, discovering the condition of the various fowles of the night*. London: Henry Shepheard and William Lay, 1646.

Mist, Nathaniel. *A collection of miscellany letters, selected out of Mist's* Journal. Vol. 2. London: N. Mist, 1722.

Monardes, Nicolás. *Primera y seguna y tercera partes de la historia medicinal: de las cosas que se traen de nuestras Indias Occidentales, que se sirven en medicina*. Seville: Alonso Escrivano, 1574.

Monardes, Nicolás. *Segunda parte del libro, de los cosas que se traen de nuestras Indias Occidentales, que sirven al uso del medicina: Donde se trata del tabacco, y de la sassafras, y del carlo sancto, y de otras muchas yervas y plantas, simientes, y licores que agora nuevamente han venido de aquellas partes, de grandes virtudes y maravillosos effectos*. Seville: Alonso Escrivano, 1571.

Moseley, Benjamin. *Medical tracts*. 2nd ed. London: John Nichols, 1800.

Moseley, Benjamin. *Observations on the properties and effects of coffee*. London: Printed for John Stockdale, 1785.

Motteux, Peter. *A poem in praise of tea*. London: J. Tonson, 1712.

Mun, Thomas. *England's treasure by forraign trade*. London: Printed by J. G. for Thomas Clark, 1664.

Mutain, Daniel. *Theses medicae. De natura, usu & abusu caffé, thé, chocolatae, & tabaci*. Besançon: Nicolai Couche, 1726.

Muzzarelli, Alfonso. "La bottega del caffè." In *Il tempio della fedeltà*, 35–45. Bologna: Ferdinando Pisarri, 1774.

Navas de Carrera, Manuel. *Dissertacion historica phisico-chimica, y analysis del cacao, su uso, y dossis*. Zaragoza: Francisco Moreno, 1751.

A new tea-table miscellany: or, bagatelles for the amusement of the fair sex. London: E. Duncomb, 1750.

Newcastle, Margaret Cavendish, Duchess of. *Observations upon experimental philosophy to which is added the description of a blazing new world*. London: A. Maxwell, 1666.

Newton, Thomas. *Approoved medicines and cordiall receiptes with the natures, qualities, and operations of sundry samples*. London: Thomas Marshe, 1580.

Nieuhof, Johan. *Het gezantschap der Neerlandtsche Oost-Indische Compagnie, aan den grooten Tartarischen cham, den tegenwoordigen kaizer van China*. Amsterdam: Jokob van Meurs, 1665.

Nokken, H. V. *Beschryving van een nieuw werktuig, om den rook van tabak in de darmen te brengen* in *Uitgegeeven door de Hollandsche maatschappye der weetenschappen, te Haarlem*. Haarlem: J. Bosch, 1765.

The occasional monitor. London: H. Cooke and E. Cooke, 1731.

Of the use of tobacco, tea, coffee, chocolate, and drams. London[?]: H. Parker, 1722.

"*De oozraak der slaaverny.*" *De vaderlander*, October 23, 1775.

L'oppio nostrale suoi effetti, e virtù. Naples: Amato Cone, 1788.

An oration, delivered before an audience of distillers, by Baalzebub. London: J. Scott, 1760.

Origoni, Pier Luigi. *Discorso contro l'abuso del tabacco*. Milan: Filippo Ghisolfi, 1643.

Ovington, John. *An essay upon the nature and qualities of tea*. London: R. Roberts, 1699.

Palmieri, Giovanni, *Il papavero sonnifero per far l'oppio superiore di efficacia al tebajco in commercio*. Foligno: G. Tomassini, 1808.

Papillon, David. *The vanity of the lives and passions of men*. London: Robert White, 1651.

Parmentier, Antoine-Augustin. "*Abus dans la fabrication du chocolat.*" In *Bibliothèque physique oeconomique*, 176–84. Paris: Chez Buisson, 1786.

Paulli, Simon. *A treatise on tobacco, tea, coffee, and chocolate*. Translated by Dr. James. London: T. Osborn, 1746.

Pers, Dirck Pieterszoon, and Gillis van Scheyndel. *Bacchus wonder-wercken: Waer in het recht gebruyck en misbruyck des wijns door verscheyden vermaecklijcke eerlijcke en leerlijcke historien wort afgebeeld ende lasteringe der dronckenschap met levende verwen afgemaelt*. Amsterdam: Dirck Pieterzsoon Pers, 1628.

Philanthropos. *The trial of the spirits: or some considerations upon the pernicious consequences of the gin-trade to Great Britain*. London: T. Cooper, 1736.

Philaretes. *Work for chimney-sweepers: or a warning for tabacconists. Describing the pernicious use of tabacco, no lesse pleasant than profitable for all sortes to reade*. London: T. Este, 1602.

Philips, John. *Sportive wit the muses merriment, a new spring of lusty drollery, joviall fancies, and a la mode lamponnes*. London: Nath. Brook, 1656.

Piccino, Giovanni. *Il petopiccino, overo eccelenza, e dote del tabacco*. Viterbo: li Diotallevi, 1635.

Pinelli, Matteo [Alessandro Sanlorini da Prunalbeta]. *La polvere schernita, overo invettiva contr'al tabacco*. Florence: Francesco Onofri, 1654.

Le porte feuille galant, contenant les entretiens des caffez, & autres ouvrages mêlez de prose & de vers. Paris: Jean Moreau, 1700.

Primrose, James. *Popular errours, or the errours of the people in physick*. London: Nicholas Bourne, 1651.

Prynne, William. *A short demurrer to the Jewes long discontinued barred remitter into England*. London: Edward Thomas, 1655.

Proposizione sulla necessità d'introdurre in Toscana la coltivazione dei papaveri in grande per estrarne l'oppio. Florence: Guglielmo Piatti, 1807.

R., P. van. *Nieuwe en naauwkeurige verhandeling van den tabak*. 1770[?]. Amsterdam: Gerrit Bom, 1785.

R. T. *Good husbandry, or the improvement of time; being a sure way to get and keep money*. London: J. G., 1675.

R. V. N. *Natuur-kundige verhandelin van de theé, koffeé, tabak en snufpoeders*. Amsterdam: J. ten Hoorn, 1701.

Rambaldi, Angelo. *Ambrosia arabica, overo della salutare bevanda café*. Bologna: per il Longhi stampatore Arcivescogale, 1691.

Ramón, Tomás. *Nueva prematica de reformacion contra los abusos de afeytes, calçado, guedejas, guardainfantes, lenguaje critic, moños, trajes; y excess en el uso del tabaco*. Zaragoza: Diego Dormer, 1635.

Ramsden, Henry. *A gleaning in gods harvest foure choyce handfuls; the gate to happinesse, wounded savior*. London: J. D. and R. M., 1639.

Rich, Barnabe. *Faultes fault, and nothing else but faultes*. London: Jeffrey Chorleton, 1606.

Rich, Barnabe. *My ladies looking glasse. Wherein may be discerned a wise man from a foole, a good woman from a bad: and the true resemblance of vice, masked under the vizard of vertue*. London: Thomas Adams, 1616.

The rise and progress of tea, &c. Dublin: n.p., 1729[?].

Rolle, Samuel. Shlohavot, *or, the burning of London in the year 1666 commemorated and improved in a CX discourses, meditations, and contemplations, divided into four parts*. London: Nathaniel Ranew and Jonathan Robinson, 1667.

Rowlands, Samuel. *A crew of kind gossips, all met to be merrie complayning of their husbands, with their husbands answeres in their owne defence*. London: John Deane, 1613.

Rowlands, Samuel. *Humors ordinarie where a man may be verie merrie, and exceedingly well used for his sixe-pence*. London: William Firebrand, 1605.

Rowlands, Samuel. *The knave of clubbs*. London: W. Ferebrand, 1609.

Rowlands, Samuel. *Looke to it: for, ile stabbe ye*. London: W. Ferbrand and George Loftes, 1604.

Rowlands, Samuel. *More knaves yet? The knaves of spades and diamonds. With new additions*. London: n.p., 1613.

Rumsey, Walter. Organon salutis, *an instrument to cleanse the stomach, as also divers new experiments of the virtue of tobacco and coffee: how much they conduce to preserve humane health*. London: D. Pakeman, 1657.

Rush, Benjamin. *An inquiry into the effects of ardent spirits upon the human body and mind: with an account of the means of preventing, and of the remedies for curing them*. Philadelphia: Thomas Dobson, 1787.

Sala, Angelo. *Opiologia: or, a treatise concerning the nature, properties, true preparation and safe use and administration of opium*. Translated by Thomas Bretnor. London: Nicholas Okes, 1618.

Sanvitale, Giacomo. *Memorie veridiche contrapposte alle memorie istoriche sull' uso del cioccolato in giorno di digiuno*. N.p., 1748.

Sassenus, J. B. *De voortreffelijkheid van de thee, en hare bewonderenswaardige verdienste in de geneeskunde*. Rotterdam: T. J. Wijnhoven Hendriksen, 1828.

A satyr against coffee. N.p., 1674.

"A satyr upon brandy." In *Directions for brewing malt liquors*, 25–28. London: J. Nutt, 1700.

Sbalbi, Giambattista. *La cioccolata, versione dal latin rime toscane del Canonico Giambattista Sbalbi*. Piacenza: Niccolò Orcesi, 1789.

Sennert, Daniel N., and Abdiah Cole. *The sixth book of pratical physick of occult or hidden diseases*. London: Peter Cole, 1662.

Serafini, Lorenzo. *Lettera in cui si esaminato le ragioni addotte dall' autore del primo parere intorno all' uso della cioccolata dedicate all' illustriss. Sig. Ca. Cosimo degli Albizzi*. Florence: n.p., 1728.

Short, Thomas. *Discourses on tea, sugar, milk, made-wines, spirits, punch, tobacco, &c., with plain and useful rules for gouty people*. London: T. Longman and A. Millar, 1750.

Short, Thomas. *The natural, experimental, and medicinal history of the mineral waters of Derbyshire, Lincolnshire, and Yorkshire*. London: F. Gyles, 1734.

Short, Thomas. Vinum Britannicum*: or, an essay on the properties and effects of malt liquors*. London: D. Midwinter, 1727.

A short history of the gin act: or, an impartial account of the conduct of some of those who have been instructed with the execution of it. London: H. Goreham, 1738.

Slare, Frederick. "A vindication of sugars against the charge of Dr. Willis, other physicians, and common prejudices: dedicated to the ladies." In *Experiments and observations upon oriental and other bezoar-stones, which prove them to be of no use in physick*, 1–64. London: Tim Goodwin, 1715.

Slyboots, Saynought. *The tavern scuffle: or the club in an uproar; occasion'd by a hot dispute, between Mr. Swell-Gut, a brewer, and Mr. Scorch-Gut, a distiller, concerning geneva, the reigning liquor now in vogue among the common people*. London: T. Warner, 1726.

Smith, Hugh. *An essay on the nerves, illustrating their efficient, formal, material, and final causes . . . To which is added an essay on foreign teas*. London: P. Norman, 1780.

Smollett, Tobias. *A dissertation on Mr. Hogarth's six prints lately publish'd, viz. Gin-Lane, Beer-Street, and the Four Stages of Cruelty*. London: B. Dickerson, 1751.

Smythson, Hugh. *The compleat family physician; or, universal medical repository*. London: Harrison, 1785.

Speculative historische aanmerkingen, dewelke op de heedendaagse nieuwe belastinge der coffy, thee, chocolaat en andere medicinale dranken van water, huy ofte melk, door het mengen met eenige kruiden ofte spetien (hoe ok bereid) en door ded doctorenveelmaalen als een huis-medicyn, tot voorkoming van verscheide ziekte geordineert, bescheidentlijktoegepast kunnen werden. N.p., 1699.

Spooner, Lawrence. *A looking-glass for smoakers: or, the danger of the needless or intemperate use of tobacco*. London: A. Baldwin, 1703.

Steele, Richard. *Spectator* 49, April 26, 1711.

Stella, Benedetto. *Il tabacco*. Rome: F. M. Mancini, 1669.

Strictures on an address to the people of Great Britain, on the propriety of abstaining from West-India sugar and rum. 2nd ed. London: T. Boosey, 1792.

Stubbe, Henry. *Indian nectar, or a discourse concerning chocolata.* London: Andrew Crook, 1662.

Surgeon, J. N. *Remarks on Mr. Mason's treatise upon tea.* London: J. Roberts, 1745.

Sylvester, Joshua. *Tobacco battered; & the pipes shattered (about their eares that idely idolize so base & barbarous a weed; or at least-wise over-love so loathsome vanitie).* London: H. Lownes, 1616 or 1617.

T. S. *A proper reply to a scandalous libel, intitulated, The trial of the spirits.* 2nd ed. London: J. Roberts, 1736.

Tate, Nahum. *Panacea, a poem upon tea in two canto's.* London: J. Roberts, 1700.

Taylor, John. *The nipping and snipping of abuses.* London: Nathaniel Butler, 1614.

Tea, a poem. In three cantos. London: Aaron Ward, 1743.

The tea drinking wife, and drunken husband. To which is added, three other songs. Newcastle-upon-Tyne: n.p., 1749.

"The Tea-table." In *A banquet of the muses: or, the miscellany of miscellanies*, 23–24. London: Jacob Bickerstaff, 1746.

Teare, Edward. *A treatise on the use and abuse of tobacco tending to shew why this plant is hurtful to the nervous system in particular, and of course to the whole human frame in general; the beneficial use of tobacco is also considered.* Doncaster: n.p., 1789[?].

Thevet, André. *The new found world, or Antarctike wherin is contained wonderful and strange things.* Translated by anonymous. London: Henrie Bynneman for Thomas Hacket, 1568.

Thorius, Raphael. Hymnus tabaci*; A poem in honour of tabaco.* Translated by Peter Hausted. London: Humphrey Moseley, 1650 [year originally 1651, but crossed out and replaced by 1650].

Tobaco-mastix or thee common use of that weed in all the wayes of preparing it, taxed by arguments from reason and experience, with all the vulgar objections discust and answered. Scotland[?]: n.p., 1677.

Tomkis, Thomas. *Lingua: or the combat of the tongue, and the five senses for superiority a pleasant comoedie.* London: Simon Waterson, 1607.

A treatise upon the herb tobacco, pointing out its deleterious pernicious quality, and its fatal effects upon the human constitution, by the great variety of disorders it occasions. London: Charles Stalker, 1789.

Trotter, Thomas. *An essay medical, philosophical, and chemical on drunkenness and its effects on the human body.* Edited by Roy Porter. London: Routledge, 1988.

Trotter, Thomas. *A view of the nervous temperament.* 2nd ed. London: Longman, Hurst, Rees, and Orme, 1807.

Trotter, Thomas. *The good housewife made doctor, or, health's device and sure friend.* 2nd ed. London: H. N. and T. S., 1692.

Tryon, Thomas. *Healths grand preservative: Or the womens best doctor.* London: printed for the author, 1682.

Tryon, Thomas. *Tryon's letters, domestick and foreign, to several persons of quality.* London: Geo. Conyers and Eliza. Harris, 1700.

Two broad-sides against tobacco. Edited by John Hancock. London: John Hancock, 1672.

De vaderlander, 1775–78. Nos. 1 (January 2, 1775) through 209 (December 25, 1778). Amsterdam: Erven van F. Houttuyn.

Valisneri, Antonio. *Dell'uso e dell'abuso delle bevande, e bagnature calde o fredde.* Modena: Pel' Capponi, 1725.

Van Helmont, Joan Baptista. *A ternary of paradoxes. The magnetick cure of wounds, nativity of tartar in wine, image of God in man.* Translated and "amplified" by Walter Charlteon. London: William Lee, 1650.

Venner, Tobias. *A briefe and accurate treatise, concerning, the taking of the fume of tobacco which very many, in these days, doe too too* [sic] *licentiously use.* London: Richard Moore, 1621.

Venner, Tobias. Via recta ad vitam longam, *or a plaine philosophical discourse of the nature, faculties, and effects, of all such things, as by way of nourishments, and dieteticall observations, make for the preservation of health with their just applications into every age, constitution of bodie, and time of yeare.* London: Edward Griffin, 1620.

Verri, Pietro. "*Considerazioni sul lusso.*" In *Scritti vari di Pietro Verri.* Vol. 2. Edited by Giuliu Carcano, 28–35. Florence: Felice le Monnier, 1854.

The vertues of chocolate East-India drink. N.p., 1660.

A vindication of the use of sugar, the produce of the West-India islands. London: T. Boosey, 1792.

Waldron, John. *A satyr against tea. Ovington's essay upon the nature and qualities of tea, &c. dissected and burlesq'd.* Dublin: Sylvanus Pepyat, 1733.

Ward, Edward. *The school of politicks or, the humours of a coffee-house a poem.* London: Richard Baldwin, 1690.

John Wesley. *A letter to a friend, concerning tea.* London: A. Macintosh, 1825.

West, Richard. *Wits A.B.C. or a centurie of epigrams.* London: Thomas Thorp, 1608.

Whipping-Tom: or, a rod for a proud lady, bundled up in four feeling discourses, both serious and merry. 4th ed. London: Sam. Briscoe, 1722.

Whitaker, Edward. "A satyr upon brandy." In *Directions for brewing malt liquors,* 25–28. London: J. Nutt, 1700.

White, Thomas. *The middle state of souls from the hour of death to the day of judgment.* N.p., 1659.

Willis, Thomas. *Dr. Willis's practice of physick.* London: Thomas Dring, Ch. Harper, and John Leigh, 1684.

Willis, Thomas. *Two discourses concerning the souls of brutes which is that of the vital and sensitive of man.* Translated by S. Pordage. London: Thomas Dring, Ch. Harper, and John Leigh, 1683.

Wilson, Alexander Philip. *An experimental essay, on the manner in which opium acts on the living animal body.* London: J. Johnson and G. G. & J. Robinson, 1795.

Wilson, Andrew. *Medical researches: Being an enquiry into the nature and origin of hysterics in the female constitution, and into the distinction between that disease and hypochondriac or nervous disorders.* London: S. Hooper and Robson, 1776.

Wilson, Thomas. *Distilled spirits the bane of the nation.* London: J. Roberts, 1736.

Wither, George. *Abuses stript, and whipt. Or satirical essayes.* London: Francis Burton, 1613.

Woodville, William. *Advice to parents on the management of their children in the natural small pox, and during inoculation; with a few cases confirming the author's opinion. To which are added, some general observations on the use of tea, and the present regimen of diet among the higher ranks of society*. Newark: S. and J. Ridge, 1797.

The women's petition against coffee representing to publick consideration the grand inconveniences accruing to their sex from the excessive use of that drying, enfeebling liquor. London: n.p., 1674.

Yates, James. *The effects of drinking spiritous, and other intoxicating liquors, described in four sermons, preached at the chapel in Union-Place, Glasgow*. Glasgow: James Hedderwick, 1818.

Young, George. *A treatise upon opium*. London: A. Millar, 1753.

Younge, Richard. *The victory of patience and benefit of affliction, and how to husband it so, that the weakest Christian (with blessing from above) may bee able to support himselfe in his most miserable exigents*. London: R. B., 1636.

Zorzi Prete, Luigi. "In lode del tabacco." In *In lode del fico, in lode del tabacco, di ringraziamento, capitoli tre*. Verona: Pietro Bisesti, 1822, 9–16.

Secondary Works

Abbott, Elizabeth. *Sugar: A Bittersweet History*. London: Duckworth Overlook, 2009.

Albritton Jonsson, Fredrik. "Natural History and Improvement: The Case of Tobacco."In *Mercantilism Reimagined: Political Economy in Early Modern Britain and Its Empire,* edited by Philip J. Stern and Carl Wennerlind, 117–30. Oxford: Oxford University Press, 2013.

Albritton Jonsson, Fredrik. "Scottish Tobacco and Rhubarb: The Natural Order of Civil Cameralism in the Scottish Enlightenment." *Eighteenth-Century Studies* 49, no. 2 (2016): 129–47.

Anderson, Jennifer L. *Mahogany: The Costs of Luxury in Early America*. Cambridge MA: Harvard University Press, 2012.

Andrews, Jonathan. "History of Medicine: Health, Medicine and Disease in the Eighteenth Century." *British Journal of Eighteenth Century Studies* 34, no. 4 (2011): 503–15.

Arcila Farias, Eduardo. *Haciendo y comercio de Venezuela en el siglo XVII: 1601–1650*. Caracas: Banco Central de Venezuela, 1985.

Arrizabalaga, Jon. "The World of Iberian *converso* practitioners, From Lluís Alcanyís to Isaac Cardoso." In *Más allá de la Leyendera Negra: España y la Revolución Cientifica/ Beyond the Black Legend: Spain and the Scientific Revolution*, edited by Víctor Navarro Brotóns and William Eamon, 307–22. Valencia: Publicaciones de la Universitat de Valencia, 2007.

Ashworth, William J. *Customs and Excise: Trade, Production, and Consumption in England, 1640–1845*. Oxford: Oxford University Press, 2003.

Atlas of the Transatlantic Slave Trade. Edited by David Eltis and David Richardson. New Haven, CT: Yale University Press, 2010.

Barker-Benfield, G. J. *The Culture of Sensibility: Sex and Society in Eighteenth-Century Britain*. Chicago: University of Chicago Press, 1992.

Barnett, Richard. *The Book of Gin*. New York: Grove, 2011.

Barr, Timothy. "Without Apparent Occasion: Recent Research on Melancholy." *Journal of the History of Ideas* 80, no. 2 (2019): 313–32.

Beatty, Heather R. *Nervous Disease in Late Eighteenth-Century Britain: The Reality of a Fashionable Disorder*. London: Pickering and Chatto, 2012.

Benedict, Carol. *Golden-Silk Smoke: A History of Tobacco in China, 1550–2020*. Berkeley: University of California Press, 2011.

Berg, Maxine. *Luxury and Pleasure in Eighteenth-Century Britain*. Oxford: Oxford University Press, 2005.

Berg, Maxine, and Elizabeth Eger. "The Rise and Fall of the Luxury Debates." In *Luxury in the Eighteenth Century: Debates, Desires and Delectable Goods*, edited by Maxine Berg and Elizabeth Eger, 7–28. Houndmills: Palgrave Macmillan, 2003.

Berridge, Virginia, and Griffith Edwards. *Opium and the People: Opiate Use in Nineteenth-Century England*. London: Allen Lane/St. Martin's, 1981.

Berry, Christopher J. *The Idea of Commercial Society in the Scottish Enlightenment*. Edinburgh: Edinburgh University Press, 2013.

Besky, Sarah. *Tasting Qualities: The Past and Future of Tea*. Oakland: University of California Press, 2020.

Biljsma, Rudmer. "Alienation in Commercial Society: The Republican Critique of Jean-Jacques Rousseau and Adam Ferguson." *Southern Journal of Philosophy* 57, no. 3 (2019): 347–77.

Blei, Daniela. "The False Promises of Wellness Culture." JSTOR Daily, January 4, 2017. https://daily.jstor.org/the-false-promises-of-wellness-culture/.

Bleichmar, Daniela. *Visible Empire: Botanical Expeditions and Visual Culture in the Hispanic Enlightenment*. Chicago: University of Chicago Press, 2012.

Blondé, Bruno, and Wouter Ryckbosch. "Material Cultures." In *Interpreting Early Modern Europe*, edited by C. Scott Dixon and Beat Kümin, 183–214. New York: Routledge, 2019.

Booth, Martin. *Opium: A History*. New York: St. Martin's, 1996.

Breen, Benjamin. *The Age of Intoxication: Origins of the Global Drug Trade*. Philadelphia: University of Pennsylvania Press, 2019.

Brennan, Thomas. *Public Drinking and Popular Culture in Eighteenth-Century Paris*. Princeton, NJ: Princeton University Press, 1988.

Brookes, Kristen G. "Inhaling the Alien: Race and Tobacco in Early Modern England." In *Global Traffic: Discourses and Practices of Trade in English Literature and Culture from 1550 to 1700*, edited by Barbara Sebek and Stephen Deng, 157–78. New York: Palgrave Macmillan, 2008.

Calhoun, Craig. *Habermas and the Public Sphere*. Cambridge, MA: MIT Press, 1992.

Campbell, Jodi. *At the First Table: Food and Social Identity in Early Modern Spain*. Lincoln: University of Nebraska Press, 2017.

Cañizares Esguerra, Jorge. "New World, New Stars: Patriotic Astrology and the Invention of Indian and Creole Bodies in Colonial Spanish America, 1600–1650." *American Historical Review* 104, no. 1 (1999): 33–68.

Capp, Bernard. *When Gossips Meet: Women, Family, and Neighbourhood in Early Modern England*. Oxford: Oxford University Press, 2003.

Cavallo, Sandra. *Artisans of the Body in Early Modern Italy: Identities, Families and Masculinities*. Manchester: Manchester University Press, 2007.

Cavallo, Sandra, and Tessa Storey. *Healthy Living in Late Renaissance Italy*. Oxford: Oxford University Press, 2014.

Chakrabarti, Pratik. *Medicine and Empire, 1600–1960*. Basingstoke: Palgrave Macmillan, 2014.

Cheney, Paul. "István Hont, the Cosmopolitan Theory of Commercial Globalization, and Twenty-First-Century Capitalism." *Modern Intellectual History* (2021): 1–29.

Clarence-Smith, William Gervase. *Cocoa and Chocolate, 1765–1914*. London: Routledge, 2000).

Clark, Peter. *The English Alehouse: A Social History 1200–1830*. London: Longman, 1983.

Clemis, David. "Medical Expertise and the Understandings of Intoxication in Britain, 1660 to 1830." In *Intoxication and Society: Problematic Pleasures of Drugs and Alcohol*, edited by Jonathan Herring, Ciaran Regan, Darin Weinberg, and Phil Withington, 33–51. London: Palgrave Macmillan, 2013.

Clendinnen, Inga. *Ambivalent Conquests: Maya and Spaniard in Yucatan, 1517–1570*. Cambridge: Cambridge University Press, 1987.

Cockayne, Emily. *Hubbub: Filth, Noise, and Stench in England, 1600–1770*. New Haven, CT: Yale University Press, 2007.

Coe, Sophie D., and Michael D. Coe. *The True History of Chocolate*. London: Thames and Hudson, 1996.

Coles, Kimberly Anne. *Bad Humor: Race and Religious Essentialism in Early Modern England*. Philadelphia: University of Pennsylvania Press, 2022.

Cook, Harold J. *Matters of Exchange: Commerce, Medicine, and Science in the Dutch Golden Age*. New Haven, CT: Yale University Press, 2007.

Cook, Harold J., and Timothy D. Walker. "Circulation of Medicine in the Early Modern Atlantic World." *Social History of Medicine* 26, no. 3 (2013): 337–51.

Coulton, Richard, ed. *Tea and the Tea-Table in Eighteenth-Century England*. Vol. 2, *Tea in Natural History and Medical Writing*. London: Pickering & Chatto, 2010.

Courtwright, David T. *Forces of Habit: Drugs and the Making of the Modern World*. Cambridge MA: Harvard University Press, 2001.

Courtwright, David T. "The Rise and Fall and Rise of Cocaine in the United States." In *Consuming Habits: Drugs in History and Anthropology*, edited by Jordan Goodman, Paul E. Lovejoy, and Andrew Sherratt, 206–14. New York: Routledge, 1995.

Cowan, Brian. *The Social Life of Coffee: The Emergence of the British Coffeehouse*. New Haven, CT: Yale University Press, 2005.

Crawford, Matthew James. *The Andean Wonder Drug: Chinchona Bark and Imperial Science in the Spanish Atlantic, 1630–1800*. Pittsburgh: University of Pittsburgh Press, 2016.

Cree, Jose Murgatroyd. "Protestant Evangelicals and Addiction in Early Modern England." *Renaissance Studies* 32, no. 3 (2018): 446–62.

Curran, Andrew S. *The Anatomy of Blackness: Science and Slavery in an Age of Enlightenment*. Baltimore, MD: Johns Hopkins University Press, 2011.

De Vries, Jan. *The Industrious Revolution: Consumer Behavior and the Household Economy, 1650 to the Present*. Cambridge: Cambridge University Press, 2008.

Debus, Alan G. *The Chemical Philosophy: Paracelsian Science and Medicine in the Sixteenth and Seventeenth Centuries*. 2 vols. New York: Science History, 1977.

Delbourgo, James. "Sir Hans Sloan's Milk Chocolate and the Whole History of the Cacao." *Social Text* 106. No. 1 (2011): 71–101.

Derks, Hans. *History of the Opium Problem: The Assault on the East, ca. 1600–1950*. Leiden: Brill, 2012.

Dillon, Patrick. *Gin: The Much-Lamented Death of Madam Geneva*. Boston: Justin, Charles, 2002.

Drayton, Richard. *Nature's Government: Science, Imperial Britain, and the 'Improvement' of the World*. New Haven, CT: Yale University Press, 2000.

Drugs on the Page: Pharmacopeias and Healing Knowledge in the Early Modern Atlantic World. Edited by Matthew James Crawford and Joseph M. Gabriel. Pittsburgh: University of Pittsburgh Press, 2019.

Earle, Rebecca. *The Body of the Conquistador: Food, Race and the Colonial Experience in Spanish America, 1492–1700*. Cambridge: Cambridge University Press, 2012.

Earle, Rebecca. "Diet, Travel, and Colonialism in the Early Modern World." In *Global Goods and the Spanish Empire, 1492–1824: Circulation, Resistance and Diversity*, edited by Bethany Aram and Bartolomé Yun-Casalilla, 137–52. Houndmills: Palgrave Macmillan, 2014.

Elias, Norbert. *The Civilizing Process: Sociogenetic and Psychogenetic Investigations*. Rev. Ed. Edited by Eric Dunning, Johan Goudsblom, and Stephen Mennell. Translated by Edmund Jephcott. Malden, MA: Blackwell, 2000.

Ellis, Markman. *The Coffee House: A Cultural History*. London: Weidenfeld & Nicolson, 2004.

Ellis, Markman, ed. *Eighteenth-Century Coffee-House Culture*. Vols. 1–4. London: Pickering & Chatto, 2006.

Ellis, Markman, Richard Coulton, and Matthew Mauger. *Empire of Tea: The Asian Leaf That Conquered the World*. London: Reaktion, 2015.

Everill, Bronwen. *Not Made by Slaves: Ethical Capitalism in the Age of Abolition*. Cambridge, MA: Harvard University Press, 2020.

Fattacciu, Irene. "Cacao: From an Exotic Curiosity to a Spanish Commodity. The Diffusion of New Patterns of Consumption in Eighteenth-Century Spain." *Food & History* 7, no. 1 (2009): 53–78.

Fattacciu, Irene. "The Resilience and Boomerang Effect of Chocolate: A Product's Globalization and Commodification,." In *Global Goods and the Spanish Empire, 1492–1824: Circulation, Resistance and Diversity*, edited by Bethany Aram and Bartolomé Yun-Casalilla, 255–73. New York: Palgrave Macmillan, 2014.

Fenster, Thelma, and Daniel Lord Smail, eds. *Fama: The Politics of Talk and Reputation in Medieval Europe*. Ithaca, NY: Cornell University Press, 2003.

Ferry, Robert. "Trading Cacao: A View from Veracruz, 1629–1645." *Nuevo Mundo, Mundos Nuevos*. Accessed September 11, 2023. https://journals.openedition.org/nuevomundo/1430.

Fertig, Christine, and Ulrich Pfister. "Coffee, Mind, and Body: Global Material Culture and the Eighteenth-Century Hamburg Import Trade." In *The Global Lives of Things: The Material Culture of Connections in the Early Modern World*, edited by Anne Gerritsen and Giorgio Riello, 221–40. New York: Routledge, 2016.

Foucault, Michel. *Discipline and Punish: The Birth of the Prison*. Translated by Alan Sheridan, 2nd ed. New York: Vintage, 1995.

Games, Alison. "Atlantic History: Definitions, Challenges, and Opportunities." *American Historical Review* 111, no. 3 (2006): 741–57.

Gentilcore, David. *Food and Health in Early Modern Europe: Diet, Medicine, and Society, 1450–1800*. London: Bloomsbury Academic, 2016.

Gentilcore, David. "The 'Golden Age of Quackery' or 'Medical Enlightenment'? Licensed Charlatanism in Eighteenth-Century Italy." *Cultural and Social History* 3, no. 3 (2008): 250–63.

Goodman, Jordan. "Excitantia, or, How Enlightenment Europe Took to Soft Drugs." In *Consuming Habits: Drugs in History and Anthropology*, edited by Jordan Goodman, Paul E. Lovejoy, and Andrew Sherratt, 126–47. New York: Routledge, 1995.

Goodman, Jordan. *Tobacco in History: The Cultures of Dependence*. London: Routledge, 1993.

Grigson, Caroline. *Menagerie: The History of Exotic Animals in England, 1100–1837*. Oxford: Oxford University Press, 2016.

Habermas, Jürgen. *The Structural Transformation of the Public Sphere: An Inquiry into a Category of Bourgeois Society*. Translated by Thomas Burger with Frederick Lawrence. Cambridge MA: MIT Press, 1989.

Hailwood, Mark. *Alehouses and Good Fellowship in Early Modern England*. Woodbridge: Boydell, 2014.

Hall, Kim F. "Culinary Spaces, Colonial Spaces: The Gendering of Sugar in the Seventeenth Century." In *Feminist Readings of Early Modern Culture: Emerging Subjects*, edited by Valerie Traub, M. Lindsay Kaplan, and Dympna Callaghan, 168–90. Cambridge: Cambridge University Press, 1996.

Hall, Kim F. "'Extravagant Viciousness': Slavery and Gluttony in the Works of Thomas Tryon." In *Writing Race across the Atlantic World: Medieval to Modern*, edited by Philip D. Beidler and Gary Taylor, 93–111. New York: Palgrave Macmillan, 2005.

Hancock, David. "Commerce and Conversation in the Eighteenth-Century Atlantic: The Invention of Madeira Wine." *Journal of Interdisciplinary History* 29, no. 2 (1998): 197–219.

Hancock, David. *Oceans of Wine: Madeira and the Emergence of American Trade and Taste*. New Haven, CT: Yale University Press, 2009.

Hannaford, Ivan. *Race: The History of an Idea in the West*. Washington, DC: Woodrow Wilson Center Press, 1996.

Harrison, Larry. "Tobacco Battered or the Pipes Shattered: A Note on the Fate of the First British Campaign against Tobacco Smoking." *British Journal of Addiction* 81 (1986): 553–58.

Harrison, Mark. *Medicine in an Age of Commerce and Empire: Britain and its Tropical Colonies, 1660–1830*. Oxford: Oxford University Press, 2010.

Hart, Carl L. *Drug Use for Grown-Ups: Chasing Liberty in the Land of Fear*. New York: Penguin, 2021.

Hartigan-O'Connor, Ellen. *The Ties That Buy: Women and Commerce in Revolutionary America*. Philadelphia: University of Pennsylvania Press, 2009.

Harvey, Karen. "Barbarity in a Teacup? Punch, Domesticity, and Gender in the Eighteenth Century." *Journal of Design History* 21, no. 3 (2008): 205–21.

Hickman, Clare. *The Doctor's Garden: Medicine, Science, and Horticulture in Britain*. New Haven, CT: Yale University Press, 2021.

Hindmarsh, D. Bruce. *The Evangelical Conversion Narrative: Spiritual Autobiography in Early Modern England*. Oxford: Oxford University Press, 2005.

Holcomb, Julie L. *Moral Commerce: Quakers and the Transatlantic Boycott of the Slave Labor Economy*. Ithaca, NY: Cornell University Press, 2016.

Hont, István. "The Early Enlightenment Debate on Commerce and Luxury." In *The Cambridge History of Eighteenth-Century Political Thought*, edited by Mark Goldie and Robert Wokler, 379–418. Cambridge: Cambridge University Press, 2006.

Jay, Mike. "Drink It, Don't Eat It or Smoke It." *London Review of Books* May 13, 2010.

Jones, Christine A. "Exotic Edibles: Coffee, Tea, Chocolate, and the Early Modern French How-To." *Journal of Medieval and Early Modern Studies* 43, no. 3 (2013): 623–53.

Kettler, Andrew. *The Smell of Slavery: Olfactory Racism and the Atlantic World*. Cambridge: Cambridge University Press, 2020.

Klerk, Saskia. "The Trouble with Opium. Taste, Reason, and Experience in Late Galenic Pharmacology with Special Regard to the University of Leiden (1575–1625)." *Early Science and Medicine* 19, no. 4 (2014): 287–316.

Kowaleski-Wallace, Elizabeth. *Consuming Subjects: Women, Shopping, and Business in the Eighteenth Century*. New York: Columbia University Press, 1997.

Kowaleski-Wallace, Elizabeth. "Tea, Gender, and Domesticity in Eighteenth-Century England." *Studies in Eighteenth-Century Culture* 23 (1994): 131–45.

Kugler, Emily M. N. *Sway of the Ottoman Empire on English Identity in the Long Eighteenth Century*. Leiden: Brill, 2012.

Kümin, Beat. *Drinking Matters: Public Houses and Social Exchange in Early Modern Central Europe*. Houndmills: Palgrave Macmillan, 2007.

Kwass, Michael. "Ordering the World of Goods: Consumer Revolution and the Classification of Objects in Eighteenth-Century France." *Representations* 82, no. 1 (2003): 87–116.

Lakshmin, Pooja. *Real Self-Care: A Transformative Program for Redefining Wellness (Crystals, Cleanses, and Bubble Baths Not Included)*. New York: Penguin Life, 2023.

Landweber, Julie. "Furnishing the Taste for Coffee in Early Modern France." In *The Mobility of People and Things in the Early Modern Mediterranean*, edited by Elisabeth A. Fraser, 49–69. New York: Routledge, 2019.

Langford, Paul. *A Polite and Commercial People: England 1727–1783*. Oxford: Oxford University Press, 1992.

Lemon, Rebecca. *Addiction and Devotion in Early Modern England*. Philadelphia: University of Pennsylvania Press, 2018.

Leong, Elaine. *Recipes and Everyday Knowledge: Medicine, Science, and the Household in Early Modern England*. Chicago: University of Chicago Press, 2018.

Levine, Harry G. "The Discovery of Addiction: Changing Conceptions of Habitual Drunkenness in America." *Journal of Studies on Alcohol* 39 (1978): 143–74.

Lifestyle and Medicine: The Six Non-Naturals in the Long Eighteenth Century. Edited by James Kennaway and Rina Knoeff. New York: Routledge, 2020.

Lindemann, Mary. *Medicine and Society in Early Modern Europe*. 2nd ed. Cambridge: Cambridge University Press, 2010.

Lippi, Donatella. "Chocolate in History: Food, Medicine, Medi-Food." *Nutrients* 5, no. 5 (2013): 1573–84.

Lloyd, Paul S. "Dietary Advice and Fruit-Eating in Late Tudor and Early Stuart England." *Journal of the History of Medicine and Allied Sciences* 67, no. 4 (2011): 553–86.

MacLean, Gerald. *Looking East: English Writing and the Ottoman Empire before 1800*. Houndmills: Palgrave Macmillan, 2007.

Maehle, Andreas-Holger. *Drugs on Trial: Experimental Pharmacology and Therapeutic Innovation in the Eighteenth Century*. Amsterdam: Rodopi, 1999.

Mäkikalli, Aino. *From Eternity to Time: Conceptions of Time in Daniel Defoe's Novels*. Bern: Peter Lang AG, 2007.

Martin, A. Lynn. *Alcohol, Violence, and Disorder in Traditional Europe*. Kirksville MO: Truman State University Press, 2009.

Martínez, María Elena. *Genealogical Fictions: Limpieza de Sangre, Religion, and Gender in Colonial Mexico*. Stanford, CA: Stanford University Press, 2008.

McCalman, Iain. *Radical Underworld: Prophets, Revolutionaries, and Pornographers in London, 1795–1840*. Cambridge: Cambridge University Press, 1988.

McCormick, Ted. "Population: Modes of Seventeenth-Century Demographic Thought." In *Mercantilism Reimagined: Political Economy in Early Modern Britain and Its Empire*, edited by Philip J. Stern and Carl Wennerlind, 25–40. Oxford: Oxford University Press, 2013.

Merritt, J. F. "Reinventing Westminster Abbey, 1642–1660: A House of Kings from Revolution to Restoration." *Journal of Ecclesiastical History* 64, no. 1 (2016): 122–38.

Merritt, Jane T. *The Trouble with Tea: The Politics of Consumption in the Eighteenth-Century Global Economy*. Baltimore, MD: Johns Hopkins University Press, 2017.

Midelfort, Erik H. C. *Mad Princes of Renaissance Germany*. Charlottesville: University Press of Virginia, 1992.

Midgley, Clare. *Women against Slavery: The British Campaigns, 1780–1870*. New York: Routledge, 1992.

Miller, Clarence H., ed. *Erasmus and Luther: The Battle over Free Will*. Indianapolis: Hackett, 2012.

Miller, Peter N. "Nazis and Neo-Stoics: Otto Brunner and Gerhard Oestreich before and after the Second World War." *Past and Present* 176 (2002): 144–86.

Miller, William Ian. "Gluttony." *Representations* 60 (1997): 92–112.

Mintz, Sidney W. *Sweetness and Power: The Place of Sugar in Modern History*. New York: Penguin, 1985.

Molineux, Catherine. *Faces of Perfect Ebony: Encountering Atlantic Slavery in Imperial Britain*. Cambridge MA: Harvard University Press, 2012.

Morrison, Robert. *The English Opium-Eater: A Biography of Thomas De Quincey*. London: Weidenfeld & Nicolson, 2009.

Muldrew, Craig. *The Economy of Obligation: The Culture of Credit and Social Relations in Early Modern England*. Houndmills: Palgrave Macmillan, 1998.

The New Wellness Revolution: How to Make a Fortune in the Next Trillion Dollar Industry. Edited by Paul Zane Pilzer. Hoboken: John Wiley & Sons, 2002.

Nicholls, Albert G. "Nicolas de Blegny and the First Medical Periodical." *Canadian Medical Association Journal* 31, no. 2 (1934): 198–202.

Nirenberg, David. "Was There Race before Modernity? The Example of 'Jewish' Blood in Late Medieval Spain." In *Neighboring Faiths: Christianity, Islam, and Judaism in the Middle Ages and Today*. Chicago: University of Chicago Press, 2014.

Norton, Marcy. *Sacred Gifts, Profane Pleasures: A History of Tobacco and Chocolate in the Atlantic World*. Ithaca, NY: Cornell University Press, 2008.

Norton, Marcy. "Tasting Empire: Chocolate and the European Internalization of Mesoamerican Aesthetics." *American Historical Review* 111, no. 3 (2006), 660–91.

Oestreich, Gerhard. *Neostoicism and the Early Modern State*. Edited by Brigitta Oestreich and H. G. Koenigsberger. Translated by David McLintock. Cambridge: Cambridge University Press, 1982.

Payne, Roger M. *The Self and the Sacred: Conversion and Autobiography in Early American Protestantism*. Knoxville: University of Tennessee Press, 1980.

Pedeliento, Giusepe, Valeria Pinchera, and Daniela Andreini. "Gin: A Marketplace Icon," *Consumption Markets and Culture*, 2020. Accessed September 11, 2023. https://www.tandfonline.com/doi/abs/10.1080/10253866.2020.1806066?journalCode=gcmc20.

Peeters, Frank. "Leven en bedrijf van Timotheus ten Hoorn (1644–1715)." *Medelingen van de Stichting Jacob Camp Weyerman* 25 (2002): 20–28.

Peirce, Leslie. "Writing Histories of Sexuality in the Middle East." *American Historical Review* 114, no. 5 (2009): 1325–39.

Phillips, Rod. *Alcohol: A History*. Chapel Hill: University of North Carolina Press, 2014.

Pincus, Steven. *1688: The First Modern Revolution*. New Haven, CT: Yale University Press, 2009.

Pincus, Steven. "'Coffee Politicians Does Create': Coffeehouses and Restoration Political Culture." *Journal of Modern History* 67, no. 4 (1995): 807–34.

Porter, David. *Ideographia: The Chinese Cipher in Early Modern Europe*. Stanford, CA: Stanford University Press, 2001.

Porter, Roy. "The Drinking Man's Disease: The 'Pre-History' of Alcoholism in Georgian Britain." *British Journal of Addiction* 80 (1985): 385–96.

Porter, Roy. *The Greatest Benefit to Mankind: A Medical History of Humanity*. New York: W. W. Norton, 1997.

Porter, Roy. "Introduction." In *George Cheyne: The English Malady (1733)*, ix–li. London: Tavistock/Routledge, 1991.

Price, Jacob M. *France and the Chesapeake: A History of the French Tobacco Monopoly, 1674–1791, and of Its Relationship to the British and American Tobacco Trades*. Vol. 1. Ann Arbor: University of Michigan Press, 1973.

Questier, Michael C. *Conversion, Politics and Religion in England, 1580–1625*. Cambridge: Cambridge University Press, 1997.

Raphael, Rina. *The Gospel of Wellness: Gyms, Gurus, GOOP, and the False Promise of Self-Care*. New York: Henry Holt, 2022.

Rappaport, Erika. *A Thirst for Empire: How Tea Shaped the Modern World*. Princeton, NJ: Princeton University Press, 2017.

Rasmussen, Dennis C. *The Problems and Promise of Commercial Society: Adam Smith's Response to Rousseau*. University Park: Penn State University Press, 2008.

Reddy, William M. *The Navigation of Feeling: A Framework for the History of Emotions*. New York: Cambridge University Press, 2001.

Reinert, Sophus A. *The Academy of Fisticuffs: Political Economy and Commercial Society in Enlightenment Italy*. Cambridge, MA: Harvard University Press, 2018.

Reinke-Williams, Tim. *Women, Work, and Sociability in Early Modern London*. Houndmills: Palgrave Macmillan, 2014.

Rendell, Jane. *The Pursuit of Pleasure: Gender, Space, and Architecture in Regency London*. New Brunswick, NJ: Rutgers University Press, 2002.

Riley, James C. *The Eighteenth-Century Campaign to Avoid Disease*. New York: St. Martin's, 1987.

Romaniello, Matthew P., and Tricia Starks. "*Tabak*: An Introduction." In *Tobacco in Russian History and Culture: From the Seventeenth Century to the Present*, edited by Matthew P. Romaniello and Tricia Starks, 1–8. New York: Routledge, 2009.

Rosenwein, Barbara H. *Emotional Communities in the Early Middle Ages*. Ithaca, NY: Cornell University Press, 2006.

Rössner, Philipp Robinson. *Freedom and Capitalism in Early Modern Europe: Mercantilism and the Making of the Modern Economic Mind*. Cham, Switzerland: Palgrave Pilot, 2020.

Saarinen, Risto. *Weakness of Will in Renaissance and Reformation Thought*. Oxford: Oxford University Press, 2011.

Santo-Tomás, Enrique García. "El dogma placentero: políticas de consume en chocolate y tabaco. Ayuno eclesiástico y natural (1645) de Tomás Hurtado." In *En Buena Compañía: Estudios en Honor de Luciano García Lorenzo*, edited by Joaquín Álvarez Barrientos, Óscar Cornago Bernal, Abraham Madroñal Durán, and Carmen Menéndez-Onrubia, 311–17. Madrid: Consejo Superior de Investigaciones Científicas, 2009.

Schiebinger, Londa. *Plants and Empire: Colonial Bioprospecting in the Atlantic World.* Cambridge MA: Harvard University Press, 2007.

Schrad, Mark Lawrence. *Smashing the Liquor Machine: A Global History of Prohibition.* New York: Oxford University Press, 2021.

Schweikardt, Christoph. "More than Just a Propagandist for Tea: Religious Argument and Advice on a Healthy Life in the Work of the Dutch Physician Cornelis Bontekoe (1647–1685)." *Medical History* 47, no. 3 (2003): 357–68.

Seth, Suman. *Difference and Disease: Medicine, Race, and the Eighteenth-Century British Empire.* Cambridge: University of Cambridge Press, 2018.

Shackelford, Joel. "Paracelsian Uroscopy and German Chemiatric Medicine in the *Medicina Pennsylvania* of George de Benneville." In *Medical Theory and Therapeutic Practice in the Eighteenth Century: A Transatlantic Perspective*, edited by Jürgen Helm and Renate Wilson, 13–35. Stuttgart: Franz Steiner Verlag, 2008.

Shahani, Gitanjali G. *Tasting Differences: Food, Race, and Cultural Encounters in Early Modern Literature.* Ithaca, NY: Cornell University Press, 2020.

Shapin, Steven. "How to Eat Like a Gentleman: Dietetics and Ethics in Early Modern England." In *Right Living: An Anglo-American Tradition of Self-Help Medicine and Hygiene*, edited by Charles E. Rosenberg, 21–58. Baltimore, MD: Johns Hopkins University Press, 2003.

Shapin, Steven. "Why Was 'Custom a Second Nature' in Early Modern Medicine?" *Bulletin of Medical History* 93, no. 1 (2019): 1–26.

Shelton, Donald C. "A Satire, Not a Sermon: Four Stages of Cruelty and Murder." *Athens Journal of History* 6, no. 3 (2020): 233–86.

Shepard, Alexandra. *Meanings of Manhood in Early Modern England.* Oxford: Oxford University Press, 2003.

Sherman, Sandra. *Imagining Poverty: Quantification and the Decline of Paternalism.* Columbus: Ohio State University Press, 2001.

Siena, Kevin. "Pliable Bodies: The Moral Biology of Health and Disease." In *A Cultural History of the Human Body in the Age of Enlightenment*, edited by Carole Reeves, 3–52. Oxford: Berg, 2010.

Smail, Daniel Lord. *The Consumption of Justice: Emotions, Publicity, and Legal Culture in Marseille, 1264–1423.* Ithaca, NY: Cornell University Press, 2003.

Smail, Daniel Lord. *Legal Plunder: Households and Debt Collection in Late Medieval Europe.* Cambridge, MA: Harvard University Press, 2016.

Smail, Daniel Lord. *On Deep History and the Brain.* Berkeley: University of California Press, 2008.

Smail, Daniel Lord. "Telling Tales in Angevin Courts." *French Historical Studies* 20 (1997): 18–215.

Smith, Mark M. *How Race Is Made: Slavery, Segregation, and the Senses.* Chapel Hill: University of North Carolina Press, 2006.

Smith, S. D. "Accounting for Taste: British Coffee Consumption in Historical Perspective." *Journal of Interdisciplinary History* 27, no. 2 (1996): 183–214.

Smith, Woodruff D. *Consumption and the Making of Respectability, 1600–1800.* New York: Routledge, 2002.

Spary, E. C. *Eating the Enlightenment: Food and the Sciences in Paris*. Chicago: University of Chicago Press, 2012.

Spary, E. C. "Opium, Experimentation, and Alterity in France." In "Intoxicants and Early Modern Globalization," special issue, *Historical Journal* 65 (2022): 49–67.

Stern, Philip J. and Carl Wennerlind. "Introduction." In *Mercantilism Reimagined: Political Economy in Early Modern Britain and Its Empire*, edited by Philip J. Stern and Carl Wennerlind, 3–22. Oxford: Oxford University Press, 2013.

Stolberg, Michael. *Experiencing Illness and the Sick Body in Early Modern Europe*. Translated by Leonhard Unglaub and Logan Kennedy. Houndmills: Palgrave Macmillan, 2011.

Sussman, Charlotte. *Consuming Anxieties: Consumer Protest, Gender, and British Slavery, 1713–1833*. Stanford, CA: Stanford University Press, 2000.

Taylor, Scott K. "Coffee and the Body: From Exoticism to Wellness in Eighteenth-Century Europe." *Eighteenth Century Studies* 54, no. 3 (2021): 633–50.

Taylor, Scott K. *Honor and Violence in Golden Age Castile*. New Haven, CT: Yale University Press, 2008.

Taylor, Scott K. "'A Miserable Captivity' or 'Happily Redeemed from Captivity to Liberty': Tobacco, Addiction, and Early Modern Bodies and Minds," In *A Linking of Heaven and Earth: Studies in Religious and Cultural History in Honor of Carlos M. N. Eire*, edited by Emily Michelson, Scott K. Taylor, and Mary Noll Venables, 191–203. Farnham: Ashgate, 2012.

Technologia 10 no. 1 (1987) from the Belgian Nationaal Centrum voor de Geschiedenis van de Wetenschappen/Centre National d'Histoire des Sciences.

Test, Edward McClean. *Sacred Seeds: New World Plants in Early Modern English Literature*. Lincoln: University of Nebraska Press, 2019.

Thompson, E. P. "The Moral Economy of the English Crowd in the Eighteenth Century." *Past & Present* 50 (1971): 76–136.

Tlusty, B. Ann. "Water of Life, Water of Death: The Controversy over Brandy and Gin in Early Modern Augsburg." *Central European History* 31, no. 1–2 (1998): 1–30.

Trivellato, Francesca. "The Moral Economies of Early Modern Europe." *Humanity: An International Journal of Human Rights, Humanitarianism, and Development* 11, no. 2 (2020): 193–201.

Trocki, Carl A. *Opium, Empire, and the Global Political Economy*. London: Routledge, 1999.

Tullett, William. "Grease and Sweat: Race and Smell in Eighteenth-Century English Culture." *Cultural and Social History* 13, no. 3 (2016): 307–22.

Tullett, William. *Smell in Eighteenth-Century England: A Social Sense*. Oxford: Oxford University Press, 2019.

Tullett, William. "State of the Field: Sensory History." *History* 106, no. 373 (2021): 804–20.

Van Krieken, Robert. "The Organisation of the Soul: Elias and Foucault on Discipline and the Self." *European Journal of Sociology/Archives Européennes de Sociologie* 31 (1990): 353–71.

Van Krieken, Robert. "Social Discipline and State Formation: Weber and Oestreich on the Historical Sociology of Subjectivity." *Amsterdams Sociologisch Tijdschrift* 17, no. 1 (1990): 3–38.

Varey, Simon, Rafael Chabrán, and Dora B. Weiner, eds. *Searching for the Secrets of Nature: The Life and Works of Dr. Francisco Hernández*. Stanford, CA: Stanford University Press, 2002.

Vickery, Amanda. "Fashioning Difference in Georgian England: Furniture for Him and for Her." In *Early Modern Things: Objects and their Histories, 1500–1800*, edited by Paula Findlen, 342–59. London: Routledge: 2013.

Vickery, Amanda. "His and Hers: Gender, Consumption, and Household Accounting in Eighteenth-Century England." In "The Art of Survival: Gender and History in Europe, 1450–2000," supplementary issue, *Past and Present*, no. 1 (2006): 12–38.

Von Hoffman, Viktoria. *From Gluttony to Enlightenment: The World of Taste in Early Modern Europe*. Urbana: University of Illinois Press, 2016.

Vos, Paula de. "The Science of Spices: Empiricism and Economic Botany in the Early Spanish Empire." *Journal of World History* 17 (2006): 399–428.

Wallis, Patrick. "Consumption, Retailing, and Medicine in Early-Modern London." *Economic History Review* 61, no. 1 (2008): 26–53.

Wallis, Patrick. "Exotic Drugs and English Medicine: England's Drug Trade, c. 1550–c. 1800." Economic History Working Papers 143, no. 10. Department of Economic History, London School of Economics and Political Science, 2010. Accessed September 11, 2023. http://eprints.lse.ac.uk/28577/.

Walvin, James. *Fruits of Empire: Exotic Produce and British Taste, 1660–1800*. New York: New York University Press, 1997.

Warner, Jessica. "Before There Was Alcoholism: Lessons from the Medieval Experience with Alcohol." *Contemporary Drug Problems* 19, no. 3 (1992): 409–29.

Warner, Jessica. *Craze: Gin and Debauchery in an Age of Reason*. New York: Basic Books, 2002.

Warner, Jessica. "'Resolv'd to Drink No More': Addiction as a Preindustrial Construct." *Journal of Studies on Alcohol* 55, no. 6 (1994): 685–91.

Wear, Andrew, "Place, Health, and Disease: The *Airs, Waters, Places* Tradition in Early Modern England and North America." *Journal of Medieval and Early Modern Studies* 38, no. 3 (2008): 443–65.

Weber, Max. *The Protestant Ethic and the Spirit of Capitalism*. With an introduction by Randall Collins. Translated by Talcott Parsons. Los Angeles: Roxbury, 1996.

Wheeler, Roxann. *The Complexion of Race: Categories of Difference in Eighteenth-Century British Culture*. Philadelphia: University of Pennsylvania Press, 2000.

Wickham, Chris. "Gossip and Resistance among the Medieval Peasantry." *Past and Present* 160, no. 24 (1998): 3–24.

Wilson, Catherine. *Epicureanism at the Origins of Modernity*. Oxford: Clarendon, 2008.

Wilson, Frances. *Guilty Thing: A Life of Thomas De Quincey*. New York: Farrar, Straus and Giroux, 2016.

Withington, Phil. "Addiction, Intoxicants, and the Humoral Body." In "Intoxicants and Early Modern Globalization," special issue, *Historical Journal* 64 (2022): 68–90.

Withington, Phil. "Intoxicants and Society in Early Modern England." *Historical Journal* 54, no. 3 (2011): 631–57.

Withington, Phil. "Where Was the Coffee in Early Modern England?" *Journal of Modern History* 92, no. 1 (2020): 40–75.

Wolff, Larry. *Paolina's Innocence: Child Abuse in Casanova's Venice*. Stanford, CA: Stanford University Press, 2012.

Working, Lauren. "Locating Colonization at the Jacobean Inns of Court." *Historical Journal* 61, no. 1 (2018): 29–51.

Working, Lauren. *The Making of an Imperial Polity: Civility and America in the Jacobean Metropolis*. Cambridge: Cambridge University Press, 2020.

Working, Lauren. "Tobacco and the Social Life of Conquest in London, 1580–1625." In "Intoxicants and Early Modern European Globalization," special issue, *Historical Journal* 65 (2022): 30–48.

Yerushalmi, Yosef Hayim. *From Spanish Court to Italian Ghetto. Isaac Cardosó: A Study in Seventeenth-Century Marranism and Jewish Apologetics*. New York: Columbia University Press, 1971.

Yıldırım, Duygu. "*Bevanda asiatica*: Scholarly Exchange between the Ottomans and Europeans on Coffee." *Osmanlı Araştırmaları/ Journal of Ottoman Studies* 56 (2020): 25–47.

Zieger, Susan. *Inventing the Addict: Drugs, Race, and Sexuality in Nineteenth-Century and American Literature*. Amherst: University of Massachusetts Press, 2008.

Zionkowski, Linda. "Mother Gin, Motherhood, and the Problem of Domestic Order." *Eighteenth-Century Women: Studies in their Lies, Works, and Culture* 4 (2006): 1–26.

Index

www.ingramcontent.com/pod-product-compliance
Lightning Source LLC
Chambersburg PA
CBHW021817210526
45486CB00019B/294/J
* 9 7 8 1 5 0 1 7 7 5 4 6 8 *